Good Housekeeping

1000 HOME REMEDIES

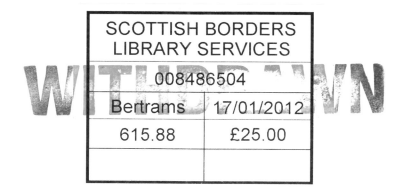
First published in the United Kingdom in 2010 by Collins & Brown
10 Southcombe Street
London
W14 0RA

An imprint of Anova Books Company Ltd

The Good Housekeeping website is
www.allboutyou.com/goodhousekeeping

This book is provided for your general information only and is not a substitute for professional medical or health recommendations. Readers should always to consult a doctor or other health professional for specific advice on personal health matters. Every effort is made to ensure that the information in this book is accurate and up to date at the time of going to press. The publishers make no representations or warranties (either express, implied or statutory) about the content of this book and to the extent permitted by law exclude all liability incurred either directly or indirectly in connection with the information it contains including but not limited to any defects, errors, mistakes or inaccuracies.

10 9 8 7 6 5 4 3 2 1

ISBN 978-1-84340-603-7

A catalogue record for this book is available from the British Library.
Produced by SP Creative Design

Repro by Rival Colour UK Ltd, UK
Printed by GRAFO, S.A.

This book can be ordered direct from the publisher at www.anovabooks.com

All images reproduced courtesy of istockphoto.com apart from p.6, 14, 22, 23 (Lucinda Symons), p.16, 17 (Caroline Molloy).

Good Housekeeping

1000 HOME REMEDIES

Safe and sensible treatments for everyday ailments

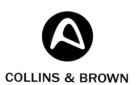

COLLINS & BROWN

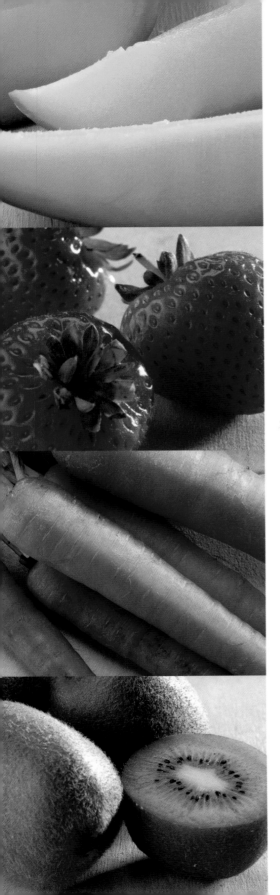

Contents

Foreword 7
Herbal remedies 8
Aromatherapy essential oils 9
Homeopathic remedies 10

1

Skin and hair problems 12
- Dry skin 14
- Oily skin 16
- Acne 18
- Eczema 20
- Wrinkles 22
- Psoriasis 24
- Dermatitis 26
- Cellulite 28
- Blisters 30
- Chapped lips 31
- Cold sores 32
- Boils 33
- Hives and heat rash 34
- Athlete's foot 36
- Nail problems 38
- Calluses and corns 40
- Warts and verrucas 41
- Body and foot odour 42
- Dry hair 44
- Dandruff 47
- Greasy hair 48
- Head lice 50

2

Ear, eye and mouth problems 54
- Ear problems 56
- Eye strain 58
- Eye irritation 60
- Styes 62
- Conjunctivitis 63
- Gum problems 64
- Toothache 66
- Mouth ulcers 68
- Bad breath 70
- Dry mouth 71

3

Musculo-skeletal problems 74
- Back pain 76
- Sciatica 80
- Trapped nerve 81
- Neck and shoulder pain 82
- Osteoporosis 84
- Shin splints 86
- Arthritis 88
- Rheumatism 90
- Repetitive strain injury 92
- Foot pain 94
- Muscle cramps 96
- Gout 98

4

Heart and circulation problems 102
- Angina 104
- Blood pressure 106
- High cholesterol 108
- Palpitations 110
- Anaemia 112
- Varicose veins 114
- Restless legs 116
- Deep vein thrombosis 117
- Chilblains 118

5

Respiratory problems 122
- Asthma 124
- Hay fever 126
- Colds 128
- Coughs 130
- Bronchitis 132
- Sore throat 134
- Tonsillitis 136
- Sinusitis 138
- Hiccups 140

6

Immune system problems — 144
- Allergies — 146
- Food allergies — 148
- Fever — 150
- Influenza — 152
- Glandular fever — 154
- Chickenpox — 156
- Shingles — 158
- German measles — 160
- Herpes simplex — 162

7

Digestive problems — 166
- Constipation — 168
- Diarrhoea — 170
- Nausea and vomiting — 172
- Gastroenteritis and food poisoning — 174
- Indigestion and heartburn — 176
- Inflammatory bowel diseases — 178
- Irritable bowel syndrome — 180
- Peptic ulcers — 182
- Wind — 184
- Intestinal worms — 186
- Haemorrhoids — 188

8

Urinary problems — 192
- Incontinence — 194
- Water retention — 196
- Cystitis — 198
- Kidney stones — 200

9

Emotional and nervous disorders — 204
- Headache — 206
- Migraine — 208
- Fatigue — 210
- Insomnia — 212
- Stress — 214
- Neuralgia — 216
- Chronic fatigue syndrome — 218
- Depression — 220
- Seasonal affective disorder — 222
- Dementia — 224

10

Men's health problems — 228
- Shaving problems — 230
- Prostate problems — 232
- Impotence — 234
- Infertility — 236

11

Women's health problems — 240
- Premenstrual tension — 242
- Heavy bleeding — 244
- Period pain — 245
- Thrush — 246
- Fibroids — 248
- Pregnancy health problems — 250
- Infertility — 252
- Menopause — 254

12

Children's health problems — 258
- Nappy rash — 260
- Infant colic — 262
- Teething — 264
- Catarrh — 265
- Colds — 266
- Infectious childhood diseases — 268
- Sleep problems — 272
- Bedwetting — 274

13

First aid and emergencies — 278
- Bites and stings — 280
- Burns and scalds — 282
- Bruises — 284
- Cuts and grazes — 286
- Nosebleeds — 287
- Fainting — 288
- Sprains and strains — 289
- Heat exhaustion — 290
- Sunburn — 291
- Shock — 292
- Splinters — 293
- Motion sickness — 294
- Hangover — 295

Glossary — 296
Useful information — 298
Index — 302

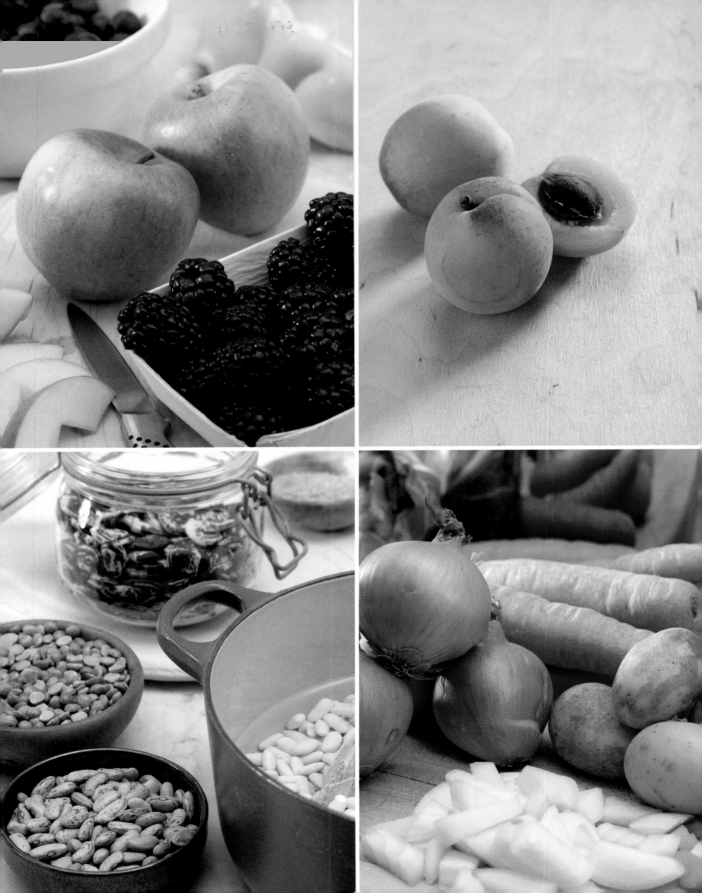

Foreword

We live in a fast-paced, high-technology world. The boundaries of medicine seem to be being pushed back at an awesome speed and there has never been a greater range and availability of medicines available to both doctors and patients alike. Laser treatments, gene therapy and body scanning are becoming almost commonplace, yet the growth in interest in natural treatments continues to grow at an even faster rate. This increasing popularity of complementary therapy has meant that health practitioners are now required to take notice as to why at least one-third of people in the Western world are now willing to consider using natural treatments ahead of prescription-based medicines (statistics based on the House of Lords Science and Technology 6th Report, Complementary and Alternative Medicine). More doctors than ever before are training in the use of complementary therapies to complement their conventional scientific background, allowing them to practise integrated medicine in which conventional and complementary treatments are used to achieve a full holistic range of therapy in a wide range of common medical conditions.

This book looks at the key areas of women's and men's health – such as medical, circulatory, urinary and skin problems, nervous disorders and first aid – from both a conventional and natural viewpoint. Laid out in easy-to-find sections, with colour coding and concise advice in all areas, each topic looks at symptoms, prevention, available remedies, and when to seek medical advice either as an emergency or as a routine appointment. There are also 'quick fix' tips, which will be a revelation to many people, and fascinating 'Did you know?' boxes to further increase your understanding of each area of health. Its aim is to help de-mystify complementary treatments and allow anyone to evaluate their state of wellbeing as well as providing the most complete answers to common medical questions. It can be read as a textbook from start to finish, or dipped into as and when required.

Over 2,000 years ago, the great physician Galen, the father of modern medicine, said that 'the doctor is only Nature's assistant'. That quotation is as true today as it was then and reminds us that it is by looking at the widest range of treatments available to us that we stand the greatest chance of remaining as healthy as possible. If we also remind ourselves that health is actually a state of complete physical, mental and social well-being rather than the absence of disease or infirmity then we should surely add home remedies to the armoury of conventional medical treatments at our disposal.

As a family doctor whose patients frequently ask for my advice on complementary treatments, I have long believed that the best doctors have an open mind but not one that is closed to science. This book is a major step forward in helping people to take a holistic approach to their wellbeing and, in doing so, promote optimum health for all – the holy grail for doctors and patients.

Dr. Roger Henderson

Common herbal remedies

ALOE VERA Clear gel from leaves is used for skin problems, acne, burns, insect bites and cuts.

BASIL Improves digestion and reduces excess mucous

BURDOCK Cleanses the blood and is used to treat arthritis, fever, infections, boils and sores.

CAYENNE Improves circulation, helps digestion, normalises blood pressure and is also used to treat stiff joints.

CHAMOMILE Traditionally used to induce sleep but also for digestive problems, poor appetite, colds, fever, flu, and for anxiety and stress due to its calming effect. Also good for sleeping problems, colic, and teething in babies and young children.

CHICKWEED Used as a diuretic to stimulate the kidneys as well as for treating wounds and itchy or inflamed skin.

CLOVES Improves digestion and clears mucous in lungs (asthma, colds and coughs) as well as relieving toothache.

COLTSFOOT Used as a cough remedy; the leaves can be made into a poultice for bites and stings.

COMFREY Soothes coughs, and heals wounds and burns, promoting new healthy tissue growth.

CRAMP BARK Used to treat menstrual cramps, asthma and heart palpitations.

DANDELION A powerful diuretic which is used to treat a wide range of conditions, including liver, gall bladder and kidney problems, constipation, dyspepsia, skin disease and rheumatism.

ECHINACEA This natural antibiotic herb is used for colds, coughs, sore throat, influenza and fever, as well as acne, athlete's foot, thrush and urinary tract infections.

GARLIC Promotes good digestion, lowers blood cholesterol, strengthens the immune system, and fights respiratory infections, colds and influenza.

GINGER Calms the digestive system, stimulates circulation and is used to treat arthritis, muscular cramps, colds, chills, nausea, vomiting and motion sickness.

GOLDEN SEAL Treats respiratory infections, digestive ailments (nausea, colitis, gastroenteritis, irritable bowel), urinary tract infections and boils. Combined with echinacea, it is a natural antibiotic.

GOTU KOLA An Asiatic herb used to cleanse the blood and to strengthen nerves; treats fevers and skin problems.

LAVENDER A sedative, calming herb, which is used for treating headaches, migraine, stress, insomnia, indigestion and burns.

LEMON BALM A calming herb for many nervous problems, depression, upset stomach, fever, premenstrual tension, and treating insect bites; a natural insect repellent.

LIQUORICE Promotes hormonal balance and used for some pregnancy and menopausal problems, as well as treating coughs and congestion.

MARIGOLD As an ointment or cream (calendula), treats cuts, grazes, burns, insect bites, stings, eczema and skin problems; also used for fevers, gum disease and to regulate menstruation.

MARSHMALLOW Good for soothing inflammations and treating boils, abscesses, infections, coughs, congestion, irritable bowel and colitis.

MEADOWSWEET A source of natural aspirin; good for headaches, arthritis, rheumatism, urinary infections and digestive problems.

MINTS Stimulating, energising and calming; aids digestion, colic and flatulence; and good for catarrh and bronchitis, and soothes headaches.

NETTLE A good blood cleanser, regulator and strengthener, which is used for treating anaemia and bleeding; also for arthritis, rheumatism and asthma.

PARSLEY Improves digestion, eases menstrual cramping and tension headaches, and is also a good diuretic herb.

PLANTAIN Good for treating wounds, abrasions, burns, insect bites and stings and skin problems, including eczema; also for urinary infections, thrush, irritable bowel, fever and gum disease.

ROSEMARY A herb used for many common health

problems, including headaches, migraine, colds, fever, influenza, congestion, stomach ache, indigestion, constipation and premenstrual tension, as well as for treating arthritis and rheumatism.

SAGE Excellent for sore throats, clearing excess mucous, and also for alleviating hot flushes during menopause.

SLIPPERY ELM All-round herb for treating wounds, ulceration, congestion, digestive problems (diarrhoea, constipation, colitis, irritable bowel, gastroenteritis), sore throat, bronchitis and asthma.

ST JOHN'S WORT Effective antidepressant used commonly for treating anxiety, stress, nervous tension, depression and night terrors in children; also used for neuralgia, sciatica, rheumatism and period pain as well as cuts, abrasions and burns.

THYME A good expectorant for coughs and bronchitis, and also used for treating colds, influenza and sore throat.

YARROW An ancient herb used for treating wounds and infection; also good for the digestion, treating colds and influenza, and easing cramps and heavy bleeding.

Aromatherapy essential oils

BASIL Clears the sinus and a good study aid, helping to focus the mind.

BERGAMOT Calming, uplifting and mood enhancing; used to treat anxiety, stress and depression, and also abscesses and boils.

CLOVE Oil is commonly used for relieving toothache.

CYPRESS Used for treating respiratory problems, especially coughs, sore throat, bronchitis and asthma; also for rheumatism and foot odour.

EUCALYPTUS Effective in treating many respiratory ailments, including colds, sinusitis and congestion, but also good for relieving muscular pain.

FRANKINCENSE A calming, soothing oil, which is used for anxiety and inducing meditation; also for asthma and lung infections.

GERANIUM Good for women's health problems and balancing hormones, especially premenstrual tension and during menopause; also used for acne, fluid retention and nervous tension.

GINGER Warming and good for digestive problems, nausea and motion sickness, as well as muscular aches and pains and arthritis.

JASMINE Uplifting and antidepressant, this is used for painful periods and to ease labour pain.

JUNIPER Cleansing and detoxifying, this is useful for treating respiratory infections, sciatica, gout and rheumatism.

LAVENDER Relaxing, sedative and calming, used to treat insomnia and headaches; also colds, sore throat and bronchitis; and insect bites and stings, cuts and minor burns.

LEMON Good for oily skin and acne as well as warts and verrucas.

LEMON GRASS Excellent for fatigue and tired, aching muscles as well as restless legs; an effective insect repellent and a digestive tonic.

MANDARIN A calming, relaxing oil, which is suitable for babies; used to treat rheumatic aches and pains, nervous tension, cellulite and water retention.

MARJORAM Calming oil for nervous tension, headaches and stress; induces sleep; eases respiratory problems, such as colds, sinusitis and bronchitis; and good for muscular pain, stiffness and sports injuries.

MELISSA Also known as lemon balm, a good antidepressant for treating shock, anxiety and depression; it is also used for irregular periods and cold sores.

NEROLI Good for stress, panic attacks and insomnia as well as stress-related irritable bowel syndrome.

ORANGE An uplifting tonic, which is used for heartburn, indigestion, constipation and colic.

PEPPERMINT A good digestive, used for treating flatulence, indigestion and colic; decongestant and effective relief for colds, blocked sinus and influenza.

ROMAN CHAMOMILE An excellent, gentle oil for soothing young children; also can be used to treat skin inflammations, acne, eczema and psoriasis; muscular aches and sprains and joint problems; digestive ailments (indigestion, flatulence and colic); and premenstrual tension, stress-related headaches, anxiety and insomnia.

ROSE Antidepressant and used to treat stress and grief; relieves premenstrual tension, headaches and hangovers.

ROSEMARY An invigorating skin toner and good for shiny hair and treating dandruff; used for treating colds, congestion, rheumatism, headaches and indigestion.

SANDALWOOD Soothing for sore throat, laryngitis and bronchitis; good for dry skin, eczema and acne; and useful in treating anxiety and depression.

TEA TREE Extremely beneficial for skin problems, including acne, cuts, cold sores, stings and minor wounds; also for treating athlete's foot, corns, callouses, warts and verrucas, as well as coughs, congestion, sinusitis and sore throats.

Homeopathic remedies

APIS MELLIFICA Often known as Apis and prepared from the honey bee, this homeopathic remedy is used for treating many skin conditions, rheumatism and swollen joints, throbbing headaches, dry coughs and irregular periods.

ARGENTUM NITRICUM Made from silver nitrate, this can treat hay fever, asthma, anxiety, depression, chronic fatigue syndrome and nervous disorders; digestive problems such as gastritis and irritable bowel; and burns and warts.

ARNICA MONTANA The most commonly used remedy for bruising and muscular pain; can also be used for treating fatigue and jet lag.

ARSENICUM ALBUM Useful for treating skin problems, especially eczema and psoriasis; digestive ailments such as vomiting, diarrhoea, food poisoning, gastritis; hay fever, asthma, sore throat, conjunctivitis, and dandruff.

BELLADONNA Sourced from deadly nightshade, this is good for treating fever, especially in the early stages, as well as rubella; and severe headaches, arthritis, tonsillitis and neuralgia.

BRYONIA Made from the climbing bryony plant, this is good for arthritis, rheumatism, sciatica and back pain as well as digestive disorders (diarrhoea, gastritis, indigestion), headaches and chest infections.

CALCAREA CARBONICA Derived from calcium carbonate, this can be helpful in treating a wide range of ailments, including colds, coughs and headaches.

CANTHARSIS Used for urinary system and skin conditions as well as treating diarrhoea, dandruff and mouth ulcers

CHAMOMILLA Sourced from the chamomile plant, this is especially good for relieving toothache, teething pain and earache; colic and painful periods; cough, arthritis and withdrawal symptoms following drug abuse or excessive caffeine consumption.

CIMICIFUGA Sourced from the North American black cohosh plant, this is often used for neck and back pain, severe headaches and rheumatism.

COLOCYNTHIS A remedy made from the bitter cucumber plant, used for sciatica, neuralgia, colic and stomach pain.

FERRUM PHOSPHORICUM A remedy sourced from iron phosphate, frequently used for treating fever, headaches and nosebleeds as well as indigestion and heavy periods.

GELSEMIUM Used for mental and emotional problems, especially anxiety, fear of the dentist or similar, and ME, influenza and diarrhoea.

HEPAR SULPHURIS Also known as Hepar sulph, can be used for skin conditions, boils, abscesses and acne; sore throat, earache, coughs and bronchitis.

IGNATIA Used to treat acute grief, bereavement

and depression; and headaches, coughs and digestive problems (diarrhoea, stomach cramps and flatulence).

IPECACUANHA Made from the dried root of a Brazilian plant, good for relief of nausea and vomiting, asthma and heavy periods.

KALI CARBONICUM Derived from wood ash, this is used for treating indigestion and nausea, asthma and puffy eyelids (as in allergies), catarrh and phlegm, arthritis and insomnia.

LACHESIS Made from the venom of a South American snake, this constitutional medicine is good for menopausal symptoms (hot flushes), heavy periods, sore throat, asthma, depression, back pain and sciatica.

LYCOPODIUM Widely used for digestive disorders, especially bowel problems, irritable bowel syndrome and heartburn; migraine, headaches and urinary tract infections.

MERCURIUS SOLUBILIS Often referred to as Mercurius, used for colds, tonsillitis, sore throat and ear infections; arthritis and digestive problems, such as colitis.

NATRUM MURIATICUM Better known as sodium chloride or common salt, this treats mouth ulcers and cold sores; eczema and psoriasis; headaches and premenstrual tension; back pain, asthma and irritable bowel syndrome.

NUX VOMICA Mainly used for digestive problems (colic, peptic ulces, irritable bowel); stress, fatigue, headaches, insomnia and sleeping problems; hay fever and asthma.

PHOSPHORUS Sourced from bone ash, this can treat digestive ailments, such as gastritis, colitis, peptic ulcers; dry, hacking coughs and bronchitis; nosebleeds and haemorrhage; and angina.

PULSATILLA Often used in pregnancy for morning sickness and nausea; period and women's hormonal problems; digestive ailments, especially irritable bowel syndrome; hay fever, cystitis, asthma and arthritis.

RHUS TOXICODENDRON Although derived from poison ivy, this is used for treating skin rashes, eczema, shingles and chickenpox; rheumatism, arthritis, sprains, stiff neck and influenza.

SABINA Good for treating arthritis and gout as well as nose bleeds, back pain and painful periods.

SANGUINARIA Usually used for treating allergies, especially hay fever and asthma; shoulder pain and joint conditions; menopausal hot flushes, migraine and coughs.

SEPIA Made from cuttlefish ink, this is very helpful for treating fatigue, exhaustion, depression, premenstrual tension and headaches, especially during a period or menopause; also used for cystitis, back pain, warts and nausea in pregnancy.

SILICA This is helpful for people who lack physical stamina; often used for treating abscesses and headaches.

STAPHYSAGRIA Good for emotional problems and ailments related to grief or suppressed anger, especially depression, psoriasis and insomnia; also warts, cystitis and premenstrual tension.

SULPHUR Especially useful for skin problems, including eczema, abscesses, acne; and digestive ailments such as diarrhoea; conjunctivitis, migraine, tonsillitis, asthma, dandruff, arthritis and hot flushes in menopause.

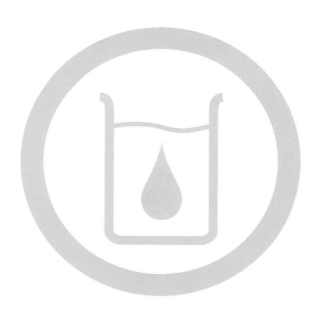

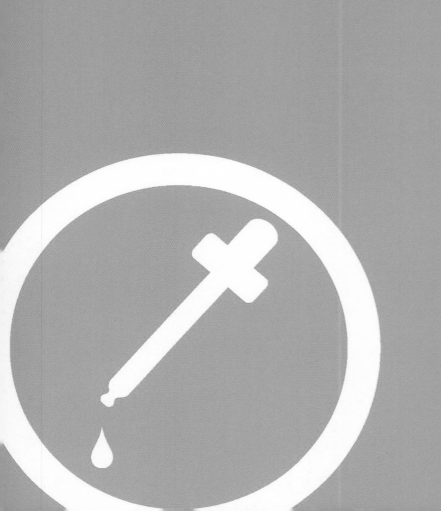

Skin and hair problems

The appearance of your skin and hair reflects your state of health and is an important barometer of your general wellbeing. In fact, skin and hair problems should be taken seriously as they are sometimes signs of underlying illness. Natural blemish-free skin and shiny, healthy hair depend as much on good nutrition and a healthy lifestyle as the conventional and natural products and remedies you use on them.

Your skin is the largest organ in your body (over 15 per cent of your body weight), and it constantly renews itself during a four-week cycle. It protects the skeletal system, muscles and organs; it helps maintain a constant body temperature; and its specialised cells perform essential functions. Vitamin D is produced when it is exposed to sunlight; and its nerve endings sense pain, itching, pressure, heat and cold. Rashes, spots, boils, inflammation, blisters and redness can all be symptoms of allergic reactions, hormonal changes or illness.

Your body is covered in hair, with the exception of the palms of your hands and the soles of your feet. Most of it is soft and downy, but it grows more profusely on your head and its condition is affected by your diet, environment and general health. On average, 100 to 150 of the 300,000 hairs on your scalp are shed every day and are replaced by new hairs as part of the natural growth cycle.

Caring for your skin and hair will keep them looking good and help you to spot tell-tale signs of underlying health problems, so you can treat them effectively before they get worse.

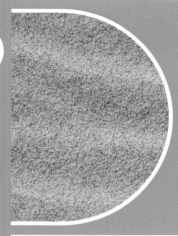

Dry skin

The skin is the largest organ in your body, accounting for over 15 per cent of your body weight. Its appearance reflects your age, health and general well-being. Dry skin tends to be fine but it can flake easily and feel tight, and it is more predisposed to developing fine lines and wrinkles than other skin types.

 SYMPTOMS

▷ Dry, close-textured and fine
▷ Flaky patches
▷ Tightness across cheeks and forehead
▷ Chaps easily
▷ Skin feels cracked and rough
▷ Thread veins, facial lines and wrinkles
▷ Prone to itching and irritation

PREVENTION

Using a moisturiser daily locks in natural moisture. Other prevention measures include:

- Use gentle cleansers and alcohol-free toners on your face
- Try to avoid soap, which tends to be very drying – liquid soaps and special cream- or oil-based soaps are gentler than conventional ones
- Always use a night cream
- Use a moisturising face mask once a week
- Protect your skin in extreme cold, heat and windy conditions
- Do not shower or take a bath more than once a day, if possible, and for no longer than 10–15 minutes
- Eat a healthy, well-balanced diet
- Drink plenty of liquids – the recommended daily intake is eight 250ml glasses of water
- Limit alcohol and caffeinated drinks, such as tea and coffee – they have a diuretic effect
- Give up smoking
- Fill your home with houseplants to add moisture, and place a humidifier in your bedroom in winter
- Protect your skin against the sun – always wear a sunscreen.

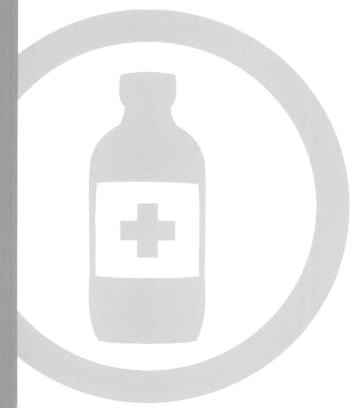

CONVENTIONAL REMEDIES

The conventional remedy for dry skin is to use a moisturiser to replace sebum – a natural skin lubricant that keeps it moist. There are so many products to choose from that you may find it difficult selecting the right one. They range from very expensive creams and serums made by international beauty companies through medicated brands to newer, more natural, cruelty-free moisturisers.

 ## NATURAL REMEDIES

Healthy skin is not so much a matter of what you use as what you do. Your lifestyle, environment, level of exercise you take and diet will all affect your skin and how it looks. For home-made remedies you can make yourself, see pages 52–53.

HERBAL REMEDIES Try applying some soothing aloe vera gel – it removes dead skin cells and helps moisturise and soften really dry skin. Make herbal tea with dandelion, chamomile or peppermint and drink a cup once every day.

AROMATHERAPY Tea tree essential oil penetrates deep into the skin – just add a couple of drops to a carrier oil and massage gently into dry areas. When taking a bath, add a few drops of lavender oil to the water.

 ## EXERCISE

Regular exercise has many beneficial effects on your skin: it increases your oxygen intake, removes toxins that can clog up your skin, boosts healthy cell renewal and helps the efficient absorption of nutrients by your body. You don't have to be a fitness fanatic or join a gym – even a brisk 20-minute walk every day can make a positive difference to your skin.

 ## NUTRITIONAL MEDICINE

A healthy, varied diet that supplies all the essential nutrients is your skin's best friend. Too few vitamins and minerals can leave your skin dehydrated and dull. You need the following:

VITAMIN A Carrots and dark green and yellow vegetables

VITAMIN B Whole-grain cereals, meat, fish, eggs, dairy products, green leafy vegetables, beans and pulses, and yeast

VITAMIN C Citrus fruits and leafy green vegetables

VITAMIN E Whole-grain cereals and eggs

ZINC Meat and dairy products

SELENIUM Meat, fish and whole-grain cereals.

 ## SEE YOUR DOCTOR

Persistent dry skin that does not respond to a healthy diet and moisturisers may need a different approach. It can even be a symptom of an underlying more serious health problem, such as diabetes. If the condition does not improve and you experience redness, crustiness, severe rashes or other irritating skin conditions, consult your doctor.

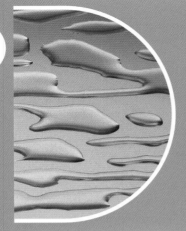

Oily skin

This skin type looks shiny and has a tendency to develop spots but, on the plus side, it does have a tendency to age better than other skin types. As with dry skin (see page 14), eating a really healthy diet will help to improve its texture and appearance. The increased sebum production is caused by the male hormone testosterone, which is also present, to a lesser extent, in women.

 SYMPTOMS

▷ Enlarged visible and open pores
▷ Overall shine
▷ Tendency to blemishes
▷ Prone to spots and blackheads
▷ Skin feels greasy

 PREVENTION

If you have a natural tendency to oily skin, it is difficult to prevent it. However, there are positive steps you can take to prevent it getting worse and becoming 'problem' skin.

- Never use harsh cleansers, which can strip away the skin's natural oils
- Use a mild pH-balanced liquid soap or cleanser
- Use an oil-free moisturiser
- Deep-cleansing face masks and facial scrubs can be beneficial
- Eat a healthy diet with plenty of fresh fruit and vegetables and less fried foods, chocolate, refined flour and sugar products
- Drink herbal teas in preference to regular tea and coffee
- Invest in some flax seed oil and take one 15ml tablespoon daily
- Don't forget to protect your skin against the sun – always wear a sunscreen.

 Did you know?

If you take an oral contraceptive pill, your skin may have a tendency to be oily. Some women also find that their skin becomes more oily in late pregnancy due to higher progesterone levels in the body. However, after the birth of their baby, it usually reverts to its normal type.

CONVENTIONAL REMEDIES

The traditional way of dealing with oily skin was to use harsh astringent toners to dry it out. However, we now know that this approach can be damaging and make the problem even worse by stripping away the natural oils and over-stimulating oil production. Instead, use gentle cleansers and toners that have been formulated specially for oily skin.

NATURAL REMEDIES

For home-made remedies you can make yourself, turn to pages 52–53.

HERBAL REMEDIES Make your own gentle toner by steeping some sage or peppermint leaves in hot water for half an hour before straining and cooling. Apply to oily skin with a cotton wool pad. Alternatively, put some eucalyptus, rosemary or thyme in a basin, pour over some boiling water and then, with a towel over your head, lean over the basin and inhale the steam.

AROMATHERAPY Sage and lemongrass essential oils may help to slow down the oil production in the skin, whereas basil, eucalyptus and lavender oils can help normalise the condition.

 ## NUTRITIONAL MEDICINE

Poor diet and junk food can make naturally oily skin even worse, leading to an increased tendency to developing spots and acne. Try cutting out all fried, greasy and high-fat foods, such as potato crisps and French fries, and also reduce your consumption of chocolate, sugary biscuits and cakes. Eat more salads, fruit and fresh vegetables.

 ## SEE YOUR DOCTOR

Oily skin should not usually necessitate a visit to your doctor. However, if you have outbreaks of spots or a tendency to acne, it would be worth consulting your general practitioner and getting some professional advice. You may even be prescribed a topical cream or some antibiotics.

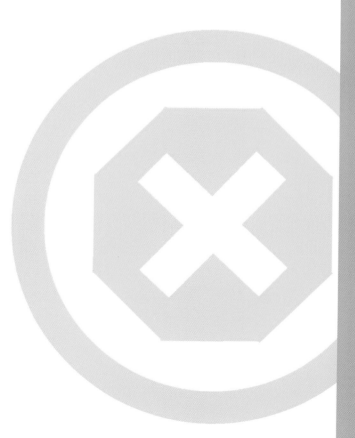

 ## Quick fix

Blot any excess oil on your face with loose face powder, not pressed, which may contain oil. Pop a little sachet of alcohol wipes into your bag and use when required.

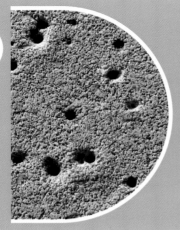

Acne

This distressing condition affects over 70 per cent of young people at some point during their adolescence. The blemishes are caused by an excessive production of sebum, which is secreted through pores in the skin. The pores become plugged, leading to blackheads or whiteheads, or infected, causing pus-filled spots.

 SYMPTOMS

▷ Blackheads – dark-pigmented blocked pores
▷ Whiteheads – small lumps with a white centre
▷ Skin feels greasy
▷ Spots filled with pus on face, neck, chest, shoulders and back
▷ Pitted, scarred skin

 PREVENTION

Acne is triggered during puberty by an increase in the hormone testosterone and is therefore impossible to prevent, especially if it runs in your family. However, you can take positive action to improve it or, at the very least, to prevent it getting worse.

• Always wash your hands before touching your face.
• Never squeeze or pick at spots – this can cause scarring.
• Cleanse your face twice a day – first thing in the morning and before going to bed.
• Use a medicated soap or cleanser or tea tree oil skin wash to remove bacteria.
• Use an oil-free, water-based moisturiser.
• Never use oil-based make-up.
• Eat a healthy diet with lots of fresh fruit and vegetables and less fried foods, chocolate, crisps, sweets and biscuits.
• Drink plenty of water.
• Regular exercise improves circulation and is beneficial for the skin.
• Tie long hair back off your face and wash greasy hair frequently.

 Did you know?

Acne can be made worse by the following: taking oral contraceptives, corticosteroids and some anti-epileptic medicines; and suffering from stress and anxiety.

CONVENTIONAL REMEDIES

Over-the-counter creams, gels and lotions are all available, and these may be effective in treating mild acne. Prescription drugs for more severe cases may be topical (applied directly to skin) or oral, including antibiotics and retinoids.

 ## NATURAL REMEDIES

Self-help measures and natural remedies can make a difference, especially in improving milder outbreaks of spots on the face.

HERBAL REMEDIES Facial steam baths can be beneficial as they help open the pores in the skin – just cover some chamomile, rosemary, thyme or sage laves with boiling water and, with a towel over your head, 'bathe' your face. Alternatively, dab the spots with a moist, warm chamomile tea bag. Drink one cup of herbal tea made with echinacea, burdock, dandelion or marigold three times a day.

AROMATHERAPY Bergamot, lavender and tea tree oils are relaxing, calming and anti-bacterial. You can apply a few drops of these essential oils to your bath water or use in a compress. Dab a drop of neat lavender oil onto spots.

 ## NUTRITIONAL MEDICINE

Contrary to popular belief, acne is not caused by poor diet and eating greasy foods, but healthy nutrition can help to combat it. Reduce your intake of animal fats, sugar and high-fat convenience foods, and try to eat more whole-grain cereals, fruit and vegetables.

 ## HOMEOPATHIC REMEDIES

Consult a qualified homeopath or, for less severe outbreaks, try the following:

Sulphur 6C: Take one tablet twice daily to relieve chronic acne with itchy, red, sore spots that are often infected and pus filled

Kali bromatum 6C: Take one tablet twice daily to relieve bluish-red spots on the face, cheeks, forehead, neck and shoulders, which leave scars

 ## SEE YOUR DOCTOR

If your acne is persistent and does not respond to over-the-counter treatments or self-help remedies within two months or becomes worse and distressing, see your doctor. You may be prescribed antibiotics or even be referred to a dermatologist if the condition is very bad or you have scarring.

Healing sunlight

Many people find their acne is worse in the winter, when there is less natural light, and that it improves in the summer, when their skin is exposed to more ultraviolet light. However, do take care not to sunbathe in the middle of the day when the sun is at its strongest and you may get burnt.

 ### Quick fix

Whenever you notice a new spot, just dab it with some witch hazel before applying your concealer in the usual way.

20

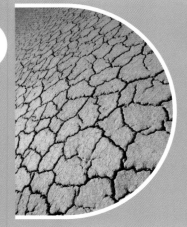

Eczema

Eczema, also referred to as dermatitis, often occurs on the fronts of the elbows, backs of the knees, ankles, wrists, neck and face. There are different types of eczema, with atopic eczema (the eczema that runs in families) being the most common. There are various conventional and natural treatments you can try to help keep outbreaks of eczema under control.

 ## SYMPTOMS

- ▷ Areas of red, inflamed skin
- ▷ Patches of dry, scaly or cracked skin
- ▷ Itching
- ▷ Thickening of the skin
- ▷ Flaky scalp
- ▷ Sore, blistering, weeping, wet or bleeding skin

 ## PREVENTION

One of the most important things you can do to prevent eczema is to stop your skin drying out by moisturising regularly.

- Don't use soap – it will dry your skin out. Use an emollient cream instead.
- Avoid over-washing your skin or using water that is too hot; this will strip your skin of its natural oils.
- Use alcohol-free and fragrance-free toiletries to reduce irritation.
- Some materials, such as synthetic fibres or wool, can irritate your skin. Always wear natural fibres, such as cotton.
- Try to avoid any extremes of temperature. Cold weather dries the skin, whereas getting hot and sweaty can cause inflammation.
- Don't scratch – scratching will make the condition worse and may lead to bleeding or infection. Keep your nails short to minimise damage.
- Try to avoid stress, as this can cause outbreaks of eczema. Taking regular exercise and practising relaxation techniques will help you to cope with stressful situations.

 ## Did you know?

Eczema is more common in childhood, and although many children grow out of it, some people continue to live with it into adulthood. Many also suffer from hay fever or asthma.

CONVENTIONAL REMEDIES

Emollients, such as aqueous cream, soften and rehydrate the skin. Corticosteroid creams reduce redness and inflammation, and antihistamines can help to ease itching. If your eczema is persistent, you may be referred to a dermatologist for a course of ultraviolet light therapy. If you have severe eczema, a skincare specialist may show you how to apply a special type of dressing.

 ## NATURAL REMEDIES

Here are some natural remedies that you may wish to consider for treating your eczema:

NUTRITIONAL MEDICINE Eczema may be associated with a zinc deficiency. Good sources of zinc include oysters, dairy products, beans, nuts, seeds (especially pumpkin seeds) and fortified breakfast cereals.

HERBAL REMEDIES Applying a cream containing St John's Wort (hypericum) to any affected areas of skin may provide some relief from eczema symptoms.

ACUPUNCTURE This treatment addresses heat imbalances within the body to treat outbreaks of eczema and provide long-term relief.

 ## HELPFUL THERAPIES

Many people find that their eczema gets better in the summer and flares up again during the winter months, and therefore your skin may benefit from a little sun exposure, but without getting sunburnt. Sunshine promotes the synthesis of vitamin D, which is necessary for healthy skin.

 ## IMMEDIATE RELIEF

A salt-water compress may help to relieve itching. Dissolve a teaspoon of pure, natural sea salt (not table salt) in one cup of warm water, soak a clean washcloth in it and apply to itchy areas of your skin.

 ## SEE YOUR DOCTOR

If your current method of treating eczema does not seem to be working, see your doctor as it may be necessary to change treatments. You should also see your doctor if:

- Your skin becomes crusty or starts oozing, blistering, or bleeding. This could be a sign of infection
- Your self-confidence is very low, you feel depressed, or your quality of life is suffering because of your eczema.

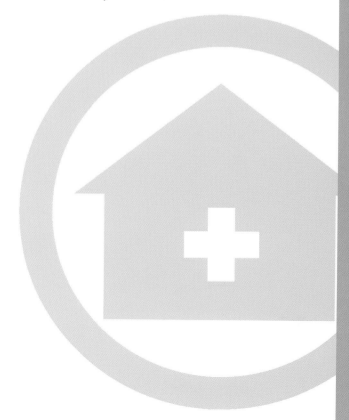

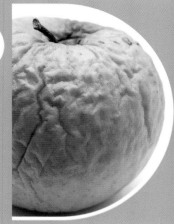

Wrinkles

As you age, your skin's natural moisture content will decrease – it becomes drier, and fine lines and wrinkles start to appear. However, you can take positive action to protect your skin from premature ageing and adapt your skincare routine accordingly. In fact, the sooner you start, the better – don't wait until you are in your 50s.

 SYMPTOMS

▷ Fine lines around the corners of the eyes and down the sides of the mouth
▷ Dry skin
▷ Skin starts to sag with loss of firmness and elasticity
▷ Uneven and dull skin tone

 PREVENTION

You cannot prevent wrinkles totally – they are part of the ageing process – but you can do a lot to slow them down and minimise the impact of the ones that appear.

- Apply a soothing eye gel or a little wheatgerm oil around the eyes first thing in the morning and at bedtime.
- Moisturise day and night to replace the loss of natural oils in your skin.
- Always wear a sunscreen or sun-block on your face to protect your skin from harmful, ageing ultraviolet light.
- Never use sunbeds.
- Always wear sunglasses in bright sunlight.
- Use a soap-free cleanser on your face – soap is too drying.
- Apply a moisturising mask once weekly.
- Eat a healthy diet with lots of fruit and vegetables, and reduce your consumption of refined and processed foods.
- Drink plenty of water.
- Stop smoking and reduce your consumption of alcohol.
- Breathe deeply to increase the amount of oxygen supplied to the skin.
- Regular exercise improves circulation and is nourishing for the skin.

 Did you know?

Antioxidants can help to prevent skin damage and ageing by neutralising free radicals – the electrically charged oxygen molecules that attack healthy cells in your skin.

CONVENTIONAL REMEDIES

An astonishing array of anti-ageing, anti-wrinkle creams, serums and moisturisers is available in your local pharmacy or from the beauty counters in large stores. Or you can even try such treatments as Botox injections, chemical peels or a facelift.

 ## NATURAL REMEDIES

Luckily, you don't have to spend a fortune on really expensive beauty products when there are so many natural remedies for combating ageing skin, fine lines and wrinkles.

HERBAL REMEDIES Apply aloe vera gel to wrinkles or, better still, take a fresh aloe vera leaf and peel back the outer skin to extract the clear gel within.

AROMATHERAPY Try diluting lavender, patchouli, tea tree, lemon, cranberry or eucalyptus essential oils in a carrier oil or cream and then massaging it gently into wrinkles.

NUTRITIONAL MEDICINE Eating a varied diet that contains all the essential nutrients your skin needs for good health will help to keep it looking youthful. Make sure that you eat oily fish, which is rich in omega-3 fatty acids, at least twice a week. You can choose from salmon, tuna, mackerel, herring and sardines.

 ## HOME-MADE REMEDIES

- You can make a nourishing face mask for very dry skin by mashing the flesh of a ripe avocado with a drop of lemon juice and smooth it over your face. Leave for at least 15 minutes
- Make an exfoliating mask that helps reduce the appearance of wrinkles by peeling a ripe papaya and mashing the flesh. Blend three 15ml tablespoons with one 15ml tablespoon oatmeal and smooth it over your face. Leave for 15 minutes, then rub vigorously into your skin and rinse off thoroughly.

Facial exercises

Exercising your facial muscles will make them stronger to support the skin and help minimise lines and wrinkles.

- For lines around the nose and mouth: curl your upper and lower lips inwards around your teeth. Press your lips together and, with your mouth closed, blow hard. Repeat 3 times.
- To tone up your cheek and chin muscles: smile with your mouth closed, raising the corners of your lips as you do so. Hold for a count of 5 and then push your jaw forwards. Hold for a count of 5. Repeat 3 times.

Harness the power of AHAs

AHAs are alpha-hydroxy acids, which occur naturally in sugar cane, sour milk, apples and acidic fruits. They help promote the shedding of dead skin cells and fight free radicals (see box opposite) as well as encouraging skin renewal and collagen growth. Many moisturising skin products you can buy contain AHAs, or you can even apply some milk, lemon juice or apple juice direct to your skin.

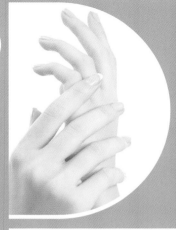

Psoriasis

Psoriasis is a chronic skin disease, which is most often characterised by inflamed, red, flaky patches of skin, known as plaques. These plaques form due to excessive numbers of skin cells collecting together on the surface of the skin. The cause of psoriasis is still not fully understood, but genes are known to be partly involved as the condition often runs in families.

 SYMPTOMS

▷ Dry, red crusty patches of skin, with silver scales that flake easily
▷ Dandruff-like flakes on the scalp
▷ Itchy skin or scalp
▷ Pitted or discoloured nails
▷ Sore or painful skin
▷ Cracked or bleeding skin
▷ Joint pain and stiffness

 PREVENTION

Psoriasis is unpredictable, coming and going as it pleases, but there are some things that you can do to help prevent it flaring up.

• Eat a balanced diet to support your general health and well-being.
• Take extra care to avoid skin injuries, such as cuts, scrapes, bruises and burns, that can lead to outbreaks of psoriasis.
• Moisturise your skin regularly to counteract dryness, and use an emollient instead of soap.
• Psoriasis can often flare up in times of stress. Some useful ways of managing stress include taking physical exercise, and relaxation and meditation techniques.
• Some medicines, such as ibuprofen and beta blockers, are known to make psoriasis worse. If you are taking any medication, ask your doctor if it will aggravate your psoriasis.
• Moderate your alcohol consumption and don't smoke.

 Did you know?

Old skin cells are normally replaced with new ones approximately once every 28 days, but in psoriasis, new skin cells are produced more quickly than usual, before they are needed.

CONVENTIONAL REMEDIES

If your psoriasis is mild to moderate, your doctor may recommend a corticosteroid, coal tar, emollient or vitamin D cream to put on your skin, and a shampoo for your scalp. If you have a more persistent case of psoriasis, you may be referred to a dermatologist for a course of ultraviolet light therapy. For more severe cases of psoriasis, there are oral medicines and injections available to help control the inflammation.

 ## NATURAL REMEDIES

You might like to try the following natural methods to see if they improve your psoriasis.

NUTRITIONAL MEDICINE EPA (a type of omega-3 fatty acid found in oily fish) may help to reduce inflammation associated with psoriasis. Try taking up to 1000mg EPA fish oil daily.

AROMATHERAPY Helichrysum essential oil is known for its anti-inflammatory effects. Add a few drops to a carrier oil, such as jojoba or sweet almond oil, and massage it into your skin.

ACUPUNCTURE This treatment is a great way of reducing stress, which, in turn, can help alleviate the symptoms of psoriasis.

 ## HEALING FOODS

A diet containing foods that are rich in beta-carotene may help reduce the risk of psoriasis. Good sources include green leafy vegetables, carrots, red peppers, mangoes and apricots. The body converts beta-carotene into vitamin A, which is important for healthy skin.

 ## SEE YOUR DOCTOR

You should see your doctor if:

- Your current method of controlling your psoriasis does not seem to be working
- Your skin becomes inflamed all over, pus-filled spots develop on your skin, or there are signs of infection
- You develop stiff or painful joints
- Your psoriasis is greatly interfering with your everyday activities at home, work or school
- You become very depressed or anxious about the appearance of your psoriasis and it affects your social relationships.

IMMEDIATE RELIEF

Try soaking in a warm, soothing oatmeal bath for 15 minutes to relieve itching and soften your skin. Apply a good moisturiser afterwards to lock in moisture.

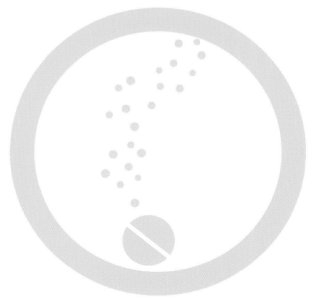

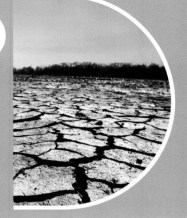

Dermatitis

Dermatitis is inflammation of the skin, most often affecting the hands and face. It occurs when the skin comes into contact either with an irritant (irritant contact dermatitis) or a substance that triggers an allergic reaction (allergic contact dermatitis). Atopic dermatitis, or eczema, runs in families and it often occurs alongside hay fever and asthma.

 ## SYMPTOMS

▷ Red rash
▷ Skin inflammation
▷ Thickened patches of skin
▷ Dry or cracked skin
▷ Blisters
▷ Itching
▷ Stinging, burning or sore skin

 ## PREVENTION

The best way to avoid irritant or allergic contact dermatitis is to identify the offending irritant or allergen and avoid coming into contact with it. This could be something in your day-to-day life, or something you come into contact with at work. Some common substances that cause dermatitis include nickel, makeup, hair dye, skin creams, perfumes, latex, adhesives, detergents, oils, solvents, acids, alkalis, dust, soil and some plants.

- Wash your skin as soon as possible after coming into contact with the substance that triggers your dermatitis.
- Wear gloves or other protective clothing when necessary to protect your skin.
- Avoid immersing your hands in water for long periods of time.
- Avoid products containing alcohol or soap, as these dry out the skin.
- Prevent your skin from drying out with a good moisturiser or an emollient, such as aqueous cream.
- Use fragrance-free products.
- Avoid scratching dermatitis; this will only make the condition worse and may lead to infection.

 ## Did you know?

If you have allergic contact dermatitis, areas of your skin that did not come into contact with the allergen may be affected as well as the areas that did. Symptoms of allergic dermatitis may take several days to appear.

CONVENTIONAL REMEDIES

While it is best to avoid the substance that is causing your dermatitis, this is not always practical or possible. Most people find they are able to improve the symptoms of dermatitis by using an emollient. Emollient creams soothe and soften the skin, and should be used frequently throughout the day if necessary. Your doctor may prescribe a corticosteroid cream to reduce inflammation. A medication known as alitretinoin is used to treat severe cases of dermatitis.

 NATURAL REMEDIES

Some natural options for treating dermatitis include the following remedies.

NUTRITIONAL MEDICINE Omega-3 fatty acids have an anti-inflammatory effect and help prevent skin itchiness and dryness. Some good sources include cold-water fish, such as salmon and mackerel, flaxseeds, walnut oil, pumpkin seeds and green leafy vegetables.

HERBAL REMEDIES Skin creams containing chamomile or witch hazel can help to soothe itching and burning, and aid healing.

ACUPUNCTURE The anti-inflammatory effects of acupuncture may relieve the itching caused by dermatitis and help to heal skin lesions.

 HOMEOPATHIC REMEDIES

Here are some homeopathic medicines that may ease the symptoms of dermatitis.

Rhus toxicodendron 6C: Take one tablet four times daily for a poison ivy type rash that itches and burns, or has swelling and blisters.

Sulphur 6C: Take one tablet three times daily for red, burning, itching, scaling skin that is irritated by heat and water.

Urtica urens 6C: Take one tablet three times daily for an itchy, stinging, blotch rash and cracked skin.

SEE YOUR DOCTOR

You should see your doctor if:

- Your current method of treating your dermatitis is not working
- You are having difficulty avoiding the substance causing your dermatitis
- Your dermatitis flares up more than usual, becomes painful, starts weeping or crusts over; you may have an infection that needs treatment with antibiotics
- Your dermatitis is making you depressed, or is significantly affecting the quality of your day-to-day life.

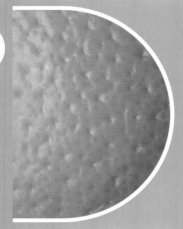

Cellulite

Cellulite is the name given to the visible pockets of fat, fluid and toxins trapped in tissue beneath the skin, and it is the bane of many women's lives (although men can get it, too). Cellulite appears most often on the buttocks, thighs, stomach, lower back and upper arms, and gives the skin a dimpled, wobbly appearance.

 SYMPTOMS

▷ Dimpling of the skin
▷ An 'orange peel' effect
▷ Cottage cheese-like lumps visible beneath the skin

 PREVENTION

The prevention of cellulite focuses on maintaining good blood circulation and preventing the build-up of fluid and toxins. This is achieved by adopting a healthy lifestyle, as listed below.

- Exercise regularly to improve circulation and encourage lymphatic drainage (the removal of fluid from tissues). Aim for about 30 minutes of aerobic activity five times a week.
- Eat a healthy diet with plenty of fibre, fruits and vegetables, and limit junk food.
- Reduce the amount of saturated fat in your diet. This causes cholesterol to clog up the walls of your blood vessels and hinders blood circulation.
- Avoid excess salt. Too much salt can lead to fluid retention and make cellulite look worse. Eat no more than 6g salt per day.
- Drink at least 1.5 litres of water every day. This will help to prevent water retention, encourage the removal of toxins and improve the appearance of your skin.
- Minimise your daily consumption of caffeine, alcohol and nicotine; these all encourage the build-up of toxins.

 Did you know?

It is not just overweight people who suffer from cellulite; anyone can get it regardless of size. As well as diet, exercise and other lifestyle factors, genetics can also play an important part in determining whether you will develop cellulite or not.

CONVENTIONAL REMEDIES

The appearance of cellulite can be improved with diet and exercise. Alternatively, specially-formulated cellulite creams may make your skin smoother and improve the appearance of cellulite. Body wrap treatments made from mineral salts and clay may tighten and firm the skin. Endermologie is a type of massage, which uses suction and rollers to improve circulation, remove toxins and soften the skin.

 NATURAL REMEDIES

Cellulite can be treated from the inside or outside. Try the following natural remedies and therapies.

NUTRITIONAL MEDICINE Increase your intake of omega-3 fatty acids (found in oily cold-water fish, such as salmon and mackerel, and flax seeds and walnuts), as they reduce inflammation and hydrate the skin cells.

AROMATHERAPY Mix three drops each of juniper, rosemary and lavender essential oils with 15ml jojoba oil. Massage regularly into your skin to improve the skin tone and circulation.

HERBAL REMEDIES Gotu kola has anti-inflammatory properties, encourages circulation and improves skin firmness. Take one to two 250mg tablets daily.

 HELPFUL THERAPIES

Dry skin brushing for a few minutes each day can improve circulation and encourage the removal of toxins. Use a brush with soft, natural bristles to brush your skin in the direction of your heart.

 EXERCISE

Try the following exercise for firming up your thighs and buttocks.

1 Stand with your feet hip-width apart.

2 Lunge back with your left leg, squeezing your buttocks as you do so.

3 Hold for one second, and then step forward with your left leg, raising your left knee in front of you.

4 Step back to the standing position and repeat with the other leg. Perform 15 repetitions each side five times a week.

 Quick fix

You can try vigorously rubbing some used ground coffee over your cellulite-inflicted areas while you are in the shower.

Caution

Liposuction is a medical procedure that vacuums away fatty deposits from underneath your skin. However, it can cause complications, such as circulatory problems and lymphatic system damage, and may make your cellulite look worse than before.

Blisters

Blisters are pockets of clear fluid between the layers of skin. They are usually caused by friction, burns or skin conditions, such as eczema or shingles. Although not serious, they may be quite painful and take time to heal.

 ## SYMPTOMS
▷ Clear fluid (sebum) beneath the skin
▷ Blister may be tinged with blood
▷ Friction blisters on hands and feet

 ## PREVENTION
You can prevent blisters by taking the following simple measures:
- Don't wear tight, badly-fitting shoes, and wear socks with new shoes
- Wear thick socks – or even two pairs – on hikes and long walks
- Keep your feet dry with powder or antiperspirants – blisters are more likely to form on damp skin
- Wear gloves when you are doing manual work, such as gardening
- Check the grip on your sports rackets
- Wear a protective sunscreen to prevent sunburn and blistering.

 ## CONVENTIONAL REMEDIES
The conventional remedy depends on where blisters occur. Do not lance or drain them; keep them clean and if they are likely to rub or get knocked, apply some antiseptic lotion or cream before covering with a plaster; or smear with petroleum jelly or dab with antiseptic lotion and leave open to the air to heal.

 ## NATURAL REMEDIES
To speed up healing and reduce itching and soreness, try one of the following therapies.
HERBAL REMEDIES Apply a little aloe vera gel or calendula cream to the blister and cover with a plaster or dressing.
AROMATHERAPY Dab a little lavender essential oil on to the blister.

 ## SEE YOUR DOCTOR
Most blisters do not merit medical attention but if you have a extremely large one or it becomes infected or does not heal within a few days, consult your doctor. Seek medical advice for blisters caused by conditions like eczema, impetigo, chickenpox and shingles.

Draining a blister
Resist popping a blister if possible as this can introduce infection. However, if you do need to drain one, only use a sterilised needle to break the skin. To do this, hold the needle with tweezers over a naked gas flame until really hot and then cool before using. Dab the blister with antiseptic and squeeze out the fluid gently. Apply a soothing antiseptic cream before covering with a plaster, dressing or special 'Second Skin' blister dressing.

Chapped lips

Your lips do not contain natural moisturising agents, so they can get dry, sore and cracked in cold or windy conditions, or hot sunshine. You need to protect them against extreme weather and moisturise them inside and out.

 SYMPTOMS

▷ Dry lips that crack easily
▷ May be sore and itchy

 PREVENTION

You can help to keep your lips smooth and moist by doing the following:

- Apply a little petroleum jelly every night at bedtime and wear it under lipstick during the day
- Always wear a protective lip screen in hot weather to prevent sunburn
- Use a creamy, moisturising lipstick
- Apply a lip salve in cold weather
- Drink plenty of water (ideally, eight glasses a day) to prevent dehydration
- Eat a healthy diet with plenty of whole-grain cereals, leafy green vegetables, fresh fruit, seeds and nuts
- Don't lick your lips too often.

 CONVENTIONAL REMEDIES

You can buy conventional lip salves and balms in most pharmacies – some are even flavoured, coloured or frosted. However, do make sure you check the labels if you tend to have sensitive skin – a minority of people can be allergic to some ingredients.

Don't lick your lips

It's very tempting to keep licking sore, dry lips but, unfortunately, this will only make them worse, as saliva dries them out even more.

 NATURAL REMEDIES

There are many tried-and-tested home remedies for soothing chapped lips. Try one of the following natural treatments.

- Rub a little honey on to sore, chapped lips – it is a natural moisturiser.
- Apply some natural beeswax lip balm.
- Break open a vitamin E capsule and apply the oil to sore lips.
- Smooth in some cocoa butter, coconut oil or even olive oil.

HERBAL REMEDIES Apply a little aloe vera gel to your lips several times a day.

 SEE YOUR DOCTOR

Most chapped lips don't necessitate a visit to the doctor, but if your lips are persistently cracked and even bleeding, then get them checked them out. You may have an allergic reaction to something or even a yeast infection.

Cold sores

Cold sores are painful blisters, which appear on the skin around the mouth and lips. They are commonly spread between people through skin-to-skin contact and are caused by the herpes simplex virus.

 ## SYMPTOMS
▷ Tingling sensation on the lips
▷ Fluid-filled blisters
▷ Redness and swelling
▷ Yellow crusty scabs

 ## PREVENTION

In the first instance, cold sores are caught through skin-to-skin contact. They can be prevented by avoiding kissing anyone with cold sores and not sharing objects they have used, such as razors or lip gloss. Flare-ups are triggered by various factors, including stress, tiredness, being run down, illness, a weakened immune system, menstruation and exposure to sun or wind.

- Take antioxidant vitamins, such as C and E, to boost your immune system.
- Take ginseng to improve your body's tolerance of stress.
- Avoid exposure to strong wind or sunlight.
- Get more sleep.
- Avoid coffee, alcohol and sugar, as they can reduce the immune response.

 ## CONVENTIONAL REMEDIES

Cold sores are treated with over-the-counter or prescribed antiviral ointments, plus painkillers for pain or discomfort. Antibiotics may be needed if cold sores become infected.

 ## NATURAL REMEDIES

There are various natural remedies you can try. The main ones are listed below.

NUTRITIONAL MEDICINE Eat foods that are rich in the amino acid lysine, such as eggs, meat, fish and kidney beans, as it may help to suppress the herpes simplex virus.

HERBAL REMEDIES Take the herb echinacea to boost your immune system. Use liquorice gel to ease inflammation and lemon balm cream to aid healing.

 ## SEE YOUR DOCTOR

If your symptoms don't ease or your cold sores become infected, see your doctor.

 ## Did you know?

Once you've caught the herpes simplex virus, it remains in your body for the rest of your life. Although you can't get rid of the virus, you can take practical steps to reduce the likelihood of getting cold sores again.

Boils

A boil is an infection that occurs in the hair follicles of the skin. It forms as a small red lump, filled with pus. Boils can develop on any area of the skin, but are particularly common on the neck, thighs, face or in the armpits.

 SYMPTOMS

▷ A small red lump on the skin, which may grow
▷ When pus forms inside, the head of the boil develops a white or yellow dot
▷ Boils that get larger can become painful

 PREVENTION

To help prevent the likelihood of boils, you can do the following:

- Regularly wash your skin and keep it clean – use an anti-bacterial soap if you wish
- If you have cuts, grazes or wounds on your skin, keep them covered with a plaster or bandage until they heal
- Exercise regularly and eat a healthy diet.

 CONVENTIONAL REMEDIES

You can have single boils, or small clusters, and they can grow bigger, but they're generally harmless. Usually, boils don't require treatment, as they burst on their own and then heal. However, on other occasions, your doctor may need to lance the boil, which involves draining out the pus with a sterilised needle. If there's risk of further infection, antibiotics may be prescribed.

 NATURAL REMEDIES

You can try using natural remedies to treat boils if they appear.

HOMEOPATHIC REMEDIES For a sudden, inflamed, red and painful boil, try Belladonna 6C.
AROMATHERAPY Lightly dab a boil with one drop of tea tree oil on a cotton wool pad. Repeat until the boil goes.

 SEE YOUR DOCTOR

If a boil does not heal after a fortnight, it's particularly large or painful, you develop a fever, or you've got a weak immune system, you should consult your doctor.

 ## Quick fix

Boils respond well to heat and it also helps the healing process, so try putting a warm flannel or cloth onto the boil for 10 to 20 minutes, twice a day.

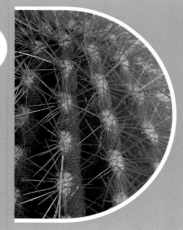

Hives & heat rash

Two skin conditions that can suddenly occur are hives (urticaria) and heat rash (also called prickly heat). With hives, red swollen weals suddenly appear on the skin and are very itchy. In many cases, they disappear after a few hours, but sometimes they can go on for longer. Unlike hives, heat rash is not an allergic reaction but is caused by blocked sweat glands in hot conditions.

 ## SYMPTOMS

HIVES

▷ Red, pink or white raised up weals

▷ A ring of red skin

▷ Itchiness

▷ Flat red marks left on the skin after an attack

HEAT RASH

▷ Itchy skin

▷ Red rash

▷ Small red or clear spots

▷ Prickling sensation

▷ Tiredness

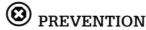 ## PREVENTION

• Avoid using a concoction of soaps and shower gels – stick to a mild or sensitive soap and only use once a day.

• Try to avoid very hot climates or, if you have to be in the heat, acclimatise yourself slowly to the temperature. Wear loose-fitting and lightweight clothing.

• Stay out of the sun if you're taking antibiotics, as some medicines can increase the risk of heat rash.

• Avoid having hot showers or baths, eating spicy food and drinking hot drinks.

• If you've managed to identify a potential allergen for your hives, then avoid it where possible.

• If you have chronic hives, avoiding stress and alcohol can prevent it from getting worse.

 ## Did you know?

Hives can often be caused by an allergic reaction to lifestyle or dietary factors, such as the washing product you are using. Diet is also important. An elimination diet, worked out with a qualified nutritionist, can help to identify the potential cause of hives.

CONVENTIONAL REMEDIES

Antihistamine tablets may be prescribed for hives, as they usually reduce the itching and help allergic reactions. Some types of antihistamines can be bought over the counter, too, but try and avoid any tablets that make you sleepy. For severe symptoms, a short course of steroids may be required, alongside antihistamine. Heat rash can be eased by cooling creams, such as calamine lotion or those containing menthol.

 ## NATURAL REMEDIES

Try the following natural remedies for alleviating the symptoms of hives and heat rash.

AROMATHERAPY Make a compress of lavender or chamomile oil (a few drops will be sufficient) and apply to heat rash. Or add a few drops of one of the oils into a warm bath and soak in it.

FLOWER REMEDIES Take four drops of Rescue Remedy or the flower remedy Impatiens to relieve itchy skin caused by heat rash or hives. Apply neat to the tongue or add two drops to a small glass of water and sip it.

NUTRITIONAL MEDICINE Vitamin C has a natural antihistamine effect, but it's more effective if combined with bioflavonoids, such as quercetin or rosehip. Take one tablet daily to reduce the symptoms of hives and prevent future attacks.

 ## HERBAL REMEDIES

- Soothe irritated, inflamed, itchy or burning skin with some aloe vera gel, nettle juice or calendula cream.
- Drink yarrow and chamomile tea to help ease the symptoms of hives. Make your own tea by adding one 15ml tablespoonful of each herb to a teapot and pouring boiling water over the top. Steep for 10 minutes before straining and drinking.

 ## HOMEOPATHIC REMEDIES

Remedies vary depending on the symptoms you have. If they don't work within 24 to 36 hours, you should consult your doctor.

Apis 30C: Take one tablet every two hours, up to a maximum of eight times through the day, as soon as heat rash develops.

Urtica 6C: Take one tablet three times a day, for up to five days, when urticaria or hives occurs.

Sol 30C: Take one table three times a day for up to three weeks if you're in a hot and humid climate and prone to heat rash.

 ## SEE YOUR DOCTOR

Heat rash will fade in cooler temperatures, but if you have hives and your rash persists or worsens, you should see your doctor.

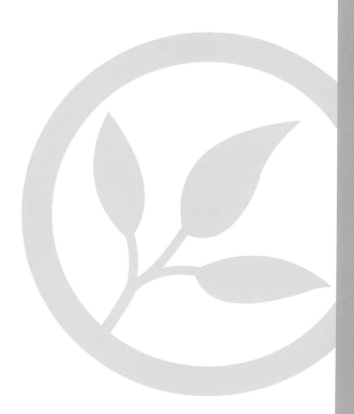

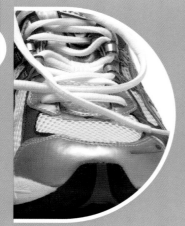

Athlete's foot

This common skin condition, which affects the feet, is caused by a fungal infection. Anyone can get it (not just athletes), although it's more common among teenagers and men, as they are more likely to wear airtight shoes. Known medically as *tinea pedis*, athlete's foot makes the skin on the foot, and between the toes, become red, itchy, dry, flaky and scaly.

 ## SYMPTOMS

▷ An itchy rash between your toes
▷ Dry, flaky or scaly skin
▷ Redness
▷ Blisters
▷ Swelling
▷ Cracked skin
▷ A burning or stinging sensation

 ## PREVENTION

The athlete's foot fungus thrives in moist, warm and dark environments, so some of your prevention strategies should focus on keeping your feet dry.
It can also spread by walking bare foot in swimming pool changing rooms, showers and saunas and from direct contact with someone who has it.

- Keep your feet clean and fresh by washing them every day.
- Dry your feet thoroughly, especially between the toes, before putting on clean socks or tights.
- Avoid sharing towels, especially with someone who has athlete's foot.
- Wash your towels and bedding regularly.
- Use talcum powder on your feet to help prevent sweating.
- Expose your feet to the air when you're at home, by taking shoes and socks off.
- Wear different pairs of shoes regularly, rather than always the same pair.
- In communal changing rooms, saunas or showers, wear flip-flops or sandals.
- Don't share or borrow other people's shoes.

 ## Did you know?

Athlete's foot is usually mild and can be successfully treated at home, but, if left untreated, it can go on for prolonged periods.

CONVENTIONAL REMEDIES

Antifungal medications are commonly used to treat athlete's foot and come in the form of creams, lotions, sprays or powder. These are applied to the affected area of the foot and the surrounding skin, and they are available over-the-counter in pharmacies. Oral antifungal tablets are sometimes required and are prescribed by a doctor.

 NATURAL REMEDIES

There are various natural remedies you can try for relieving athlete's foot.

AROMATHERAPY Tea tree essential oil can be effective for treating fungal infections. Try soaking your feet in a bowl of water with a drop of tea tree oil added. Alternatively, put one or two drops of oil onto a piece of cotton wool and dab directly onto the affected area.

NUTRITIONAL REMEDIES Cutting out caffeine and sugar from your diet may help reduce the risk of fungal infection developing. Eat garlic, which is packed with antifungal and antibacterial properties.

 HERBAL REMEDIES

- Use some marigold or calendula cream to help soothe itching.
- Soak your feet in an infusion of goldenseal, which is known for its antifungal properties, and dust your dry feet with goldenseal powder.
- Help support your immune system by taking echinacea tablets or tincture during an athlete's foot outbreak.

 HOMEOPATHIC REMEDIES

Homeopathic remedies can be useful in relieving some symptoms of athlete's foot:

Silica 6C: If you're prone to sweaty feet, this can help reduce the sweat and dampness that the infection loves. Take one tablet twice a day until the condition improves.

Sulphur 6C: To help aid the dry, cracked and itchy skin of athlete's foot, take one tablet twice daily.

SEE YOUR DOCTOR

If none of the remedies work and athlete's foot persists, see your doctor, as fungal infections can sometimes be an underlying sign of diabetes. In severe cases, it can spread to the toenails and, where the skin becomes very cracked, bacterial infections can develop, too.

Caution

Always wash your hands before and after treating your feet. If you don't, the fungal infection can spread to your hands, too, causing tinea manuum, a condition where your hands become dry, itchy and red.

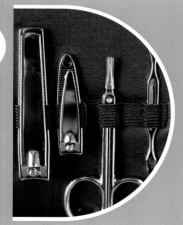

Nail problems

Like other parts of your body, your nails can be subject to their own health complaints. Nail problems, such as fungal nail infections, in-growing toenails and brittle nails, are all common. They can sometimes be a sign of nutritional deficiency or a hint of an underlying health condition, but most are easily treated once they are correctly diagnosed.

 SYMPTOMS

FUNGAL NAIL INFECTIONS
▷ Thick, discoloured and crumbly nail
▷ Pain and inflamed skin under the nail
▷ Nail may fall off
▷ Discomfort when walking

IN-GROWING TOE NAILS
▷ Pain and discomfort
▷ A nail where the edge or corner grows into the skin
▷ Hard skin
▷ Swelling and pain
▷ Tenderness
▷ Bleeding
▷ Discharging pus

BRITTLE NAILS
▷ Nails that easily break, split and chip
▷ Vertical splits

 PREVENTION

- If you have, or suspect you could have, athlete's foot, then treat it, as if left, it can spread and cause fungal nail problems.
- Keep your feet clean and dry, as damp, hot and sweaty feet encourage fungi to grow and cause nail fungal infections.
- To prevent re-occurrence of fungal nail problems, look after your nails properly.
- If you do a lot of washing up, or frequently have your hands in hot water, wear rubber gloves, as this can help prevent fingernail infections.
- Avoid biting your nails or using artificial nails, as this reduces fingernail infections.
- Avoid wearing tight shoes.
- Always cut your toenails straight across to help prevent in-growing toenails. Avoid cutting them too short, though.
- To help avoid brittle nails and to prevent nail problems as a whole, always eat a healthy, balanced and nutrition-filled diet.
- If you suffer from nail problems or have difficulty cutting your toe nails, you should visit the chiropodist regularly.

CONVENTIONAL REMEDIES

FUNGAL NAIL INFECTIONS are treated with a paint-on, anti-fungal nail lacquer or through the use of prescribed antibiotics.

IN-GROWING TOENAILS can be softened by soaking your foot in warm water, three to four times a day. Painkillers can help alleviate the discomfort. The small part of the nail that's digging into the skin may have to be removed. For bad cases, all or part of the nail may need to be surgically removed under local anaesthetic. This is usually done as day surgery at a hospital outpatients department or clinic.

BRITTLE NAILS, along with other symptoms, can sometimes be a sign of an underactive thyroid, so if your doctor suspects this, then blood tests may be required.

 ## NATURAL REMEDIES

If you suffer from nail problems, try the following alternative remedies.

HERBAL REMEDIES To help your nails become stronger, take evening primrose oil capsules daily or try the herb horsetail, which is rich in silica. Aloe vera gel or neem oil can be applied to nails that are affected by fungal infections.

HOMEOPATHIC REMEDIES Silica 6C can be taken to help fight fungal nail infections and also to aid brittle nails.

Aromatherapy

- Put a drop of tea tree oil on a piece of cotton wool and dab onto nails affected by fungal infections, or soak your feet in warm water with two drops of tea tree oil.
- A foot soak with a few drops of soothing lavender oil can ease the discomfort of in-growing toenails.

 ## NUTRITIONAL MEDICINE

Brittle nails can be a sign that you lack vitamins, such as vitamin B complex, and minerals, such as zinc and iron. Eat plenty of asparagus, broccoli, yeast extract and meat for vitamin B; a handful of pumpkin seeds for zinc; and some red meat, pulses or green leafy vegetables for iron. For an extra boost, you can take a multivitamin and mineral supplement. The overall effect of improved nutrition should be visible within three months or as the nails grow.

 ## SEE YOUR DOCTOR

If you have a painful in-growing toe nail which does not respond to self-treatment or visits to the chiropodist, see your doctor. You may need a course of antibiotics to clear up any infection. If brittle nails or fungal infections persist and do not heal, you should consult your doctor.

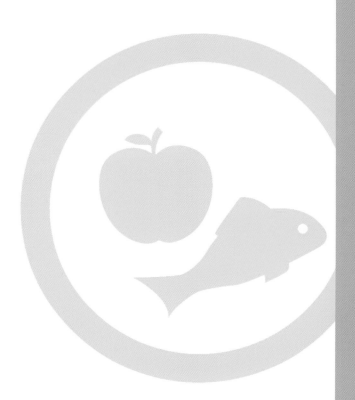

Corns and calluses

Corns and calluses both involve skin that thickens and becomes painful on the feet. Corns appear on or between the toes, usually due to badly-fitting shoes; calluses appear on the soles, often caused by pressure when walking.

 SYMPTOMS

CORNS
▷ Small, round hard area of skin
▷ A hard 'plug' in the centre
▷ Corns between the toes can be softer and are white and rubbery
▷ Pain
▷ Swelling

CALLUSES
▷ Hard, wide area of skin
▷ Undefined edge
▷ Pale or yellow colour

 PREVENTION
• Check your feet regularly and keep them in good condition.
• Soak your feet in warm water and gently remove hard skin with a foot file or pumice.
• Regularly moisturise with foot cream.
• Wear comfortable shoes that fit and don't put your toes or feet under pressure.
• Change your socks or tights every day.

 CONVENTIONAL REMEDIES

Corn plasters, padding or insoles in shoes are the usual remedies for corns and calluses. A chiropodist may cut away the corn or callus to relieve the pressure. If soft corns become infected, antibiotics may be prescribed.

 NATURAL REMEDIES

You can also try the following natural methods of dealing with these problems.

AROMATHERAPY Soften hard skin by soaking your feet in an aromatherapy footbath. Add a few drops of lavender, thyme and rosemary essential oils to soothe and cleanse the skin. Once the skin is softened, gently rub it with a pumice stone or foot file.

HERBAL REMEDIES Moisturise your feet daily using herbal foot creams, such as calendula, to keep the skin soft and reduce the likelihood of painful cracking.

AYURVEDA Mix together one 5ml teaspoon aloe vera gel with half a teaspoon of turmeric and apply nightly to your feet. Cover with cotton socks, and wash off in the morning.

FELDENKRAIS METHOD Learn awareness of how you walk and stand, as incorrect movements may increase pressure on your feet and toes.

Warts and verrucas

Warts are small, rough benign lumps that appear on the skin, and verrucas (plantar warts) occur on the feet. Although warts are normally painless, verrucas can be painful to walk on as they get pushed up into the foot.

 ## SYMPTOMS

COMMON WARTS
▷ Firm, raised up and skin-coloured
▷ Rough surface

VERRUCAS
▷ A white, hard area on the foot, with a black dot in the centre

 ## PREVENTION

Warts and verrucas are both caused by the human papilloma virus (HPV). They are contagious and skin-to-skin contact can easily pass them on, so preventative methods are very important.
- Avoid sharing flannels, towels or shoes.
- Avoid touching someone's warts or verrucas.
- Wear flip-flops or sandals in communal changing rooms, saunas or showers.

 ## CONVENTIONAL REMEDIES

Creams, gels and medicated plasters are available over-the counter. Most contain an ingredient called salicylic acid and, although it helps warts and verrucas, it can also damage healthy skin. Anyone with diabetes or circulation problems needs to be especially careful and should speak to a doctor before using salicylic acid remedies. Some warts are treated with cryotherapy, whereby a cold liquid is sprayed on to the affected area to freeze the wart and destroy it.

 ## NATURAL REMEDIES

The following natural remedies may be helpful in treating warts and veruccas.

HERBAL REMEDIES Being susceptible to warts and verrucas can signify that your immune system is low, so you could try some immune-boosting remedies, such as echinacea. Thuja cream can be rubbed into the affected area daily.

AROMATHERAPY Oregano oil is packed with antiseptic properties and can help warts. Put a drop on a piece of cotton wool and dab it on the wart daily until cleared.

 ## HOMEOPATHIC REMEDIES

Homeopathic remedies that can help warts and verrucas include the following.

Causticum 30C: For getting rid of the infection, take one tablet daily.

Thuja 30C: For hard, misshapen warts, take one tablet daily.

 ## SEE YOUR DOCTOR

For severe and persistent cases of warts or verrucas that do not improve with over-the-counter or natural remedies, you should see your doctor.

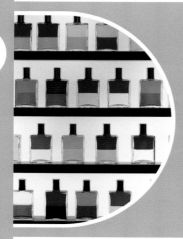

Body & foot odour

Everyone sweats, but some people have a tendency to sweat more than others and men tend to sweat more than women. Body and foot odour occur when the bacteria living on your skin causes sweat to break down into acids, which create a strong or unpleasant odour. Body odour can be an embarrassing health problem, but there are natural and conventional and natural remedies to help beat it.

 SYMPTOMS

▷ Sweating
▷ An odour under the armpits
▷ Smelly feet

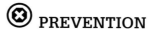 PREVENTION

- Body odour can be made worse if you are overweight or obese, so losing weight may help to prevent it.
- Dietary factors play a role in body odour – avoid eating very spicy foods and you may be saved from body odour.
- Foot odour can be prevented by not wearing trainers or any shoes that have a plastic lining, as they encourage your feet to sweat. Instead, opt for shoes that have a more foot-friendly leather lining.
- Make sure you change your socks every day and choose ones that are made from a mixture of wool and man-made fibres. These fibres will enable any sweat on your feet to evaporate.

Caution

Avoid using foot deodorants if you have a fungal foot infection – in this case, an anti-fungal foot spray or athlete's foot treatment is required.

CONVENTIONAL REMEDIES

- Warm water helps kill the bacteria on your skin, so have regular showers or baths.
- Use antibacterial soap and a deodorant or antiperspirant. Deodorants are designed to make the skin acidic, which helps ward off bacteria, whilst antiperspirants help block sweat glands and reduce sweating. Foot deodorants and antiperspirants are also available to purchase.
- Wear clothing made of natural fibres, such as cotton, wool or silk, as these allow your skin to breathe and sweat to evaporate more easily.
- Using an extra-strong antiperspirant, such as aluminium chloride, may be recommended by your doctor.
- In severe cases, a cosmetic treatment with Botox injections may be recommended. These are injected near the armpit and help to destroy the nerves that are involved in sweating.

 NATURAL REMEDIES

You can try some of the following natural remedies to combat body and foot odour.

HERBAL REMEDIES Use the herb marigold to help reduce sweating and body odour. Brew yourself a pot of marigold tea, by adding one to two teaspoons of dried marigold to a teapot and pouring boiling water over it. Drink the tea twice a day.

 NUTRITIONAL MEDICINE

Your diet can have an important effect on the smell of your sweat, so try adapting it as follows:

- Avoid eating garlic, spices or meals such as hot curries, as they could make your sweat smell stronger
- Try cutting back on eating red meat and dairy products – this may also help
- A zinc deficiency can contribute to sweating and body odour, so consider taking a daily zinc supplement.

 SEE YOUR DOCTOR

Although they are usually harmless and fine to treat at home, sometimes a change in body odour, or suddenly getting it, can be a sign of an underlying medical condition, such as diabetes, liver disease or kidney disease. If you suddenly begin to sweat a lot, have cold sweats, start sweating at night or notice that your body odour begins to smell fruity or like bleach, then please see your doctor.

Aromatherapy

- Put a few drops of antibacterial tea tree essential oil into a bowl or bath of warm water and bathe your feet in it. After washing, dry your feet thoroughly.
- For body odour, add up to six drops of essential oil to a warm bath; choose lemon, clary sage or lavender essential oils, or even a mix of all three, as they have deodorising properties.

44

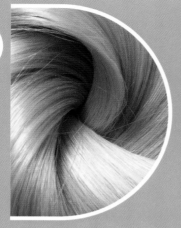

Dry hair

Silky, healthy-looking hair depends as much on good nutrition and how you feed it from the inside as the range of hair products you use and your hairdresser's skill. Indeed, your hair is an external barometer of your internal health, and its appearance and condition can be affected by many underlying medical problems as well as your lifestyle and environmental factors.

 SYMPTOMS

▷ Dry, rough and brittle hair
▷ Split, frayed ends
▷ Hair looks lacklustre
▷ The texture feels harsh like string

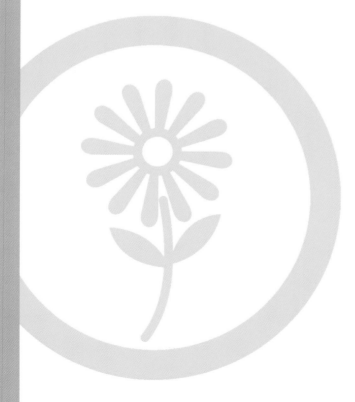

PREVENTION

The good news is that there are lots of effective remedies for dry hair and you don't have to suffer any more bad hair days. Better still, try to keep your hair well-nourished and in good condition to prevent it becoming dry and brittle. Here are some practical steps you can take to have healthy, shiny hair.

- Eat a healthy, balanced diet, which contains all the essential nutrients. Make sure you get your 5-A-Day portions of fresh fruit and vegetables, and foods that are good sources of Viamins C (citrus fruits, peppers, strawberries, tomatoes and leafy green vegetables) and E (avocados, whole-grain cereals and leafy green vegetables).
- Don't expose your hair to excessive sun – always wear a sun hat in hot weather.
- Use a swimming cap in chlorinated swimming pools.

 Did you know?

Stress, hair colourants, heat from hair dryers and straighteners, sun and chlorine, and poor nutrition can all damage your hair and dry it out. You need to consider all these factors.

- If you colour your hair yourself, always try to avoid chemical hair dyes and opt for natural colourants instead (see page 46).
- Visit the hairdresser for a trim at least once every six to eight weeks to keep the ends healthy and stop them splitting (see opposite).
- Keep the use of heated hair appliances, such as hair dryers, hot rollers, curling tongs and hair straighteners, to an absolute minimum.
- Try not to overdo applications of hairspray, mousse or styling gel – bombarding your hair with chemicals weakens and dulls it.
- Do not wash your hair every day. In reality, too-frequent washing can strip out the natural oils.
- Always rinse your hair thoroughly in warm, not hot, water to get rid of all shampoo residues
- Use a good-quality natural bristle brush, rather than a harsh nylon one, to prevent damaging your hair.
- Whenever possible, do allow your hair to dry naturally rather than use a hair dryer.

CONVENTIONAL REMEDIES

- After shampooing in the usual way, always use a conditioner that is specially formulated for dry hair and carefully comb it through from the roots to the ends of the hair. Leave for a few minutes or for the time specified on the container before rinsing it out thoroughly.
- To make an intensive-treatment conditioner more effective, apply it to your hair, then wrap your head in a hot damp towel and leave for 10–15 minutes before rinsing. Alternatively, you can use a stay-in conditioner with an in-built thermal protector – apply before blow-drying.

NATURAL REMEDIES

The natural remedies you select will depend on whether you wish to treat the condition from the inside or outside.

AROMATHERAPY Mix together one drop each of geranium, patchouli, rosemary and sandalwood essential oils with two 5ml teaspoons of jojoba oil. Massage into your scalp and hair with your fingertips and then wrap in a towel and leave for at least 15 minutes before washing out.

YOGA Some devotees of yoga believe that practising head and shoulderstand asanas can help keep hair healthy by boosting blood flow and nutrients to the scalp.

HERBAL REMEDIES

- If your scalp is very itchy, then add a soothing chamomile infusion to the final rinse.
- Make a cleansing herbal tea by infusing one 5ml teaspoon of dried burdock or marshmallow in near-boiling water. Steep for at least 5 minutes, then drain and drink.
- Make a pre-shampoo oil pack by heating some olive, almond or jojoba oil in a basin set over a pan of boiling water. Massage the warm oil into your dry hair and scalp and wrap in a towel or foil. Sit in a steamy bath for 15 minutes before rinsing and shampooing.

Split ends

To prevent split ends, you can try massaging a natural commercial brand of mayonnaise into clean, dry hair or make your own by whisking one 5ml teaspoon each of almond or vegetable oil and vinegar with a large egg, until smooth and emulsified. Leave for at least 1 hour before rinsing out.

NUTRITIONAL MEDICINE

- Make sure you include some foods that are rich in Vitamin E in your daily diet. Good sources are avocados, nuts, seeds, olive oil and leafy green vegetables.
- The most important nutrients of all for healthy hair are the B-complex group of vitamins, as deficiencies can lead to lacklustre, dry hair and dandruff (see opposite). Every day, try to eat some of the following foods: whole-grain cereals, meat, poultry, fish, eggs, cheese, bananas, brewers yeast, nuts and dark green leafy vegetables.
- Zinc and sulphur will also help to keep your hair glossy, silky and smooth.

 SEE YOUR DOCTOR

If none of the remedies seem to work and your hair remains stubbornly dry despite all your efforts, perhaps you should consult your doctor. In rare instances, dry hair can be a symptom of a more serious underlying medical condition, such as an under-active thyroid gland or even psoriasis if it is accompanied by a dry, scaly, itchy scalp. You may even be referred to a specialist or trichologist for treatment.

 HOME-MADE REMEDIES

- Add a 15ml tablespoon of cider vinegar to the rinsing water to add shine and soothe an itchy, dry scalp, which often accompanies dry hair.
- To add moisture and a healthy shine to your hair, mash up a ripe avocado with an egg yolk and a spoonful of olive oil. Massage into your hair and scalp and leave on for 20 to 30 minutes before washing out and shampooing.
- If you have any over-ripe discoloured avocados and black bananas, don't throw them away. Mash them up with a fork and smooth into your hair, rubbing the mixture into the roots. Rinse off after 15 minutes and wash in the usual way.
- Another kitchen remedy is to beat up an egg with a cup of yoghurt and the juice of a lemon. Mix in a 5ml teaspoon of coconut or olive oil and then massage into your hair and cover with a hot towel. Leave on for at least 30 minutes before rinsing and shampooing.

Natural hair colourants

Instead of using drying chemical hair colourants, try a herbal rinse for a soft and subtle effect.

- Chamomile flowers add sheen to blonde hair. Add a handful to a pan of simmering water and simmer for 20 minutes before straining and cooling. Use as a herbal rinse after shampooing and then rinse out thoroughly. Diluted lemon juice will make it shine.
- Elderberries will add a subtle, deep mahogany colour to dark hair. Prepare a herbal rinse in the same way as for chamomile above. Rinse it with a vinegar solution for extra shine.

 Did you know?

Your hair is a non-living tissue made of a protein called keratin. The hair shaft in every individual strand is coated with a layer of protective cells. Hair grows at a rate of 12mm (1/2in) per month and has a lifespan of three to six years.

Dandruff

This common scalp problem can vary in severity. Your skin cells are constantly being renewed and the old ones are shed. When this process is faster, the dead skin is more noticeable and is referred to as dandruff.

 SYMPTOMS

▷ Flaking scalp

▷ Small white flakes falling from hair onto shoulders

▷ In acute cases, may be yellowish waxy scales on scalp with large greasy flakes

 PREVENTION

- Eat a healthy, varied diet.
- Regular exercise will stimulate circulation and maintain hair health.
- Brush your hair regularly with a natural bristle brush, working from the scalp outwards.
- Wash your hair at least twice a week.
- Don't colour your hair with harsh chemical dyes.

 CONVENTIONAL REMEDIES

Dandruff is usually treated with conventional dandruff shampoos or lotions, but some can be very harsh and irritate sensitive scalps. Ideally, opt for a mild, non-detergent based one. Ask your pharmacist for advice on anti-dandruff and anti-fungal shampoos.

 NATURAL REMEDIES

For a more natural approach, wash and rinse your hair and then gently massage half a cup of warm olive oil into your scalp. Cover with a towel and leave for 30 minutes before shampooing and rinsing.

 NUTRITIONAL MEDICINE Include B vitamins and sulphur in your diet by eating whole-grain cereals, wheat germ, eggs and plenty of dark green leafy vegetables, such as cabbage. Cutting down on dairy foods may help alleviate dandruff.

 HERBAL REMEDIES

- Try a simple rosemary rinse: put a few sprigs of fresh rosemary in a saucepan, cover with water and simmer gently to 15 minutes. Cool and strain, then add a few drops of olive oil. After shampooing, use the rosemary water as a rinse before rinsing again with tepid water.
- Make an infusion of stinging nettles and add it to the final rinse.

 HOMEOPATHIC REMEDIES

Choose the appropriate remedy for your symptoms.

Oleander 6C, for an itchy, dry scalp with white flakes falling from the hair.

Kali sulphuricum 6C, for moist or sticky flaky dandruff.

SEE YOUR DOCTOR

You can usually treat dandruff yourself at home, but if it is persistent, excessively flaky and becomes acute, you should see your doctor for an accurate diagnosis. It could be a symptom of psoriasis, seborrhoeic dermatitis or a fungal infection.

Greasy hair

Healthy hair should be clean, manageable and glossy with plenty of bounce and natural shine. However, it is exposed on a daily basis to environmental pollution, wind, cold, heat, humidity and air conditioning, and all these factors can affect your hair type and condition. If you have greasy hair, do not despair – there are many natural beauty remedies as well as conventional ones.

 SYMPTOMS

▷ Hair looks and feels oily
▷ It needs frequent washing
▷ It looks dirty soon after it is washed
▷ It is limp, lank and lacks body

 PREVENTION

If you have a natural tendency towards excessively oily hair, you can take preventive measures to stop the condition getting worse.

- Eat a healthy diet with lots of fresh fruit and vegetables, and cut down on greasy, fried and high-fat, sugary foods.
- Exercise regularly to increase the oxygen supply to your scalp.
- Do not use too much conditioner, or even try cutting it out altogether – some conditioners can leave an oily residue on the hair, making the problem worse.
- Taking oral contraceptive pills can worsen the condition for some people – if you suspect that this may be the case, discuss it with your doctor who may suggest swapping to another pill.
- Use mousse to style your hair – it does not contain oil and it will add volume.
- Don't use hair sprays – they attract dust and dirt from the air and will make your hair appear even more greasy.
- Wash your hair brushes and combs regularly in tepid soapy water to avoid brushing grease back into your hair.

 Did you know?

Greasy hair is caused by over-active sebaceous glands beneath your scalp producing too much sebum (oil). Your diet, genetic inheritance, hormones, stress levels and general state of health may all contribute.

CONVENTIONAL REMEDIES

Greasy hair is usually treated by washing it frequently with a specially formulated shampoo for oily hair types. It is advisable to shampoo and rinse it twice to thoroughly remove all traces of oil and leave it squeaky clean. You may not need to use a conditioner.

 NATURAL REMEDIES

There are many natural treatments for the problem of oily hair, so why not try one of the following?

HERBAL REMEDIES Oily hair can benefit from lavender, peppermint and white dead-nettle herbs, used fresh or dried, in herbal teas, infusions and other preparations.

AROMATHERAPY Mix a massage oil by combining eight drops each rosemary, lavender, ylang ylang and lime oils. Massage gently into your scalp at bedtime. Wash with a natural shampoo the following morning and then rinse out thoroughly.

 HOME-MADE REMEDIES

- Add two beaten eggs and one 15ml tablespoon bicarbonate of soda to 600ml (1 pint) warm water. Pour over your hair and massage gently but firmly into your scalp. Leave for 10 to 15 minutes before rinsing. Shampoo and then rinse again.
- Another effective old-fashioned kitchen remedy is to add some cider vinegar to the final rinse to de-grease your hair.
- Like vinegar, lemon juice is acidic and can help control oil production. Try adding the freshly squeezed juice to a cup of warm water and pouring it over your hair after shampooing and rinsing. Leave for 5 minutes and then rinse again with some tepid water.

 SEE YOUR DOCTOR

Obviously, annoying as it may be, greasy hair is not a serious medical condition and there should be no need for you to consult a doctor. However, if it is persistent and affects your self-esteem, you may wish to make an appointment with a dermatologist or trichologist to get some specialist advice.

 Quick fix

If you have an important meeting or a date and don't have time to wash your hair, just apply some dry shampoo or even gently shake a little fine talcum powder or baby powder onto the hair roots, leave for a minute and brush through thoroughly to absorb excess oil.

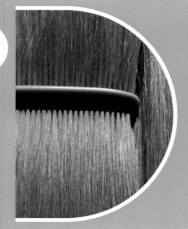

Head lice

Head lice (or nits) are small, pin-head-sized parasitic insects that live on the head where they suck the blood and lay eggs. They can spread quickly, usually among young schoolchildren, and are then transmitted to other members of their family. Contrary to popular myth, dirty hair is not a cause – head lice always prefer clean, shiny hair and healthy scalps.

 ## SYMPTOMS

▷ Itching scalp – not usually an early symptom
▷ Lice look similar to dandruff in the host's hair
▷ The eggs are oval, yellowish-white and pearl-like in appearance

 ## PREVENTION

It is difficult to prevent head lice as they do not respect good hygiene and cleanliness, but if your child does come home with nits, you can try to stop other family members becoming infested, too.

- Do not share hair brushes and combs.
- Avoid cross-infection by asking everyone to use only their own personal towels.
- Do not share a bed or bedlinen.
- Check children's hair regularly by combing with a fine nit comb.
- Keep hair tied back and avoid head-to-head contact.

 ## CONVENTIONAL REMEDIES

The conventional treatment for head lice is to use a specially formulated chemical insecticide shampoo or lotion. However, these are quite harsh and they should not be used too frequently, especially on very young children or people who suffer from asthma and allergies.

 ## Did you know?

Head lice cannot jump between heads; there has to be contact to enable them to crawl onto a new host. They lay their eggs on the sides of hair shafts close to the scalp. The eggs take seven to ten days to hatch, and the lice live for about 30 days, laying an average of 10 or so eggs per day.

NATURAL REMEDIES

Because insecticides can have unwanted side-effects, many people are seeking out more gentle natural remedies for treating head lice.

- Dampen your child's hair, adding conditioner if wished, and comb through in sections with a special fine-toothed metal nit comb (available from pharmacies) to remove the eggs, wiping the comb clean on some tissue or kitchen paper between strokes. Repeat once every three days for two to three weeks until there are no signs of any lice or eggs.
- Try rinsing the hair in cider vinegar and rubbing some lemon juice into the scalp to destroy the eggs and combat oiliness.

HERBAL REMEDIES Make an infusion of bitterwood bark by adding the chips to freshly boiled water. Leave to stand and cool before straining into a bottle. Add witch hazel and spray on to the hair. You can also scatter wormwood in your linen cupboard and drawers of clothes to kill lice and fleas. Both these herbs are available from herbalists, some pharmacies and health food stores.

 ## AROMATHERAPY

- Put a few drops of neat thyme or tea tree essential oil on a fine metal comb and comb in sections, at least twice a day, preferably first thing in the morning and at bedtime.
- Alternatively, mix five 15ml tablespoons of a carrier oil, such as vegetable oil, with 20 drops tea tree oil, 15 drops each thyme and lavender oil, and 10 drops rosemary oil. Smooth onto the hair and massage gently into the scalp and hair. Cover for at least an hour and then rinse and shampoo as normal.
- Or you can make up a simple but effective home-made treatment by putting 10 drops of each of the following oils – eucalyptus, lavender, peppermint, rosemary and tea tree – in a clean 60ml bottle or container. Fill to the top with a carrier oil, such as almond, apricot kernel or olive oil. Seal and then shake gently to mix well together. Use this mixture to rinse your hair twice daily.

 ## SEE YOUR DOCTOR

Most cases of head lice can be treated quickly and effectively with natural remedies or over-the-counter products. However, if you do not respond to these treatments or suffer allergic reactions, you should consult your doctor.

Spring clean

It is not enough to treat the infected person's head. You must wash all their towels and bedding and even, in some cases, treat the furniture, including sofas and chairs where they recline and their heads may have rested.

 ## Quick fix

Before going to bed, smear some petroleum jelly over your scalp and hair and then cover with a shower cap. It will trap the lice. Shower off the following morning.

TOP 10
Skincare recipes

If you care about what you put on your skin, and want to avoid harsh chemicals, then natural skincare is the way to go. As well as buying natural products, it's quick and easy to make your own. Here are 10 skincare recipes to try at home – all need to be washed off after use.

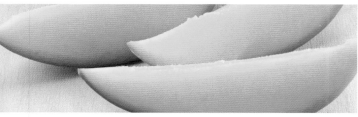
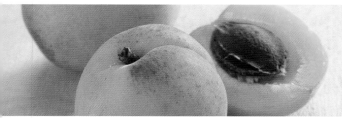
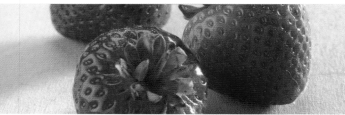
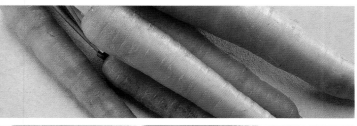
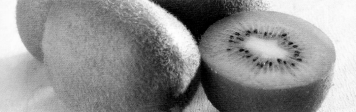

RETINOL-RICH MANGO SCRUB
BENEFITS

Mango contains retinol, or vitamin A, which helps regenerate collagen in skin.

INGREDIENTS

1 ripe mango, 1 tablespoon honey, 2 tablespoons milk and ½ cup sugar.

METHOD

Blend all the ingredients together, then apply to your face or body. Leave on for 10 minutes.

SUPER KIWI SKIN FIRMER
BENEFITS

Kiwi is rich in vitamin C and can rejuvenate tired looking skin.

INGREDIENTS

1 ripe kiwi and 1 teaspoon honey.

METHOD

Blend the ingredients, then drain off any excess liquid to leave a paste. Apply to your face for 15 minutes.

REFRESHING CUCUMBER TONER
BENEFITS

Cucumber is refreshing and witch hazel is cooling and astringent.

INGREDIENTS

½ cucumber, 3 tablespoons witch hazel.

METHOD

Chop and blend the cucumber, hen strain off the juice. Mix the juice with the witch hazel. Dab onto your face with cotton wool.

AVOCADO MOISTURIZER

BENEFITS

Avocados are packed with oily unsaturated fat, vitamins and minerals. They nourish dehydrated or damaged skin.

INGREDIENTS

1 avocado, 1 cup warmed live or almond oil.

METHOD

Mash the ingredients together, then chill. Apply to the skin for 20 minutes.

APRICOT SHOWER SCRUB

BENEFITS

Apricot moisturizes the skin and sea salt exfoliates.

INGREDIENTS

3 fresh apricots, 3 tablespoons apricot kernel oil, 2 cups sea salt.

METHOD

Blend the apricots and oil, then stir in the sea salt. Use as a scrub in the shower.

FINE LINE REDUCER

BENEFITS

Eggs contain the protein albumin and have amino acids that smooth fine lines.

INGREDIENTS

2 egg yolks, 1 teaspoon sugar.

METHOD

Whisk the egg yolks until firm, then add the sugar and mix well. Apply to your face for 20 minutes.

STRAWBERRY FACE MASK

BENEFITS

Strawberries cleanse the skin and help remove excess oil.

INGREDIENTS

½ cup strawberries, 1 tablespoon double cream.

METHOD

Blend the strawberries and then add the cream. Apply this mixture to your face and neck for 10 minutes.

SIMPLE BANANA FACE MASK

BENEFITS

Banana nourishes the skin.

INGREDIENTS

2 ripe small bananas.

METHOD

Mash the bananas, then apply to your face for 20 minutes.

CREAMY CARROT FACE CREAM

BENEFITS

Carrots contain retinol, which is important for anti-aging.

INGREDIENTS

1 large cooked carrot, 2 tablespoons cream cheese.

METHOD

Mash the ingredients together. Apply to the face and neck for 15 minutes.

ZESTY WINTER SKIN MASK

BENEFITS

The Vitamin C in the fruit rejuvenates winter skin and the scent is uplifting.

INGREDIENTS

Juice of 2 lemons and 1 orange, 1 cup powdered milk, a drop of water.

METHOD

Mix the ingredients together, adding enough water to make a thick, but spreadable, paste. Apply to your skin; leave on for 15 minutes.

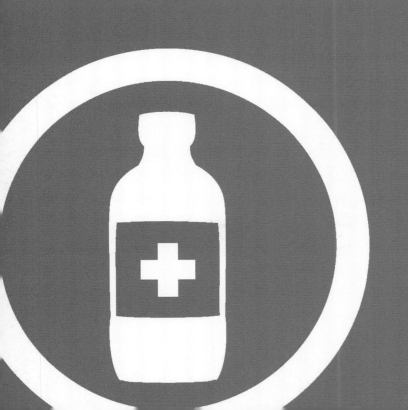

Ear, eye and mouth problems

Your ears, eyes and mouth are not only the sensory gateways to hearing, sight and taste but are also distinctive characteristics that are individual to you and your appearance. They all have important functions in the body and mirror your general health.

Your ears enable you to hear and govern your sense of balance. They consist of an outer ear (outside the body up to your eardrum), middle ear (between your ear drum and the hearing nerve) and inner ear (containing the receptor hair cells, which convert sounds to nerve impulses). Common problems range from bacterial and viral infections to build-up of wax.

Your eyes are your body's organs of vision, detecting light and sending messages to the brain via the optic nerve. Eye health is very important and is affected by many factors, including your diet, your lifestyle and state of health. Common problems include infections, inflammation (often due to allergies), visual disturbances and focusing difficulties.

Your mouth is the entry point to your digestive and respiratory systems: you eat with it, and breathe through it when your nose is blocked. Inside are your teeth for chewing food, thousands of taste buds, and three pairs of salivary glands, which moisten the food. It is also where the vibrations produced by your vocal cords are converted into speech. Effective dental care is essential both for keeping your teeth and gums healthy and preventing problems elsewhere in the body. New research suggests that there may be a link between gum disease and the incidence of heart disease and stroke.

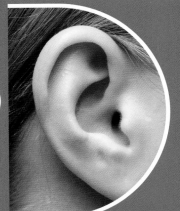

Ear problems

Ears play an important role in helping you hear clearly and also maintaining your sense of balance. Common problems affecting the ears include a build-up of excessive ear wax, which blocks the ear and affects hearing, earache and ear infections, where an infection develops in the middle ear.

 SYMPTOMS

EARWAX BUILD-UP

▷ Dulled hearing

▷ Ringing in the ear

▷ Mild dizziness or vertigo

EAR INFECTION

▷ Earache

▷ Dulled hearing

▷ Fever

▷ Feeling generally unwell

▷ Discharge from the ear

 PREVENTION

- However tempted you may be to stick a cotton wool bud in your ear to clean and remove wax, don't do it! The cotton bud will push the wax back even more and will make it become compacted, which only increases the risk of blockage from a wax build-up.

- Earache can be brought on by exposure to icy cold winds, so wear a hat that covers your ears on cold winter days.

- Frequent swimmers are sometimes prone to ear infections. Wearing ear plugs can help to prevent water getting into the ear and also reduce the risk of infection.

 Did you know?

One of the best ways of softening ear wax is olive oil. Use cooking olive oil, or buy special dropper medicinal bottles from chemists and insert a couple of drops in each ear. Often, this is the only treatment needed to clear ears from a wax build-up, although badly blocked ears may take a week to clear.

CONVENTIONAL REMEDIES

BLOCKED EARS AND EARWAX Over-the-counter eardrops can be purchased to apply to your ears, for three to four days. Many drops contain an active ingredient called urea hydrogen peroxide, which creates a fizzing sensation in the ears. Sometimes drops can make the ears irritated or painful. For bad cases, and if ears are completely blocked, syringing may be required by a practice nurse at your doctor's surgery (don't ever try to do this yourself).

EARACHE Painkillers are used to help relieve ear discomfort.

EAR INFECTION Antibiotics may be prescribed to relieve ear infections. For associated ear pain, painkillers may be required.

 ## NATURAL REMEDIES

There are various natural remedies you can try to relieve ear problems.

HOMEOPATHIC REMEDIES Aconite 6C can be taken to aid earache that is brought on by being out in a cold wind. Belladonna 6C can help ear infections, especially when there is a lot of pain and fever. Take one tablet of each, twice daily.

NUTRITIONAL MEDICINE Take vitamin C tablets daily to boost your immune system, or eat foods that are rich in vitamin C, such as oranges, broccoli, kiwi fruit or strawberries.

 ## Quick fix

Hold a warm hot water bottle, or heat pad, against your ear to relieve the distressing symptoms of earache.

 ## HERBAL REMEDIES

- Garlic oil drops can be used to help the symptoms of ear infections. Add one or two drops into each ear, ideally with a different dropper to minimise the risk of spreading the infection.
- A liquid extract of St John's Wort, which has antiseptic properties, can also be used for treating ear problems.
- Echinacea tablets or liquid can support your immune system during an infection.

 ## HELPFUL THERAPIES

HOPI EAR CANDLING This unusual therapy uses special hollowed candles, which are lit at one end, while the other end is placed just inside the ear for short periods to help clear wax. This needs to be done by a qualified practitioner and may help to relieve ear problems without the need for other remedies.

CRANIAL OSTEOPATHY A build-up of fluid in the ear occurs with ear infections, but gentle manipulation of the skull by a cranial osteopath may help to drain this fluid. Only go to a properly qualified practitioner.

SEE YOUR DOCTOR

If you have severe and persistent earache you should seek your doctor's advice – you may have an ear infection and need prescribed medication, such as antibiotics.

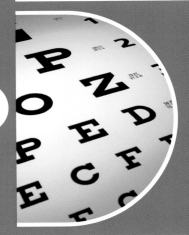

Eye strain

You may experience eye strain after focusing on a visual task for a long time, such as when reading, driving or using a computer. However, although your eyes will feel uncomfortable and tired, eye strain is unlikely to be anything serious and can be helped with a few simple measures. Eye strain is also known as asthenopia.

SYMPTOMS

▷ Tired, itchy, burning, stinging or sore eyes
▷ Dry or watery eyes
▷ Headaches
▷ Blurred or double vision
▷ Sensitivity to light
▷ Difficulty focusing
▷ Problems concentrating
▷ Fatigue

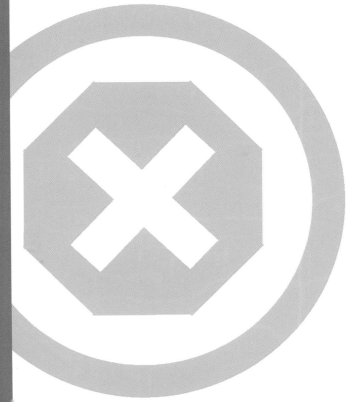

⊗ PREVENTION

You can help to prevent eye strain by making a few adjustments when you are doing close-up work. Here are some practical examples.

- Use good lighting – dim light can cause your eyes to strain in order to see what you are doing. Make sure sunlight or artificial light is not shining directly at you or on your computer screen.
- Check that the contrast and brightness, text size and resolution of your computer screen are all set at comfortable viewing levels for you.
- Sit at least one arm's length away from your computer screen.
- Occasionally look up from what you are doing and glance out of the window, or at things further away from you in the room. This will relax your eye muscles.
- Take frequent breaks. Get up and move around, stretch out your arms, shoulders, neck and back.
- When driving for a long time, glance at the speedometer or fuel gauge every now and again to shift your focus. If it's sunny, wear sunglasses to avoid squinting.

CONVENTIONAL REMEDIES

Taking frequent breaks to rest your eyes should be enough to relieve eye strain. Use over-the-counter eye drops several times daily if eye strain is causing dryness. Glasses may be prescribed for driving, reading or computer use.

 NATURAL REMEDIES

The following natural remedies may help to prevent and soothe tired eyes.

HERBAL MEDICINE To relieve eye strain, take one to two 470mg eyebright capsules daily, or drink as a herbal tea.

AROMATHERAPY Soak a clean flannel in a bowl of cold water, to which two drops of lavender essential oil have been added. Place over your eyes for 10 minutes.

NUTRITIONAL MEDICINE Kale, spinach, peas, courgettes, Brussels sprouts and broccoli are all good sources of lutein, a nutrient that is beneficial for eye health.

 HOMEOPATHIC REMEDIES

These remedies may help to ease symptoms:

Ruta graveolens 6C: Take two tablets four times daily to relieve aching eye muscles

Apis mellifica 6C: Take two tablets four times daily for stinging or burning eyes.

 EXERCISE

The following simple exercises may help to relieve eye strain and tension:

- Hold your thumb up 15cm (6in) away from your nose and focus on it. Then focus on an object in the distance. Bring your focus back to your thumb. Repeat 15 times.
- Keeping your neck and shoulders relaxed, drop your chin to your chest. Lift your head up, and then drop your head backwards. Return to the starting position. Repeat six times.
- Turn your head to the left, then back to the centre. Turn your head to the right, and then back to the centre. Repeat six times both sides.

 SEE YOUR DOCTOR

If your eye strain symptoms do not resolve themselves with any preventative or self-help measures, see your doctor or optician. You may have a vision problem or another condition that needs correcting. You should also seek medical advice if you experience pain in your eyes or loss of vision.

 IMMEDIATE RELIEF

Close your eyes, and use your fingers to massage your temples in a circular motion for 60 seconds.

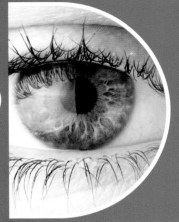

Eye irritation

Eye irritation is uncomfortable and can be caused by dust, smoke or other airborne irritants, eye makeup, tiredness, dry eyes or infection. Equally irritating is a foreign body in the eye, such as grit, sand, dust, or fragments of wood, plastic, paint, or metal.

 SYMPTOMS

▷ Watery or dry eyes
▷ Itching, burning or stinging eyes
▷ Red eyes
▷ A sensation of something being stuck in your eye
▷ A rust stain in your eye if the foreign body is metal
▷ Eye pain
▷ Sensitivity to light
▷ Blurred vision

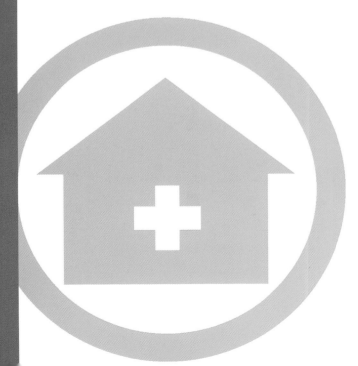

PREVENTION

Here are some simple, practical measures that you can take to avoid eye irritation and foreign bodies in your eyes.

- Wear sunglasses on windy days to protect them from airborne particles.
- Avoid smoky places.
- Replace your eye makeup regularly; if you keep it too long it will harbour bacteria.
- Spray household cleaning products and other eye-irritants well away from your face, and always use only in a well-ventilated area.
- Don't rub your eyes, especially if you have been handling irritants.
- Wear safety goggles where there is a risk of stray objects or fluids hitting you in the eye, such as: when doing DIY, strimming, hammering, mixing chemicals, sawing, sanding, drilling or welding.

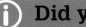 **Did you know?**

In order to examine your eye, a doctor may use a special dye that is called fluorescein. This will stain the damaged areas of your eye bright green for easy identification.

CONVENTIONAL REMEDIES

Eye drops or eye baths are used to soothe irritated eyes, but if the irritation is persistent or due to infection, anti-inflammatory medications or antibiotics may be necessary. If there is a foreign body trapped in your eye, it will need to be washed out with clean water to dislodge it. If the object won't budge, it will need removal by a doctor, who may also prescribe eye drops to prevent infection. Painkillers, such as ibuprofen or paracetamol, can be taken to ease pain.

NATURAL REMEDIES

The following remedies may make your eyes feel more comfortable.

HERBAL REMEDIES Mix one teaspoon dried eyebright with 500ml boiling water. Leave to infuse for 30 minutes, then strain. Soak a clean flannel in the solution and place over closed eyes for 10 minutes.

NUTRITIONAL MEDICINE For dry eyes, take 1000mg flaxseed oil twice daily. This helps to encourage tear production and moisturise eyes.

AROMATHERAPY Add one drop of chamomile essential oil to a cup of warm water. Soak two cotton wool pads in the solution, squeeze them out and then apply to your closed eyes for 10 minutes.

 ## HOMEOPATHIC REMEDIES

Symphytum 6C: Take one or two tablets three times daily to relieve pain after injury to the eye.

Aconitum napellus 30C: Take four tablets four times daily to soothe irritation from a foreign body in the eye.

Sulphur 30C: Take two tablets four times daily to reduce redness, inflammation and itching.

 ## SEE YOUR DOCTOR

You should see your doctor if:

- You have an object in your eye and you can't remove it
- Your eye hurts continuously
- You have distorted vision
- You can see spots or other random shapes in your field of vision
- You have cut your eye
- There is redness in your eye
- Bright light is painful
- A foreign body entered your eye when travelling at high speed.

Caution

Do not attempt to dislodge an embedded foreign body by poking it with cotton buds or other objects. You risk doing more harm than good.

Styes

A stye is a boil-like infection at the base of an eyelash on the upper or lower eyelid. Fortunately, most styes, although painful and annoying, do not warrant special treatment and they will usually burst or dry up within a week.

 SYMPTOMS

▷ Irritation of the eyelid
▷ Redness and swelling
▷ Throbbing pain
▷ Small inflamed bump appears on the eyelid
▷ Feels as though you have something in your eye
▷ May discharge pus

 PREVENTION

Styes may be a sign of general poor health and a low resistance to infection. Eating a healthy diet, regular exercise and staying relaxed and stress-free will all help to prevent them occurring.

- Take vitamin C and zinc supplements or eat foods that contain these nutrients. They will help boost your immune system.
- Eat foods that contain beta-carotene and vitamin A, such as oily fish, liver, dairy produce, eggs, dried apricots, carrots, and dark green leafy and yellow vegetables.
- If you already have a stye, always wash your hands after touching it.

 Did you know?

If a stye bursts, wipe away the pus with some moistened cotton wool. Use a clean pad each time so as not to spread infection.

- Don't rub the stye or you may spread the infection to other follicles on your eyelid.
- Use separate towels and flannels from other family members, and change them often.

 CONVENTIONAL REMEDIES

Pain-relievers may be taken for painful styes. If they do not clear up, however, they may require a course of antibiotics.

 NATURAL REMEDIES

The time-honoured natural remedy for styes is to place a warm used tea bag on your closed eye for 10 minutes. This is soothing and helps the stye to come to a head or point.

HERBAL REMEDIES Make a herbal tea (see page 142) of marigold or eyebright and, after straining and cooling, use to bathe the affected area. Take echinacea capsules to boost your immune system.

HOMEOPATHIC REMEDIES Take pulsatilla 6C for styes on the upper lid; and staphysagria 6C for recurrent styes.

 SEE YOUR DOCTOR

If your stye fails to heal within a week, consult your doctor as the infection can spread to your eye.

Conjunctivitis

Also known as pink-eye, conjunctivitis is the inflammation of the membrane that lines the inner eyelids and covers the eye itself. It may be caused by infection, an irritant or an allergic reaction, and it is highly contagious.

 SYMPTOMS

▷ Eye looks red, swollen and inflamed
▷ Eye may be itchy
▷ Feels gritty – like sand in the eye
▷ Burning sensation in eye
▷ Sensitivity to light
▷ Sticky or watery discharge
▷ Eyelids may stick together after sleeping

 PREVENTION

Although you cannot prevent conjunctivitis, you can stop it spreading to your other eye.

- Try not to rub your eye, however itchy, as this will make the condition worse.
- Always wash your hands after touching the affected eye. Dry them with disposable paper towels or a hot hand dryer.
- When wiping away discharge from the affected eye, use a different tissue or cotton wool for each wipe and dispose of them.
- Use separate towels and flannels from other family members, and change them often.
- Don't wear contact lenses or eye makeup until the infection clears up.
- Eat foods that contain beta-carotene and vitamin A, such as oily fish, liver, dairy produce, eggs, dried apricots, carrots, and dark green leafy and yellow vegetables.

 CONVENTIONAL REMEDIES

Conjunctivitis is usually treated with antibiotic eyedrops or ointment. Taking antihistamines may relieve the symptoms of allergic conjunctivitis.

 NATURAL REMEDIES

You can soothe the itching and relieve inflammation by bathing the eye(s) with boiled, cooled water (salty, if wished), or placing a used teabag or thin slice of cucumber over the closed affected eye.

HERBAL REMEDIES Use a herbal eyebath of marigold or chamomile. Take echinacea capsules every day to fight the infection and boost your immune system.

 SEE YOUR DOCTOR

Conjunctivitis can be potentially serious and unless the symptoms are very mild and disappear within a few days, you must consult your doctor – do not try to treat it yourself. Seek immediate medical help if you experience blurred vision.

 Did you know?

Allergic conjunctivitis can be triggered by a reaction to pollen, eye makeup or even the cleaning solution used by contact lens wearers.

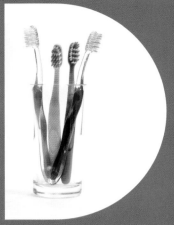

Gum problems

Gum disease is a major cause of tooth decay and there are two main types: gingivitis and periodontal disease. Both conditions are caused by poor dental hygiene and, if left untreated, they can lead to painful abscesses and even loose teeth, which will fall out eventually.

 ## SYMPTOMS

▷ Gums are inflamed, red and swollen
▷ They bleed easily when brushing, flossing or even eating
▷ Your breath may smell unpleasant
▷ Your teeth may become loose and wobbly
▷ You may develop a painful abscess

 ## PREVENTION

You may not even realise that you have gum disease as it may not be painful or evident in the early stages. However, most of us are affected, and if you visit your dentist regularly, brush and floss your teeth every day and don't consume lots of sugar, you can slow down the rate at which the disease develops and you will not lose your teeth.

- Brush your teeth with toothpaste twice daily, especially around the gum line.
- Use an electric toothbrush for more effective brushing around the gum line.
- After brushing, always floss.
- Stop smoking now – it produces more plaque and can make gum disease worse.
- Eat a healthy diet with lots of crunchy, fibrous vegetables and daily vitamin C, found especially in citrus fruits.
- Sugar is your gums' worst energy, so cut out sugary soft drinks and high-sugar foods.
- Always brush your teeth after high-sugar food and drink.
- Visit your dentist regularly for check-ups.
- Get the hygienist to show you how to clean your teeth properly to remove all the plaque.

 ## Did you know?

Gum disease is caused by plaque, a film of food and bacteria on your gums and teeth. Most can be removed by brushing and flossing; if not, it builds up around the gum line, tartar forms on the surface of teeth, your gums shrink and the resulting pockets cause abscesses and loose teeth.

CONVENTIONAL REMEDIES

You can buy specially formulated over-the-counter gels and mouthwashes in most pharmacies and supermarkets to bring instant relief to sore gums.

 ## NATURAL REMEDIES

If your gums are sore, painful and swollen, try these natural remedies.

- Gargle with saltwater to reduce germs in your mouth – dissolve one 5ml teaspoon salt in a tumbler of hot water. Allow to cool before using.
- Make a paste of bicarbonate of soda and water and apply sparingly to the gums.
- Gently massage your gums to boost circulation and blood flow.
- If your gums are swollen and painful or you have an abscess, you can apply an ice pack to your cheek over the painful area.

AROMATHERAPY Cypress, myrrh, rose, thyme and tea tree oils can all be helpful in treating gum disease. Use them in mouthwashes.

 ## HERBAL REMEDIES

- Make up some chamomile or thyme tea, then strain and cool. Use as a soothing mouthwash.
- Apply a little aloe vera gel to soothe inflamed gums.
- Add a few drops of echinacea liquid extract to a glass of warm water and rinse your mouth out three times a day.
- Rub a little calendula tincture on to sore gums to reduce inflammation.

 ## HOMEOPATHIC REMEDIES

The remedy used will depend on the symptoms presented.

Merc sol 6C: Take one tablet three times a day to relieve inflamed, bleeding gums with bad breath.

Kreosotum 6C: Take one tablet three times a day for swollen gums that bleed easily and painful teeth.

See your dentist

If your gums are sore, bleeding or receding and you notice a build-up of yellowish tartar around your teeth, you must visit your dentist. The scale can be removed and you will be given advice on how to take care of your teeth and keep your gums healthy. Make an appointment if you have a loose tooth or painful gums with a fever or swollen glands in your neck – these may be symptoms of an abscess that requires urgent treatment.

 ## Quick fix

There is no quick fix for gum disease – you have to be eternally vigilant – but if your gums are very painful, you can rub in some soothing babies' teething gel.

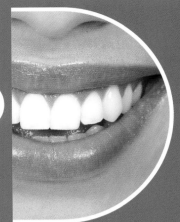

Toothache

Most toothache is caused by dental decay, gingivitis (gum disease) or an abscess, often due to poor dental hygiene. If your gums become inflamed and infected, they can recede, exposing the root of the tooth. The affected tooth can be sensitive to hot and cold food or liquids and may start throbbing.

 ## SYMPTOMS

▷ Pain around a tooth – throbbing or severe
▷ Sensitivity to extremes of temperature
▷ Red, swollen gums
▷ Bleeding when brushing or flossing

 ## PREVENTION

Good oral hygiene, regular visits to the dentist and eating a healthy diet that is low in sugar are the best ways to keep your teeth and gums healthy and prevent toothache, gum disease and dental problems.

- Brush your teeth with toothpaste twice daily, especially before going to bed.
- Brush in a circular motion.
- After brushing, floss carefully around each tooth – gum disease is the major cause of tooth decay and loss, and flossing can help prevent it.
- Eat a healthy diet with plenty of foods containing vitamin C, especially citrus fruits and leafy green vegetables.
- Cut out sugary soft drinks ¬ check the labels carefully to ensure no sugars have been added to fruit juices.
- Reduce your sugar intake and always brush your teeth after consuming high-sugar foods.
- Visit your dentist regularly for dental check-ups.
- Make regular appointments with an oral hygienist.

 ## Did you know?

If you have an abscess, with sensitive swollen gums, intense pain and even a fever, your dentist may prescribe a course of antibiotics to fight the infection before treating it.

CONVENTIONAL REMEDIES

The conventional treatment for toothache is to take painkillers and make an appointment to see your dentist. However, do read the instructions carefully to ensure that you do not exceed the recommended dose.

 ## NATURAL REMEDIES

Conventional painkillers are not always very effective and may have side-effects, so you may prefer to try natural remedies instead to deal with the nagging pain of tooth and gum disease while you wait to see your dentist.

- The traditional way to ease the pain is to dab the painful tooth and the gum surrounding it with some cotton wool soaked in clove oil.
- Alternatively, you can chew on a clove with the affected tooth – biting into it will release the oil.
- Chewing a peeled garlic clove may also bring some relief.
- A soothing warm saltwater mouthwash can be repeated several times a day to fight infection – use one 5ml teaspoon salt to a cup of hot water.

HERBAL REMEDIES Add 5 drops tincture of myrrh (available from herbalists) to a small glass of warm water and then use as a mouthwash. A tincture of calendula can be applied to swollen gums to ease the pain and swelling.

AROMATHERAPY Rub a little clove or chamomile oil around the affected tooth.

ACUPRESSURE Try applying pressure to the area between your thumb and forefinger (point 4) for up to a minute.

HOMEOPATHIC REMEDIES

The remedy used will depend on the symptoms presented.

Chamomilla 30C: Take one tablet every two hours to relieve pain aggravated by coffee and warm drinks.

Magnesia carbonica 30C: Take one tablet every two hours for pain that is worse at night and aggravated by cold.

Staphysagria 30C: Take one tablet every two hours for pain that is aggravated by cold and by eating.

 ## Quick fix

If you don't have any oil of cloves, you could try rubbing a little brandy around the affected tooth to deaden the pain.

See your dentist

Even if the remedies you try are effective at relieving the pain of toothache, you must make a dental appointment without delay to deal with the root of the problem and try to save the affected tooth.

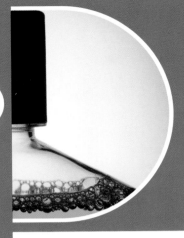

Mouth ulcers

Although mouth ulcers look small and insignificant, they are sore, painful and irritating. They may occur inside the lips and cheeks, on the roof of the mouth, the tongue and gums. They are usually nothing to worry about and are the result of injuries, such as biting your lips, ill-fitting dentures or a jagged, sharp-edged tooth.

 SYMPTOMS

▷ Small white or yellowish craters
▷ They may have a red border
▷ Appear singly or in clusters

 PREVENTION

Recurrent mouth ulcers may signal stress, poor diet or underlying health problems. You can help prevent them by doing the following.

- Eating a healthy diet containing vitamins B and C: meat, poultry, whole-grain cereals, beans, wheatgerm, leafy green vegetables, citrus fruits, tomatoes and peppers.
- Taking a daily vitamin supplement.
- Putting aside some time every day to relax if you have a hectic, stressful lifestyle or taking up yoga or meditation.
- Eating some live probiotic yoghurt every day to replace friendly bacteria in your mouth.
- Avoiding salty, hot, spicy and acidic foods.
- Checking that your toothpaste does not contain sodium lauryl sulphate, a substances that may cause ulcers in some individuals.
- Taking garlic capsules every day.
- Checking your diet as some foods can trigger outbreaks of ulcers, notably wheat and other cereals, shellfish, citrus, fruits, strawberries and chocolate.

 Did you know?

Mouth ulcers can be caused by some drugs, toothpastes, smoking, alcohol, heavily spiced and salted foods. If you suspect that one of these is the culprit, try avoiding or eliminating them, or talk to your doctor about it.

CONVENTIONAL REMEDIES

Most ulcers clear up quite quickly of their own accord but you can apply a soothing teething gel (sold for babies) or try sucking pain-relieving pastilles or lozenges that contain local anaesthetic.

 ## NATURAL REMEDIES

There are many traditional remedies that you can make yourself for treating mouth ulcers.

- Peel a clove of garlic, then cut in half and dab the cut surface on to the ulcer. Repeat three or times a day.
- Cut the top off a vitamin E capsule and squeeze out the contents on to the ulcer.

AROMATHERAPY Dab a drop of tea tree oil on to the ulcer, or make a mouthwash by adding 2 drops myrrh oil or myrrh tincture to a glass of warm water.

 ## HERBAL REMEDIES

- Cover some fresh or dried sage with boiling water, stand for 10 minutes, and then strain and use as a mouthwash when cool. Alternatively, you can make a mouthwash with some raspberry leaves, marigold, rosemary, myrrh or chamomile.
- Dab the ulcer with goldenseal tincture or add a few drops to a glass of warm water and use as a mouthwash.
- Use a little aloe vera gel on the ulcer – apply frequently to soothe and heal it.

 ## HOMEOPATHIC REMEDIES

Do not use the following remedies if you suffer from anaemia. Take them for a maximum of five days and stop as soon as the condition improves.

Borax 6C: Take one tablet twice a day for painful ulcers that bleed on touch or when eating.

Mercurius sol 6C: Take one tablet twice a day for ulcers on the tongue, mouth and throat with a metallic taste in the mouth.

Nitric acid 6C: Take one tablet twice a day for ulcers on the tongue and soft palate that bleed easily.

 ## SEE YOUR DOCTOR

If you have painful and recurrent mouth ulcers, it is worth consulting your doctor as there may be an underlying medical disorder that merits investigation.

 Quick fix

Chewing liquorice is thought to be beneficial; you can buy special DGL liquorice wafers in some health food stores.

Bad breath

If you suffer from bad breath (halitosis), you will probably be the last to know, and many friends may be too polite to tell you. It is rarely a sign of more serious medical conditions but it can be difficult identifying the cause.

 SYMPTOMS

▷ Breath smells unpleasant

 PREVENTION

Bad breath is usually caused by poor dental hygiene or an unhealthy diet. Luckily, there are lots of things you can do to prevent it.

- Brush and floss your teeth twice a day, preferably after every meal, and brush or scrape your tongue – gum disease is the most common cause of bad breath.
- Change your toothbrush every two to three months and keep it clean.
- Avoid sugary soft drinks or even sugar-free carbonated ones.
- A dry mouth can contribute to bad breath, so drink eight glasses of water a day.
- Avoid using minty mouthwashes, which can dry up breath-freshening saliva.
- Visit your dentist regularly.

 Did you know?

Bad breath is caused by bacteria in your mouth on your gums, teeth and tongue. The best way to combat it is to develop a good oral hygiene routine.

- Eat plenty of fibre to improve digestion and avoid constipation, which may contribute to bad breath.
- Onions, garlic, alcohol, smelly cheeses and spicy food may be the cause, so try eliminating them.
- Stop smoking and you will notice an immediate improvement in breath freshness.

 CONVENTIONAL REMEDIES

Choose from a wide range of over-the-counter breath fresheners and antiseptic mouthwashes.

 NATURAL REMEDIES

- Chew on some mint leaves, fennel, dill or caraway seeds, or even a coffee bean.
- Swap to a tea tree oil toothpaste.
- For a quick breath deodoriser, chew a sprig of parsley or sugar-free gum after meals, or eat an orange to stimulate the production of saliva.

HERBAL REMEDIES Make a cup of thyme tea with fresh or dried herbs and boiling water. Stand for 10 minutes, then strain.

AROMATHERAPY Use lemon, peppermint or tea tree oil in a mouthwash or gargle.

 SEE YOUR DOCTOR

There should be no need to see your doctor if you improve your dental hygiene and eat healthily. However, make an appointment if your breath smells sweet as this could indicate diabetes.

Dry mouth

If you suffer from a dry mouth, which is caused by a lack of saliva, you can make it feel moist and more comfortable by trying the remedies below. You need saliva to lubricate your mouth, break down food and help you swallow.

 SYMPTOMS

▷ Mouth feels parched, dry and lacks saliva
▷ Frequent thirst
▷ May be bad breath, mouth ulcers and sores
▷ Difficulty in tasting, chewing and swallowing food
▷ Prickly or burning sensation in the mouth

 PREVENTION

There are many possible causes but the most likely one is that your dry mouth is a side-effect of a medication you are taking. Check the label or any accompanying instructions to see if dry mouth is listed and consult your doctor.

- Drink plenty of water – carry a bottle around with you and sip some whenever you feel parched.
- To stimulate saliva production, suck sugar-free boiled sweets or chew on sugar-free gum.
- To prevent dehydration, cut down on caffeine-containing drinks, such as coffee, alcohol and carbonated drinks.

- Visit your dentist regularly to prevent increased risk of gum disease.
- Stop smoking now – saliva is reduced by cigarette smoke.
- Try not to breathe with your mouth open.
- Put a humidifier in your bedroom and don't sleep in air conditioning, which can be very drying.

 CONVENTIONAL REMEDIES

These include over-the-counter and prescription-only oral rinses and artificial saliva substitutes.

 NATURAL REMEDIES

- Munching celery stimulates the saliva glands and makes your mouth feel moist.
- Suck on a small piece of peeled fresh root ginger to boost saliva production.
- Switch from regular tea and coffee or Chinese green tea or chamomile tea.

 SEE YOUR DOCTOR

Dry mouth can be a side effect of certain diseases, infections, medical treatments, medication and medication, so talk it over with your doctor.

 Quick fix

You can try sucking an ice cube or a frozen chunk of melon for instant relief.

Chiropractic and osteopathy

These two complementary therapies involve touch and movement to treat disorders of the spine, joints and muscles, as well as a variety of other conditions, but each has its own characteristics and healing approach. Here are the key facts about chiropractic and osteopathy.

CHIROPRACTIC

The term chiropractic comes from the ancient Greek words cheiro, which means hand, and prakitikos, which means 'done by hand' or manipulation. Various forms of spinal manipulation have been practised for centuries, but chiropractic itself was developed in 1895 by Canadian Daniel D Palmer. He claimed to have managed to restore the hearing of his office caretaker, who had been deaf for 17 years due to a back and neck injury. After manipulating his back, there was a noticeable 'click' and the man's hearing was restored.

Key ideas

Chiropractors view the spine as the main structure of the body. The spinal cord carries essential nerves around the body and links the brain as well. When any problems with the spine occur, it has an effect on other parts of the body too, including internal organs and blood vessels. When the spine is properly aligned and in its natural position, the rest of the body's systems can work in harmony, which helps the body's self-healing ability to work effectively.

Which conditions can chiropractic help?

Chiropractors can help a range of conditions, as well as back problems:

- Spine problems
- Neck and shoulder problems
- Leg pain
- Sciatica
- Sports injuries
- Muscle, joint and postural disorders
- RSI
- Headaches and migraines
- Menstrual problems
- Asthma

Chiropractic treatment

Chiropractic treatment is individually tailored to your needs, but involves special adjustments – controlled techniques that slowly, and sometimes rapidly, move joints. Sometimes a 'click' can be heard, as the joint change occurs.

OSTEOPATHY

The word osteopathy also stems from Greek origins and is formed from the words osteon, which means 'bone', and pathos, which means 'suffering.' This therapy was developed in the late nineteenth century by Dr Andrew Taylor Still, an American doctor. His wife and three children died from meningitis and he developed osteopathy whilst seeking a way to encourage the body's self-healing abilities.

Key ideas

At the heart of osteopathy is the holistic idea that, if your muscular-skeletal system is in good working order and structurally balanced, then the rest of your body will work well too. The muscular-skeletal system supports and protects the main organs of the body and any physical or emotional stress, injuries or incorrect posture puts strain on the system.

Not only are osteopaths concerned with treating health problems, but they are also keen to find out what caused them in the first place.

Which conditions can osteopathy help?

An osteopath can help treat a variety of health conditions:

- Spine and neck problems
- Muscle, joint and posture problems
- Sports injuries
- Sciatica
- Headaches and migraines
- RSI
- Tinnitus
- Vertigo
- Menstrual problems

Osteopathy treatment

Osteopathy treatment is also tailored to your own unique needs but may involve stretching techniques, manipulation of the joints, muscle energy techniques or massage.

Musculo-skeletal problems

The musculo-skeletal system consists of bones, joints and muscles, which, in turn, are linked by ligaments, tendons and cartilage. While the skeleton supports the body and protects the vital organs, the joints and muscles (the locomotor system) provide our ability to move.

The skeleton consists of 206 bones, supplemented by cartilage. The bones have several functions: some act as levers, operated by muscles, to aid movement (the limbs); some protect internal organs; and others contain bone marrow where red blood cells are made. The spine is made up of 33 bones (vertebrae) and it provides a protective casing for the spinal cord, which connects with the brain. To keep your bones healthy and strong, you need to exercise regularly and eat a healthy diet, which contains protein, calcium and Vitamin D.

A joint is the area where two bones meet. Joints may be fixed to promote stability (as in the skull); cartilaginous allowing some flexibility (as in the spine); or synovial providing greater mobility and flexibility (as in the shoulders, elbows or knees). Ligaments hold the ends of the bones together.

Muscles, which enable the body and its internal organs to move, are arranged in overlapping layers. They work in pairs, contracting and relaxing in opposition to one another. Voluntary muscles (which control body movement) are connected to the bones via bands of fibrous tissue called tendons. Involuntary muscles (within the major organs, arteries and veins) control functions within the body, such as digestion. To build and maintain strong muscles, you need to use them regularly – exercise is the key.

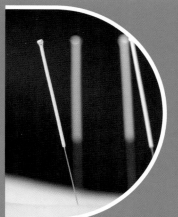

Back pain

Most of us suffer from back pain at some time in our lives; it affects four out of five people and is the largest single cause of sickness absence from work. However, precise diagnosis is difficult and there is no simple universal treatment. The pain may occur along any part of the spine with the lower back being most common.

SYMPTOMS

▷ A sharp pain in a localised area
▷ Stiffness in part of the back
▷ A general aching in the lower back
▷ Difficulty in bending
▷ Pain is often worse after standing or sitting for long periods

PREVENTION

Prevention is always the best treatment and if you have ever suffered from back pain you will become more aware of your body, your posture and your habits. Problems may occur from sitting or standing in an unnatural or uncomfortable position, straining the back muscles when lifting heavy objects or twisting awkwardly in the process, or simply from being overweight. Luckily, there are some lifestyle changes and positive measures that you can take to prevent this painful and debilitating condition.

CHECK YOUR POSTURE Is your posture putting your back at risk? You should maintain good posture at work, at home, driving your car and in your leisure interests.

CHECK YOUR FURNITURE Do your chairs and sofas have firm seats and good upright back support? Try using a lumbar support or foam wedge behind your lower back. Is your desk or work station the correct height? Are you hunched over your computer? Do you have a firm mattress on your bed that supports your spine?

CHECK YOUR HABITS Don't wear very high heels or carry a heavy bag on one side – split the load evenly between two lighter bags. Do not twist as you bend, and make sure you keep your back straight and bend your knees when reaching down to lift anything heavy.

Did you know?

Extending down the back from your head to your coccyx, the spine is designed to keep your head and body upright. Its 33 bones (vertebrae) are supported by muscles and ligaments, and separated by discs (cartilage). The spine also protects the spinal cord.

CHECK YOUR FITNESS If you are fit and supple, you are less likely to get low back pain or you will reduce the chances of it recurring. Cycling and swimming are both beneficial, but do not over-exercise as this may lead to pulled and torn muscles.

VARY YOUR MOVEMENTS When you are performing household chores, cleaning or gardening, do not make the same repetitive movements for a long time. Stop and do something else and then go back to the original task later. Do everything in moderation.

 CONVENTIONAL REMEDIES

You can ease the pain and discomfort by taking painkillers, such as ibuprofen, as soon as the pain occurs and then regularly thereafter. It is best to remain as active as possible – going about your normal daily routines may help recovery, but your doctor can advise you about this. In addition, you can apply hot and cold compresses to the affected area or take a prescribed muscle relaxant or non-steroidal anti-inflammatory drugs (NSAIDs).

 NATURAL REMEDIES

These fall into two main types: remedies that ease the symptoms; and natural therapies that improve posture, stabilise and strengthen the spine, and help prevent the pain recurring.

ALEXANDER TECHNIQUE This therapy can improve posture and balance to prevent putting pressure on the spine, joints and musculature. It teaches you a more balanced and efficient way of using your body. See a qualified practitioner.

REFLEXOLOGY Work on the medial longitudinal arches of the feet where the spinal reflexes are located. Use firm pressure along the bony ridges.

CHIROPRACTIC This can help some people with chronic back pain. The joints of the spine are manipulated by the practitioner to ease pain and facilitate movement. Your doctor may refer you to a chiropractor.

ACUPUNCTURE This is another form of treatment for relieving back pain that is now being offered via general practitioners.

Caution

Always read the small print and instructions regarding recommended dosages on any over-the-counter or prescription pain relief packaging. Never exceed the stated dose.

Quick fix

Try rubbing some deep heat ointment (available in tubes from most pharmacies) into the area for instant pain relief, or use a custom-made heating pad or heat spray.

78

 HOMEOPATHIC REMEDIES

The remedy you use will depend on the type of pain you experience and its location. Here are some common symptoms and remedies for back pain.

Aesculus hippocastanum 12C: Take one tablet three times a day until the pain subsides for continuous, severe, dull pain in the lower back and hips.

Bryonia alba 12C: Take one tablet three times a day until the pain subsides for stiffness and pain in the small of the back.

Pulsatilla 12C: Take one tablet three times a day until the pain subsides for lower back pain with tiredness.

Kali carbonicum 12C: Take one tablet three times a day until the pain subsides for severe back pain shooting down into the buttocks; a back that feels weak and stiff; back pain when feeling cold or lying on the affected side.

Rhus toxicodendron 12C: Take one tablet three times a day until the pain subsides for back stiffness, pain deep in the back muscles, which feel bruised and hurt on movement, and pain that feels worse in bed but is better for warmth.

 HERBAL REMEDIES

To ease back pain and sciatica, you can try taking one of the following herbal remedies.

- Gently massage some St John's Wort oil into the affected area for temporary relief.
- Apply a warm paste to the painful area made by blending two teaspoons ginger with one teaspoon turmeric.
- Drink some willow bark, nettle or chamomile tea.
- Take one 200mg capsule devil's claw (an anti-inflammatory) six times a day.
- Take one 250mg capsule valerian four times a day.
- Add a cup of rosemary, chamomile or peppermint tea to a warm bath.

 AROMATHERAPY

Use warming, soothing oils for muscular problems; and calming, soothing oils for painful disc problems.

- For muscular pain, use lavender, marjoram or ginger essential oils in a carrier oil to massage the affected area, or add a few drops to a hot bath and then lie back and relax your aching muscles.
- For disc pain and to relieve inflammation, you can use chamomile, marjoram or lavender, either in a compress or the bath.

 Did you know?

For many people, back pain can become a chronic, long-lasting problem with at least 50 per cent of sufferers experiencing some recurring pain.

Posture checklist

1 Stand up straight and pull your stomach muscles
in to help straighten your spine.
2 Your weight should be distributed equally between both feet.
3 When seated, don't slouch – keep your back straight and sit equally on both buttocks. Do not cross your legs.

IMMEDIATE RELIEF

Ice and heat will bring immediate relief when you experience a twinge of back pain.

ICE Apply an ice pack or a bag of frozen peas that has been wrapped in a towel to the affected area, and leave it there for 15–20 minutes. Repeat several times during the first couple of days until the swelling subsides and the pain goes.

HEAT If the pain persists, however, you should use heat instead of ice. You can apply a heat pack (available from pharmacies) or immerse a small towel in hot water, then wring it out and use to cover the painful area. Leave it on until it loses its heat.

 ## SEE YOUR DOCTOR

You should see your doctor if you experience any of the following symptoms:

- The back pain persists and it does not respond to any of the remedies you try
- You experience numbness in a limb
- You have difficulty in controlling your bowel or bladder functions
- The pain is associated with extreme weight loss
- If you also have fever, chest pain, laboured breathing or stomach cramps.

If you experience any of the above, there may be a serious underlying cause and you must consult your doctor immediately.

Old-fashioned remedies

The time-honoured way of relieving back pain is to rub in a liniment. You can choose from old favourites like mustard poultices to modern versions, such as capsaicin cream. To make a mustard poultice, blend one-third mustard powder with two-thirds flour and a little water to a paste. Put it on a clean cotton cloth and fold the ends over, so the filling is completely enclosed before placing it on the affected area for a short period – no more than 30 minutes' maximum. The paste must never be applied directly to the skin as it can burn and cause painful blisters.

Yoga

This ancient holistic system of exercises, postures, relaxation and breathing will help to relieve back pain, improve posture and make your back more flexible and supple.

- For instant relief, lie flat on your back on a mat on the floor with your arms at your sides, knees bent and shoulder-width apart, and feet flat on the floor.
- Breathe in deeply and slowly, then exhale and repeat 20 times.

Sciatica

Sciatica is any compression or irritation of the sciatic nerve, which runs from your pelvis through your buttocks down the back of each leg to your feet. Sciatica is usually due to a prolapsed disc, putting pressure on the nerves.

 ## SYMPTOMS

▷ Pain along the sciatic nerve
▷ Sharp pain radiates down the back of the leg to the foot
▷ May be numbness or tingling
▷ Pain can range from mild to severe
▷ May be due to a slipped disc

 ## PREVENTION

The fitter and healthier you are, the less likely it is that you will suffer from sciatica.

- Exercise regularly – at least three times a week. Swimming, cycling and walking briskly are all beneficial.
- Improve your posture with yoga, Pilates or the Alexander Technique.
- Eat a healthy varied diet that contains all the essential nutrients you need for good health. Poor diet can contribute to blood and lymph stagnation and accumulation in the tissues of the lower back.

 ## CONVENTIONAL REMEDIES

Acute sciatica can last for up to six weeks and may not need medical attention. If over-the-counter painkillers do not work, you may need prescription painkillers, physiotherapy or even surgery.

 ## NATURAL REMEDIES

Applying alternate hot and cold compresses to the painful area may be helpful in relieving the pain temporarily.

HERBAL REMEDIES Drink willow bark, nettle or chamomile tea to relieve sciatic pain. Evening primrose oil can be an effective anti-inflammatory. To relax the nerves, try rubbing St John's wort oil, mixed with olive oil, into painful areas at bedtime.

AROMATHERAPY Massage the lower back with a carrier oil to which is added three of the following essential oils: chamomile, lavender, rosemary, eucalyptus, peppermint and wintergreen.

 ## SEE YOUR DOCTOR

If the pain persists for several weeks, see your doctor. You may be prescribed stronger painkillers, advised on the best types of exercise, or referred to a physiotherapist or back specialist. Acupuncture, chiropractic or osteopathy may even be suggested.

Trapped nerve

This term refers to a nerve that is pinched or compressed. It is most commonly felt in the neck, mid and lower back areas, and may also cause pain in the parts of the body to which the nerve leads, such as arms, hands, legs and feet.

 ## SYMPTOMS

▷ Intense pain in a localised area
▷ Numbness or tingling in other areas
▷ Most commonly occurs in lower back

 ## PREVENTION

You cannot avoid suffering from a trapped nerve at some time in your life, but you can improve your posture and lifestyle to reduce the likelihood of this painful condition happening.

- Don't wear very high heels or always carry a bag or shoulder bag on one side only. Always bend your knees when lifting heavy weights.
- Practise good posture when you are standing, sitting or lying down – don't slouch and support your back. Yoga, Pilates or the Alexander Technique can also be helpful.
- A healthy diet with B vitamins is essential for nerve tissue health. Good sources are poultry, fish, eggs, nuts, seeds, whole-grain cereals, legumes, brown rice, dried fruit and green vegetables.

 ## CONVENTIONAL REMEDIES

Ice packs, anti-inflammatories, muscle relaxants and painkillers are the usual conventional treatments for a trapped nerve.

 ## NATURAL REMEDIES

Although exercise may be painful, try to stay mobile and walk a little each day. Apply heat packs to the affected area and relax in a warm bath.

HERBAL REMEDIES St John's wort oil is often used for spinal nerve pain. Apply to the affected area in a carrier oil.

CHIROPRACTIC This therapy, which involves manipulating the joints in the spine, can be very useful in treating a trapped nerve.

 ## SEE YOUR DOCTOR

If the pain lasts for several weeks and over-the-counter pain-relievers are not helpful, see your doctor. Likewise if you experience chest pain, numbness in your legs or the pain is getting progressively worse, not better.

Caution

Always read the directions on over-the-counter or prescription-only painkiller packages carefully and never exceed the stated dose.

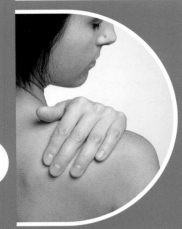

Neck and shoulder pain

There are many possible causes of this pain, including injury, arthritis, wear and tear in spinal bones and discs, tendinitis and bursitis. Even just sitting in an awkward position for too long can cause problems.

 ## SYMPTOMS

▷ Pain in the neck and when moving your head
▷ Stiffness and pain in the shoulder
▷ You cannot lift your arms above your head
▷ Difficulty in performing simple everyday tasks

 ## PREVENTION

As with all other back problems, adopting good posture is the best means of preventing neck and shoulder pain.

- When standing or seated, your ears, shoulders and hips should all be in a straight line – don't slouch.
- Keep your weight anchored evenly on both legs and feet – don't favour one leg over the other.
- Make sure that the chairs you use (including your car seat) support your back and neck. If necessary, fit a lumbar support or use a small pillow or cushion.
- Don't sit for too long in one position, especially at a computer. Get up, have a stretch and walk around occasionally.
- Don't hold the phone in the crook of your neck with your head on one side.
- Wrap a scarf around your neck in cold, damp weather.
- Don't wear high heels that tilt you forwards out of line.
- Split heavy weights or groceries between two bags, one in each hand, to spread the load more evenly.
- Don't wear a heavy shoulder bag – a rucksack is better.

 ## Did you know?

Neck ache may be one of the first symptoms of a migraine coming on or, indeed, it can be caused by tension headaches.

- Don't sleep in a draft under an open window, and always make sure that your head and neck are supported properly by a firm pillow.
- Keep your neck and shoulder muscles flexible and strong by performing regular gentle stretches and rotations.

CONVENTIONAL REMEDIES

Painkillers, heat pads and gels containing ibuprofen are the usual over-the-counter remedies for neck or shoulder pain. Non-steroidal anti-inflammatories, such as ibuprofen, can also be helpful.

NATURAL REMEDIES

For quick and effective pain relief, nothing beats heat. It helps relieve stiffness, relaxes muscles and promotes healing. You can hold a hot water bottle, a heat pad or even a towel soaked in hot water and then wrung out against the affected area. Or just treat yourself to a relaxing warm bath or an invigorating shower with the jets of water trained on your neck and shoulders.

HERBAL REMEDIES Make a hot compress to boost blood circulation, or massage the area with a soothing massage oil to which you have added a few drops of lavender oil. You could try taking devil's claw (available from health food stores in capsule form) for its anti-inflammatory properties.

OTHER THERAPIES Acupuncture, chiropractic or osteopathy may also bring some relief to many neck and shoulder problems. Manipulation can alleviate pain in the area, especially after injury.

HOMEOPATHIC REMEDIES

The remedy used will depend on the exact symptoms, but shoulder pain may improve if it is treated with Sanguinaria (right shoulder) or Sulphur (left shoulder). Cimicifuga is sometimes used for muscular neuralgic pain affecting the neck, while Rhus. tox is helpful for general neck pain and stiffness.

SEE YOUR DOCTOR

Neck and shoulder pain are very common and at least half of us will be affected at some time or another in our lives. Although it is seldom long-term or serious, it can make you feel miserable and affect every aspect of your daily routine. If the pain persists in your neck and/or shoulders for several days and does not improve after treatment with painkillers, anti-inflammatories, heat and massage, see your doctor. If you also have a fever, headache, sensitivity to light or cannot lift your arms above your head, you must seek medical advice

Quick fix

For instant relief for stiffness and soreness in your neck, try using a hairdryer to blow warm air directly onto your neck.

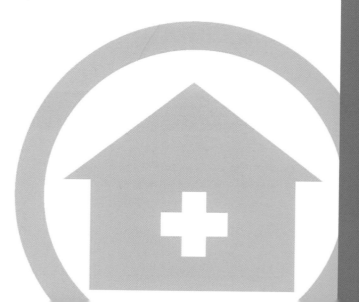

83

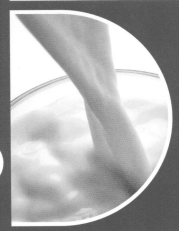

Osteoporosis

Osteoporosis is when our bones become less dense, more fragile and increasingly likely to break if we have a fall. This happens because our bone cells begin to break down faster than they are being replaced. Osteoporosis is a common problem, usually seen in people aged 50 and over, but you are unlikely to know if you have it until you experience a bone fracture.

 SYMPTOMS

▷ Joint pain
▷ Bone fractures, particularly of the wrists, hips or spine
▷ Problems standing or sitting upright
▷ Curvature of the spine
▷ Loss of height

 PREVENTION

Following a healthy lifestyle from a young age is key to keeping your bones strong and preventing osteoporosis in later life.

- Eat a well-balanced diet containing plenty of fruit and vegetables, and high-quality protein. This will ensure you get enough vitamins, minerals and amino acids to build healthy bones.
- Make sure you get enough calcium, which is found in dairy products, green leafy vegetables, nuts, beans, small-boned fish, such as sardines, and fortified foods.
- Get a few minutes of sunlight exposure each day (without getting sunburned). Sunlight allows us to make vitamin D, which is necessary for the absorption of calcium. Vitamin D is also found in oily fish, fortified foods and supplements.
- Exercise regularly. Weight-bearing and resistance exercises, such as walking, running, aerobics and weight-lifting, stimulate bone growth.
- Avoid excess alcohol, coffee and sodium consumption. These substances cause calcium to be lost from the body.
- Don't smoke. Smoking encourages calcium loss and slows bone growth.
- Maintain a sensible body weight. Extreme dieting or exercising excessively can increase your risk of osteoporosis.

 Did you know?

Bone growth happens during our early life, but from our mid-thirties onwards we begin to lose bone mass. Therefore the more bone we can build when we are young, the better.

CONVENTIONAL REMEDIES

Treatment for osteoporosis focuses on strengthening your bones, and on decreasing the risk of further fractures. Dietary changes may be necessary to increase calcium and vitamin D levels, or high-dose supplements may be recommended. You may be offered medications, such as bisphosphonates or calcitonin, to slow down the rate of bone loss. Some people may need to wear hip protectors in case they have a fall.

NATURAL REMEDIES

Here are some natural therapies that may help to prevent osteoporosis.

NUTRITIONAL MEDICINE Omega-3 fatty acids, found in cold-water fish and flax seeds, may increase calcium absorption and reduce calcium loss, and help to maintain bone mass.

HERBAL REMEDIES Black cohosh contains phytoestrogens, which may have an effect that is similar to oestrogen and help protect against bone loss. Try taking 80mg twice daily.

ACUPUNCTURE A practitioner will stimulate points that restore the flow of energy from the kidneys, which may help prevent bone loss.

Exercise

Although some rest may be necessary after a fracture, resting for a long time will reduce your bone strength further. Stay as mobile as possible, starting with a little gentle exercise at first and working up gradually to a greater intensity. For example, just going for a gentle stroll for a few minutes each day will make a difference until you are able to go for longer walks.

HEALING FOODS

- Onions contain a compound that, according to research, may inhibit bone loss and help to prevent osteoporosis.
- Green leafy vegetables contain vitamin K, which is also needed for strong bones.

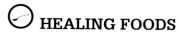 SEE YOUR DOCTOR

The long-term use of corticosteroids, thyroid or blood-thinning medications can increase the risk of osteoporosis. See your doctor if this applies to you.

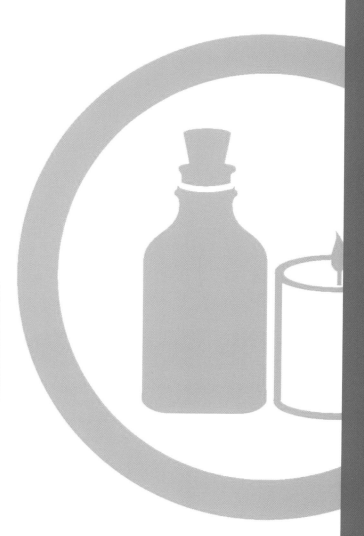

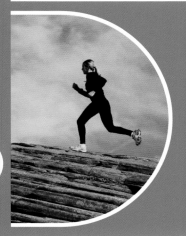

Shin splints

As an increasing number of people are taking up jogging and running, shin splints are becoming more common, especially among new, inexperienced runners. This painful condition is an overuse injury, arising from constant strain on the muscles along the front of the lower leg. People who are training for marathons may get shin splints if they increase their weekly mileage too rapidly.

 SYMPTOMS

▷ Shooting pains in the shins while out running
▷ May get worse with pain when walking

 PREVENTION

You don't have to suffer from shin splints – they are preventable. Your running style, the surface you run on and the shoes you wear can all make a difference and help to keep you fit.

- Make sure that your running shoes have adequate cushioning to provide essential shock absorption. Discard old shoes that make the problem worse and buy new ones.
- Put padded insoles in your running shoes.
- Always purchase good-quality shoes in a specialist running store and get the assistant to check that you do not over-pronate as this can make shin splints worse. The shoes you choose can compensate for this tendency.
- Run on grass – not hard roads and pavements – to protect your shins from the impact. Grass is softer and you are less likely to injure yourself.
- Don't overdo it and try to run too far too fast too soon. Progress gradually and build days of rest into your schedule.
- Listen to your body and alternate days of running with cross-training, gymwork or whatever exercise you enjoy.

 Did you know?

Shin splints can affect footballers, ballet dancers and people who engage regularly in any form of strenuous exercise that puts pressure on the muscles of the lower legs.

CONVENTIONAL REMEDIES

Aspirin and ibuprofen will help ease the pain of shin splints, while you can aid and speed up recovery with anti-inflammatory drugs. If the condition persists, you should consult a sports physiotherapist.

 ## NATURAL REMEDIES

For quick, effective pain relief, try the time-honoured sports medicine remedy known as RICE:

REST As soon as you feel any pain in your shins, rest. Take a rest from running or sport while the condition improves and heals

ICE Apply an ice pack to reduce pain and swelling. Use every four or five hours for no longer than 15–20 minutes.

COMPRESSION Wrap a bandage or towel around the ice pack to secure it in place. You can also wear an elastic compression bandage after removing the ice pack.

ELEVATION Raise your legs above your heart whenever possible. Lie on the floor or bed with your legs resting on the wall above.

 ## HERBAL REMEDIES

Make a hot compress with some comfrey tea (see page 142) and apply to the affected area.

 ## HOMEOPATHIC REMEDIES

Arnica montana ointment or gel can be rubbed gently into the shins to help speed up your recovery.

 ## SEE YOUR DOCTOR

If you rest and abstain from running, shin splints will usually heal up of their own accord. However, if rest and ice do not do the trick and the condition persists for more than a couple of weeks, ask your doctor for advice – you may have a stress fracture, which will get worse if it is not treated.

Stretching

This can be very helpful in preventing and relieving shin splints. Always make time to stretch and ease out your calf muscles after running. To stretch the muscles in your shins, lie on your back and wrap a towel or belt around the ball of your right foot. Raise your leg, holding on to the ends of the towel or belt, and then pull it down with your left hand, so your foot and leg are pulled down over your body to the left. Feel the stretch in your lower leg and hold for a count of 5. Repeat 3 times, change legs and repeat on the right.

 ### Quick fix

Ease shin pain and bring instant relief if you kneel with your toes flat on the ground, heels together. As you slowly sit back on your feet, you will feel a soothing stretch in your shins.

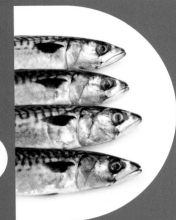

Arthritis

Arthritis is the collective term for over 200 conditions that affect the joints and bones. In osteoarthritis, the most common form, cartilage degenerates as a result of wear and tear on joints, causing pain and stiffness. Rheumatoid arthritis is a more serious, long-term disease in which the body's immune system attacks and destroys joints, causing pain and inflammation.

 SYMPTOMS

▷ General fatigue
▷ Pain in the joints, especially the knuckles of the hand
▷ Joints are swollen, red, stiff and sore
▷ Inflammation and pain are worse early in the morning
▷ Periods of improvement are followed by a relapse
▷ Joints may look abnormal in shape
▷ Hands and feet may feel cold

 PREVENTION

You can help to protect yourself against osteoarthritis as you get older. However, we do not know for sure what causes rheumatoid arthritis and it cannot be prevented. It may be triggered by a virus or an infection, but this cannot be proven.

- Being overweight puts additional stress on weight-bearing joints, especially the knees, hips, ankles and feet. If you are significantly overweight, go on a weight-reducing diet or join a slimming club.
- Whatever weight you are, eat a healthy diet with plenty of calcium (dairy foods, preferably low-fat ones) and omega-3 fatty acids (found in oily fish). These help build strong bones and healthy joints.
- If you like to pound the streets out running, wear good-quality trainers with shock-absorbing features and run on grass and soft surfaces. This reduces the impact on weight-bearing joints. Overuse of joints in sport and old sports injuries often cause arthritis in later life.
- Engage in sports that are more gentle on your body, such as swimming or cycling, where your joints are supported.
- Regular exercise will keep you active, mobile and make your muscles stronger to help support your joints. If possible, exercise four or five times a week.
- Wear comfortable shoes that fit properly with plenty of room for your feet – avoid high heels and pointed toes, which can lead to bunions (arthritis in the big toe).

 Did you know?

Gout is another form of arthritis, and it is caused by uric acid crystals accumulating in the joints, especially the big toe, and creating swelling, pain, heat and tenderness.

CONVENTIONAL REMEDIES

Arthritis cannot be cured but you can relieve the symptoms with many over-the counter analgesics and NSAIDs, taken orally or as creams and gels. Your doctor may prescribe stronger painkillers or capsaicin cream, which blocks the nerves that send pain messages. In serious cases, physiotherapy with TENS, intra-articular injections or even surgery may be offered. Rheumatoid arthritis will require specialist care and treatment.

 ## NATURAL REMEDIES

Severe arthritis is difficult to treat yourself with home remedies, but you can ease the symptoms. Heat can be helpful – keep your joints warm and use heat pads or a hot water bottle.

ACUPRESSURE AND ACUPUNCTURE Both these therapies can help control pain levels. Only go to a qualified therapist.

AROMATHERAPY Some essential oils can soothe localised pain. Massage lavender, chamomile, eucalyptus, rosemary, ginger or wintergreen oils into inflamed joints.

YOGA This aids suppleness and mobility, but only move or stretch as far as the affected joint will permit without pain.

Supplements

Many people believe that a daily supplement of chondroitin or glucosamine is helpful in alleviating stiffness and keeping joints mobile.

 ## HERBAL REMEDIES

The traditional remedy for arthritis is devil's claw. Teas made with anti-inflammatory herbs, such as bogbean, meadowsweet, birch and willow, can be taken, as can ginger tea.

 ## HOMEOPATHIC REMEDIES

It is wise to consult a qualified homeopath before treating your symptoms yourself. The usual remedies are Rhododendron (smaller joints susceptible to cold), Rhus tox (damp weather aggravates the condition) and Ruta (wrists and ankles). Take one 6C tablet twice a day until you notice an improvement.

 ## HEALING FOODS

Diet may play a role in relieving arthritis and you can try eating healthy, anti-inflammatory foods to see if they make a difference.

- Eat a variety of fresh vegetables an fruit.
- Eat foods that contain omega-3 fatty acids, such as oily fish and flaxseeds.
- Eat less processed, high-refined and sugary foods.
- Eat less polyunsaturated vegetable oils and partially hydrogenated oils.

You may also find that cutting out red meat, caffeine, acidic fruits and tomatoes is helpful.

 ## SEE YOUR DOCTOR

It is important to get a correct diagnosis, and if you suspect that you have arthritis, you must see your doctor as soon as possible.

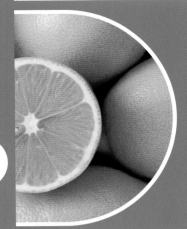

Rheumatism

Rheumatism is not a specific disease but a vague collective term we use to cover a wide range of aches and pains affecting joints, muscles, tendons and connective tissues. It does not include arthritis (see page 88). When no arthritis or specific disease can be diagnosed, the problem is often referred to as 'rheumatism'.

SYMPTOMS

▷ Swollen, stiff joints
▷ Aching joints that look red and inflamed
▷ Joints are swollen, red, stiff and sore
▷ Recurring or constant joint pain
▷ Pain is worse in cold or damp weather

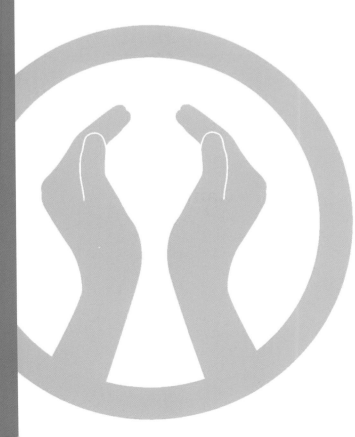

PREVENTION

Rheumatism tends to affect people as they get older and their joints age. It is more common among women and people who have experienced sports injuries. As with arthritis, eating a healthy diet and exercising regularly can help to minimise your risk of developing rheumatism and alleviate painful symptoms.

- Eat a varied diet that contains all the essential nutrients, especially vitamins A, C and E, and selenium and zinc.
- Abstain from foods that may raise levels of uric acid: yeast, yeast extracts, liver and kidney.
- Cut down your alcohol intake and choose white wine rather than red.
- Switch to herbal or green tea and reduce your coffee consumption.
- Eat oily fish (salmon, tuna, sardines, herring, mackerel) containing omega-3 fatty acids at least twice a week.
- Eat less red meat or cut it out altogether.
- Exercise regularly to boost circulation and build strong muscles to support your joints. Choose a non-weight-bearing activity that is appropriate for you.
- Lemon juice may be beneficial. Try drinking the squeezed juice of half a lemon added to a tumbler of warm water three times a day.
- Wrap up warmly in cold weather and avoid air conditioning.

CONVENTIONAL REMEDIES

The usual advice is to rest until the symptoms clear up or improve, and to take pain relief or anti-inflammatories as required, to alleviate the pain.

 NATURAL REMEDIES

There are many self-help treatments you can try. The following natural remedies may bring effective relief from rheumatic aches and pains.

HERBAL REMEDIES Anti-inflammatory massages, cleansing teas and warm compresses can all be helpful. The herbs you choose depend on your symptoms; consult a herbalist. Add rosemary or two handfuls of Epsom salts to a warm bath.

AROMATHERAPY Experiment with different essential oils, using them in a carrier oil for a massage or adding a few drops to a warm bath. Choose from chamomile, ginger, lavender and rosemary.

 SEE YOUR DOCTOR

To avoid any doubt and to obtain a precise diagnosis of your particular problem, you should consult your doctor, especially if the symptoms last for longer than three weeks.

 HOMEOPATHIC REMEDIES

Rheumatism affects people in so many ways and the homeopathic remedy selected must be applicable to the symptoms. To be on the safe side, you should seek advice from a qualified homeopath.

Bryonia alba 6C: Take one tablet three times daily for acute pain with hot, red joints which is aggravated by movement or relieved by external heat.

Colchicum 6C: Take one tablet three times daily for severe pain, which is worse in the evening or at night.

Ranunculus bulbosus 6C: Take one tablet three times daily for rheumatism which is worse in cold and damp conditions.

Caution

Always follow the packet instructions for taking pain relievers carefully, and never exceed the recommended dose in any 24-hour period.

Yoga

Many stretches and postures can be beneficial if you suffer from aching, stiff joints. You will develop better body awareness and increased suppleness and mobility. Find a local yoga class and tell the instructor that you suffer from rheumatism. They will be able to devise a custom-made programme for you.

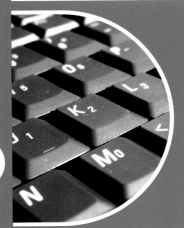

Repetitive strain injury

Repetitive strain injury (RSI) is an extremely debilitating musculo-skeletal condition that commonly affects the arms, wrists, elbows, hands, neck, shoulders and upper back, and involves chronic pain.

 SYMPTOMS

▷ Sudden onset of bad pain
▷ Painful spasms
▷ Stiffness
▷ Numbness
▷ Tingling
▷ Weakness
▷ Cramp
▷ Some swelling

 PREVENTION

- If you have a desk-based job, particularly typing, working at a computer or data entry, then be sure to take regular breaks.
- Changing your job and taking up different work is a good way of eliminating the problem, but if you can't do that, take time to stretch your arms.
- Make sure your working environment allows you to work with an upright body, so that you don't have to twist or stretch too much.
- Learn to touch type, as using all your fingers to press the right keys and looking straight ahead at the computer screen can help to prevent RSI.
- Work at reducing stress in your life, as this can increase the risk of RSI pain.
- Regular massage can help to relieve any tension and stress in your upper body, neck, shoulders and arms.

ⓘ Did you know?

RSI is caused by overuse of a particular area of the body, often due to repetitive work, such as using a computer for long periods of time in the same position, or working in a factory and repeating movements again and again.

CONVENTIONAL REMEDIES

Over-the-counter painkillers can help, and your doctor may prescribe non-steroidal anti-inflammatory drugs. Bandages or splints, for example worn on the wrists to ensure they remain straight, can offer support and relieve symptoms. For bad RSI, steroid injections may be recommended. If the pain and discomfort of RSI is interrupting your sleep, then medication to help you sleep may be prescribed for a short time. You may be referred to a physiotherapist, who will suggest exercises you can do to build up your strength in the muscle affected by RSI.

 ## NATURAL REMEDIES

The following natural remedies may help to relieve pain and other symptoms.

NUTRITIONAL MEDICINE Shiitake mushrooms are often used as a herbal remedy for RSI, as they are good for easing inflammation and helping the body to cope with stress. You can make a nutritional soup from 90g (3oz) fresh shiitake mushrooms and eat for lunch.

AROMATHERAPY Mix together two drops of black pepper and two drops of rosemary essential oils, with 30ml of a carrier oil, such as sweet almond, to create an anti-inflammatory RSI blend. Very gently rub it into the affected area – don't initially try and massage your wrist, neck, shoulder, arm or hand much at all, as it may well be very painful.

HELPFUL THERAPIES Body and movement therapies, such as yoga, Pilates and the Alexander Technique, can help bring relief from stress, develop better posture and ease strain from your muscles. See a qualified practitioner for individual guidance.

RELAXATION AND MEDITATION

If stress could be at the heart of your RSI, then try out relaxation and meditation techniques to fully relax your body.

1 Use a guided meditation or relaxation CD to help you relax, or try a DIY meditation.

2 Sit quietly with your back supported and allow all your muscles to relax.

3 Breathe slowly and deeply and forget about any stress in your life.

NOTE It may help to visualise a blackboard with your stresses written on it – and then imagine you are wiping them away.

 ## HERBAL REMEDIES

- Take a tincture of the herb meadowsweet. It contains salicylates, which help to reduce inflammation and pain. Add one 5ml teaspoon tincture to a glass of water and take three times a day until your symptoms improve.
- Make a compress from yarrow, as it helps reduce inflammation in joints and muscles and reduces pain. Soak a piece of muslin in 10 drops of yarrow oil and apply to the affected area.

 ## SEE YOUR DOCTOR

If changing your lifestyle and rest do not ease the symptoms of RSI, see your doctor. You may be referred to a specialist or physiotherapist.

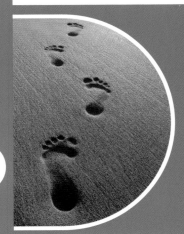

Foot pain

Feet can easily be taken for granted, but they need as much care and attention as the rest of your body. You rely on them being healthy and fine for walking and moving around, but when foot pain occurs, everything goes out of kilter. Pain is usually due to injury, disease or a health condition, or how the foot is interacting with external factors, such as the shoes you wear.

 ## SYMPTOMS

▷ Pain or discomfort in the foot
▷ Rubbing, blisters or bleeding
▷ Painful to put your foot on the floor
▷ Swelling

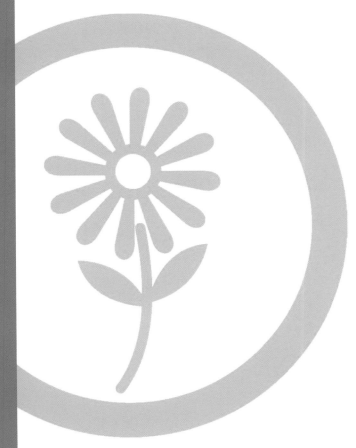

✖ PREVENTION

There are plenty of steps you can take to keep your feet in tip-top condition. Here are some suggestions.

- Wear shoes that fit well and don't rub your feet. High heels are a big culprit for causing foot problems. If you can't resist wearing them, choose a thicker heel, as this can give more stability and more evenly distribute the weight on your feet. It also helps to choose shoes without such a steep 'slope', and open toes can relieve the pressure on your toes.
- Wear in new shoes before wearing them for long periods of time, as this can help prevent them rubbing and causing sores, blisters or bleeding.
- Add orthotics or insoles to your shoes to aid comfort and prevent foot pain.
- Wear the right type of recommended shoe or boot for walking, running, playing football or other sports activities. If you are running, avoid surfaces that are too soft (sand), too hard (concrete) or very uneven, as all these can put unwanted pressure on your feet. Also, remember to warm up properly before exercising.

CONVENTIONAL REMEDIES

The RICE method – Rest, Ice, Compression and Elevation – is commonly recommended for foot pain caused by injuries. Never apply ice directly to the foot – put it in a plastic bag and wrap in a cloth before applying to your foot for 20 minutes at a time.

Large blisters on the foot, filled with pus, which are caused by rubbing, may be drained by a doctor. Covering them with a large plaster or blister pad can prevent further rubbing. Over-the-counter painkillers can help ease pain and discomfort in the foot.

 NATURAL REMEDIES

Among the most common natural remedies for foot pain are the following.

HERBAL REMEDIES If your feet are bruised or tender, apply arnica ointment to help aid healing. Rub it in well, but don't use on broken skin. Take five drops of cayenne tincture in a glass of water to help ease foot pain caused by nerve damage.

ACUPUNCTURE This can help to relieve foot pain. Depending on the location of the pain, an acupuncturist can work on areas of the foot and lower leg, helping to relieve pain and discomfort. Book an appointment with a qualified practitioner.

ALEXANDER TECHNIQUE Sometimes poor posture can put increased pressure on your feet, causing pain and discomfort. An Alexander Technique practitioner can work with you to identify old habits that are harming your health and develop new ones that relieve pain.

 AROMATHERAPY

- Relieve tired, painful or aching feet by adding a few drops of aromatherapy oils to a bath or footbath and soaking your feet. Try using anti-inflammatory peppermint, soothing lavender, refreshing lemon or antibacterial eucalyptus.
- If your foot pain is related to rheumatic aches and pain, try rosemary, which is a mild stimulant.

 HELPFUL THERAPIES

Try practising exercises, such as yoga or Pilates. They'll work by increasing the strength and stability in your foot, improve muscle strength and aid flexibility. When your muscles are stronger and more flexible, you will reduce the risk of further foot injuries.

 SEE YOUR DOCTOR

If your feet are very painful and none of the remedies you try seem to work, you should either see your doctor or visit a chiropodist.

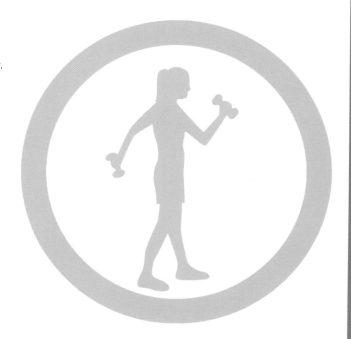

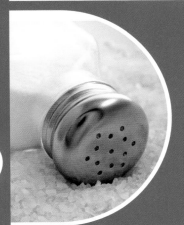

Muscle cramps

Muscle cramps can come on suddenly, usually lasting from a few seconds to several minutes, and they are caused by a spasm of a muscle. Cramp commonly occurs in the calf muscles of the legs, or in the feet, and can happen when you're sitting still, standing up, exercising or lying in bed. The amount of pain felt varies, but the affected muscle can remain uncomfortable for up to 24 hours.

SYMPTOMS

▷ A sharp or sudden pain in your leg or foot
▷ The muscle affected by cramp feels rigid and hard to move
▷ The muscle is tender for some time afterwards

PREVENTION

To prevent muscle cramp from occurring, it helps to do the following.

- Drink plenty of fluids each day, including six glasses of water.
- If you're exercising, always warm-up properly beforehand and avoid doing excessive exercise involving a lot of repetitive movements, as this can trigger muscle cramp.
- Avoid drinking too much alcohol, as this can cause cramp.
- Sometimes cramp can be linked to stress or exhaustion, so make sure you get plenty of sleep and try to avoid stressful situations.
- Drinking some tonic water, which contains quinine, before going to bed may help to prevent night-time muscle cramps.

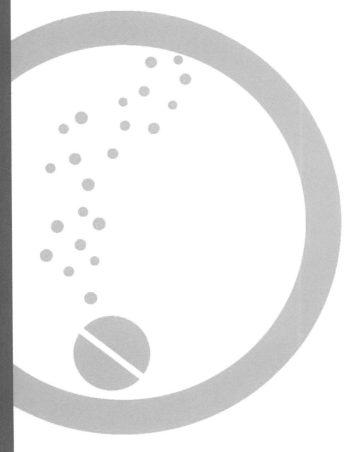

(i) Did you know?

Cramp can sometimes be caused by losing salt through sweating, such as when you're exercising. Drinking a glass of water with a little added salt can help rebalance the loss of salt and relieve muscle cramp.

CONVENTIONAL REMEDIES

To relieve the after-effects of cramp, such as a tender calf muscle, painkillers can be taken. In instances of bad, recurring cramp, then quinine sulphate tablets may be prescribed.

 NATURAL REMEDIES

There are several natural remedies that help to ease the symptoms of cramp.

NUTRITIONAL MEDICINE Muscle cramps can sometimes be caused by a lack, or imbalance, of minerals in your diet. Zinc and magnesium are two key culprits. Eat foods such as shellfish, corned beef, whole grains or nuts to increase your levels of zinc. To boost levels of magnesium, eat foods such as dark leafy vegetables, shellfish, nuts, seeds, lentils or whole-grain cereals.

HOMEOPATHIC REMEDIES The homeopathic remedy Mag Phos 8C can provide relief for cramp. For instant relief, take four tablets every 30 minutes until the effects wear off. If you have regular cramp, take three doses daily.

 HERBAL REMEDIES

- Take cramp bark tincture to help relieve the discomfort of muscle cramps. Add one teaspoon to a glass of water and take three times a day during a bad bout of cramp. Cramp bark lotion can also be rubbed into the affected muscle.
- Mexican wild yam has muscle relaxant properties. Take 1ml tincture when cramp occurs. In bad cases of persistent cramp, repeat the 1ml dose every 15 minutes until the cramp eases.
- Guelder rose has anti-inflammatory and relaxant properties. Add 25ml tincture to 75ml rosewater, or to an unscented skin cream, and gently massage it onto the affected muscle.

 SEE YOUR DOCTOR

If you have recurring cramp or it does not ease out, you should seek medical advice. It could be a sign of an underlying or serious condition, such as a blood clot or under-active thyroid, and further tests and investigations will be carried out. In some cases, medications that have been prescribed for other conditions, such as diuretics or water tablets, can result in cramp. If this is the case, your doctor may need to review your medication.

 IMMEDIATE RELIEF

- For cramp in your foot, put your bare foot on a cold floor.
- For cramp in a calf muscle, stand an arm's width away from a wall, put your feet flat on the floor and lean towards the wall, stretching your calf muscle.
- If you're prone to cramp in bed, sleep on your back and prop your feet up on a pillow – this helps prevent your toes from pointing downwards when sleeping, which is a position linked to cramp.

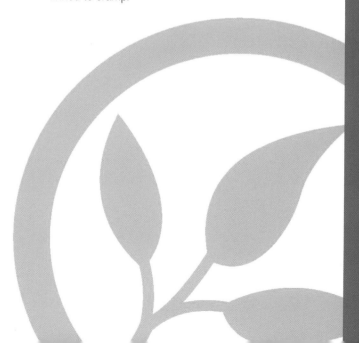

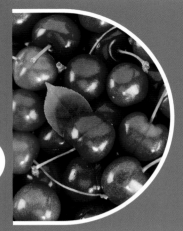

Gout

Gout is an extremely painful form of arthritis, and while it can occur in any joint, it most often affects the big toe. The condition is caused by a build-up of uric acid in the blood, which leads to crystals forming in the joints, but, fortunately, there are many things that you can do to help yourself if you suffer from gout.

 SYMPTOMS

▷ Inflammation and swelling of joints
▷ Extreme pain in your joints that comes on very suddenly
▷ Red, shiny, hot, itchy skin around the joints
▷ Visible lumps underneath the skin
▷ Difficulty walking or moving about
▷ Fever

 PREVENTION

You can help prevent gout by leading a healthy lifestyle. In particular, you should avoid foods that are high in purines, as these increase uric acid. Here are some things you can do to prevent gout.

- Limit your consumption of red meat, liver, kidney, oily fish such as mackerel and sardines, shellfish, and some vegetables, including beans, asparagus, mushrooms and spinach.
- Reduce your alcohol intake, especially beer, stout, fortified wines and port.
- Keep conditions, such as high blood pressure, diabetes, psoriasis, high cholesterol, obesity, kidney disease and vascular disease, under control, as these can increase uric acid.

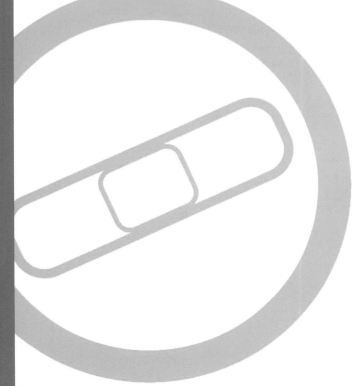

 Did you know?

Although gout is more common in men over forty, anyone can suffer from gout at any age. Some people will only experience gout once in their lifetime.

CONVENTIONAL REMEDIES

Treatment for gout focuses on reducing pain and inflammation in your affected joints, and controlling blood uric acid levels to prevent further attacks. It is important to elevate and rest the affected joint, and you may like to keep it cool with an ice pack. Don't apply ice directly to your skin, as this can cause damage. You can also take non-steroidal anti-inflammatory drugs, such as ibuprofen, to reduce inflammation and pain. In some cases, medications such as colchicine or steroids, may be prescribed to reduce uric acid. Sometimes a medication known as allopurinol may be given to reduce uric acid in the blood and prevent any further attacks of gout.

Change your lifestyle

Focusing on a healthy lifestyle will reduce the likelihood of developing gout.

- Cut down on the amount of alcohol you drink or, better still, eliminate it altogether. Avoid binge-drinking.
- Stay well hydrated by drinking plenty of water and herbal teas. Try to avoid sugary soft drinks.
- Exercise regularly (but never with an inflamed and painful joint) to improve your circulation and overall health.
- Eat a healthy, balanced, diet (not one that is high in protein), and minimise your consumption of processed, refined foods.
- Lose weight sensibly and gradually if you are overweight.

 NATURAL REMEDIES

Here are some natural remedies you might consider for treating gout.

NUTRITIONAL MEDICINE Try to eat a handful of tart cherries each day. They contain anthocyanins which have anti-inflammatory properties. You can also try taking cherry concentrate, capsules or teas.

HERBAL MEDICINE Take devil's claw extract three times daily to help reduce the pain and inflammation. You may also like to try extracts of green tea or turmeric.

AROMATHERAPY Add five drops of juniper oil to massage oil, and massage it into painful joints several times daily. Or try adding juniper, rosemary, lavender or eucalyptus oils to a footbath.

SEE YOUR DOCTOR

Although gout is relatively common, you should see your doctor if:

- You have frequent attacks of gout, as this may increase the risk of permanent joint damage
- You develop lumps in your joints that are particularly bothersome or painful
- You have difficulty getting about and gout is severely affecting your day-to-day life
- Your gout symptoms are making you depressed.

Alexander Technique and Pilates

The Alexander Technique and Pilates are two popular body and movement therapies. The two approaches share similarities, as they both aim to help you improve your posture, correct muscle imbalances, help specific health concerns and generally aid overall health and vitality.

ALEXANDER TECHNIQUE

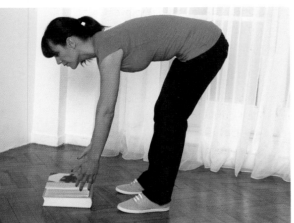

Top The incorrect technique for picking up heavy objects; this should be avoided

Bottom The correct technique for picking up heavy objects that will protect your back

The Alexander Technique was developed by the Australian actor Frederick Matthias Alexander. He made the discovery that he could stop his voice from becoming strained by improving his posture and relaxing his throat muscles. He subsequently moved to London in 1904 and worked on developing his technique further.

Key ideas

One of the key ideas behind the Alexander Technique is the idea that, as we go through life, we develop poor postural habits and they are difficult to break. Alexander believed that bad posture affects the body and mind, resulting in health problems, such as back pain, headaches, muscle strain or stress.

By relearning a series of basic movements, such as the movements needed to go from a sitting position to a standing position, or standing up straight, it is possible to become more aware of the bad habits and re-align the body in such a way that movement becomes more natural and harmonious.

Learning the Alexander Technique

To gain proper insight and expertise into the Alexander Technique and how it can help you, book a series of sessions with an experienced practitioner. One-to-one sessions are ideal for helping you discover your bad postural habits and how they could be affecting your health. An Alexander Technique teacher will help you to become aware of these habits when you're active and resting and will provide you with a series of exercises to practise to help you change your posture. It can be hard to recognize that your lifetime habits are not healthy and learn to change them, but the benefits are worth it.

PILATES

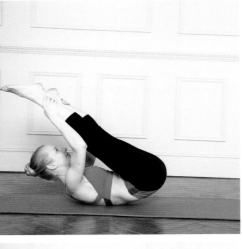

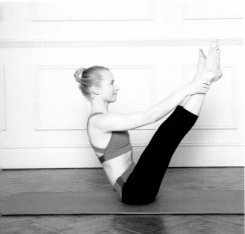

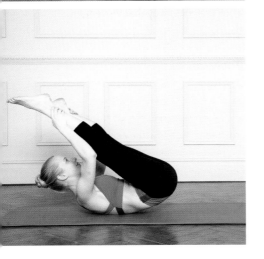

Pilates was created by Joseph Pilates, a German fitness trainer. During his childhood, Joseph was often ill and started practising gymnastics to try to improve his health. He studied yoga and tai chi before inventing his own form of exercise, which became known as pilates, in the early 1900s.

Key ideas

Joseph Pilates noticed that other exercises paid attention to the outer muscles, but he believed that it was important to focus on the deeper, inner muscles as they hold the key to all movements.

Pilates focuses on the core muscles in the centre of the torso, such as the lower back, abdomen, buttocks and hips. Precise movements help you to gain control over muscles while breathing exercises help circulate oxygen and improve your energy levels.

Learning Pilates

If you would like to try out this holistic approach to movement and posture, go along to a session with a qualified pilates teacher. Sessions are available on a one-to-one basis, or in small groups. Some simply involve mat work, whilst others use special apparatus to help you with the exercises. Regularly practising pilates can help alleviate many health conditions, such as back problems, arthritis and pain. It also results in longer and leaner muscles, more stability, strength and flexibility.

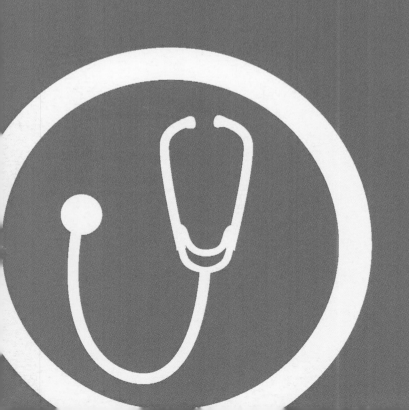

Heart and circulation problems

A healthy heart and circulatory system are essential for our wellbeing. Eating a varied, nutritionally balanced diet, not smoking and taking regular exercise will help to keep them strong and healthy and prevent relatively minor problems, such as chilblains, restless legs and varicose veins, as well as more serious ailments, including high or low blood pressure, palpitations and angina. And even if you suffer from heart problems, there are positive steps you can take to embrace a healthy lifestyle, and useful home remedies to prevent any further damage and help repair the system.

A properly functioning heart muscle and efficient blood circulation are vital for the health of every organ. Your blood transports oxygen and nutrients around your body and carries away waste products. The pressure of the circulating blood must not be too high or too low, and the blood vessels must remain free from obstructions, including clots and fatty deposits.

Cardiovascular disease is increasing but you can minimise the risk of developing it by making simple lifestyle choices and changes, as outlined in the following pages. Many natural therapies, such as herbal remedies, aromatherapy, homeopathy, reflexology and yoga, can be used to complement conventional medicine in this area. If you are unsure about their safety or are receiving medical treatment, always check with your doctor first.

Learn how to recognise the early-warning symptoms of heart and circulation problems and you may be able to take some simple steps to relieve them now and prevent them becoming more serious in the future.

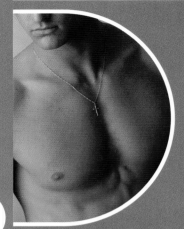

Angina

Angina is a sudden, acute pain in the chest and is due to restricted oxygen-rich blood flow to the heart. This is usually caused by hardening and narrowing of the arteries that supply the heart with oxygenated blood. Fatty deposits can gather inside these arteries and block them, a condition that is known as atherosclerosis. Angina increases the risk of having a heart attack or stroke.

 SYMPTOMS

▷ Sudden pain, squeezing or pressure in the chest
▷ Pain in the jaw, neck, left arm or back
▷ Breathlessness
▷ Tiredness
▷ Feeling sick
▷ Dizziness
▷ Burping

 PREVENTION

There are some lifestyle factors you need to address in order to prevent angina and reduce your risk of having a heart attack or stroke.

• Obesity, stress, high blood pressure and diabetes cause damage to the artery walls, so these conditions need to be managed properly.

• Exercising five times per week for 30 minutes at a time can strengthen your heart, lower blood pressure, reduce cholesterol and improve blood circulation.

• Excessive alcohol consumption increases cholesterol levels and raises blood pressure, so only drink in moderation.

• Don't smoke. Smoking increases blood pressure, damages artery walls and also increases the risk of blood clots.

• Try to reduce the amount of saturated fat in your daily diet, as it increases blood cholesterol and blocks the arteries.

 Did you know?

There are two main types of angina: stable and unstable. Stable angina is caused by triggers, such as strenuous exercise and stress, and lasts for only a few minutes. Unstable angina happens even when resting, and needs immediate medical attention.

CONVENTIONAL REMEDIES

Healthy lifestyle changes are important for treating angina, including eating less saturated fat, limiting alcohol consumption, exercising regularly and giving up smoking. Your doctor may prescribe nitroglycerin to relieve the pain during an angina attack. Other medications that slow the heart rate, increase blood flow to the heart, lower blood pressure or lower cholesterol may also be recommended. Anti-platelet drugs, such as aspirin, help to prevent blood clots. If your angina does not improve as a result of these measures, surgery may be required.

NATURAL REMEDIES

Here are some suggestions for how you can treat your angina naturally.

HERBAL REMEDIES Hawthorn may help to increase blood circulation and benefit your heart. Try taking 150mg three times daily.

NUTRITIONAL MEDICINE Increase the amount of 'good' cholesterol in your diet. This is found in avocados, oily fish, nuts and seeds, olive oil and sunflower oil.

YOGA Practising yoga may help to lower your blood pressure, improve blood circulation and help you to cope with stress and anxiety.

SEE YOUR DOCTOR

Do not attempt to treat your angina on your own without medical supervision; it could lead to serious health consequences. Only take supplements and herbal remedies to treat your angina after discussing it with your doctor. You should also see your doctor if you feel particularly anxious, stressed or depressed because of your angina.

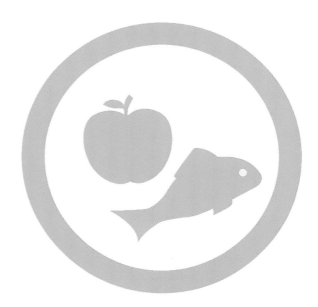

Lifestyle changes

You should make the following changes to your lifestyle if you have angina.

- Your diet should contain lots of fresh fruits, vegetables and whole-grain cereals. Keep saturated fats to a minimum.
- Reduce your salt intake as this raises blood pressure. Aim for a maximum of 6g per day.
- Drink alcohol in moderation. Men should consume no more than four units a day, and women no more than three.
- Exercise regularly. If you have angina you will need to avoid vigorous exercise, so, to begin with, keep to gentler forms of exercise, such as swimming and walking.
- Lose weight if necessary. You should be able to accomplish this with regular exercise and eating a healthy low-fat diet.
- Quit smoking.

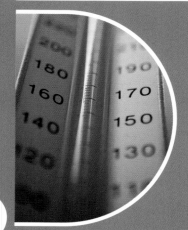

Blood pressure

High blood pressure (hypertension) is when the force of the blood being pumped around your body is greater than considered normal. Although it rarely has symptoms, if this condition is left unchecked, prolonged high blood pressure can damage the blood vessels and increase the risk of developing serious health conditions, such as kidney disease, heart disease and stroke.

 SYMPTOMS

▷ Vision disturbances
▷ Nose bleeds
▷ Breathlessness
▷ Headaches
▷ Black-outs
▷ Seizures

 PREVENTION

Diet, exercise and general lifestyle factors all play a major part in preventing high blood pressure.

- Take regular exercise: 30 minutes of moderate to vigorous intensity exercise five times per week will strengthen your heart, improve your blood circulation and help you to manage stress.
- Avoid becoming overweight or obese – concentrate on maintaining a healthy weight for your height.
- Ensure you have a healthy, balanced diet consisting of plenty of fruit, vegetables and whole-grain cereals. Minimise your intake of processed foods and foods high in sugar.
- Watch your cholesterol levels. Foods high in saturated fat increase blood cholesterol, causing narrowing of the arteries and contributing to high blood pressure.
- Drink alcohol in moderation. High alcohol consumption increases blood pressure, especially binge-drinking. Men should consume no more than 21 units of alcohol a week, and women 14.
- Pay attention to your stress levels – large amounts of stress increase blood pressure.
- Reduce your salt intake to no more than 6g per day.
- Reduce your daily caffeine intake to no more than five cups of coffee; go easy on caffeinated drinks.
- Avoid smoking.

 Did you know?

High blood pressure is defined as 140/90mmHg. The first figure represents systolic blood pressure (when the heart beats), and the second represents diastolic blood pressure (when the heart is at rest in between beats). 120/80mmHg is normal.

CONVENTIONAL REMEDIES

A few simple lifestyle changes can have a huge effect on your blood pressure levels. Exercise regularly, eat healthily, watch your salt and caffeine intake, drink sensibly, stop smoking and lose weight if necessary. Your doctor may prescribe medications that widen your arteries or slow down your heart rate in order to lower your blood pressure. They may also treat any underlying medical conditions that are contributing to your high blood pressure.

 ## NATURAL REMEDIES

Here are some natural remedies you could try for high blood pressure.

NUTRITIONAL MEDICINE Add more fish to your diet, such as salmon and halibut. These contain omega-3 fatty acids, which help to reduce blood cholesterol levels. Alternatively, you could take a fish oil supplement.

HERBAL REMEDIES Try taking 60mg ginkgo biloba daily to improve blood circulation and reduce blood pressure.

RELAXATION TECHNIQUES Transcendental meditation may be helpful to reduce stress, relax your mind and lower your blood pressure.

 ## SEE YOUR DOCTOR

If you are over 40 years of age, you should have your blood pressure checked regularly, especially if you have a family history of high blood pressure, or other factors that increase your risk of hypertension.

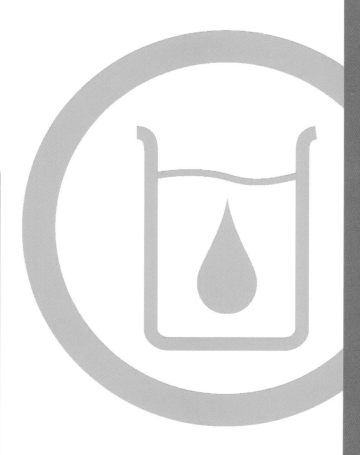

Low blood pressure

If you have low blood pressure (hypotension), which is classified as 90/60mmHg or less, you are unlikely to need treatment. To a degree, low blood pressure protects you against some of the things that cause high blood pressure, such as too much salt in your diet and weight gain. Low blood pressure can simply be a result of being particularly relaxed or physically fit. However, it can sometimes cause dizziness, light-headedness, fainting and weakness. Beta-blockers, diabetes mellitus, adrenal gland problems, dehydration, injury or shock can cause low blood pressure, but it is often nothing to worry about.

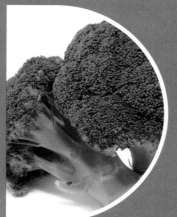

High cholesterol

Cholesterol is a type of fat, which is important for cell membranes and other functions within the body. However, high levels of blood cholesterol can cause health problems. Excess cholesterol builds up inside the walls of the arteries, restricting blood flow and increasing the risk of developing heart disease and stroke.

 ## SYMPTOMS

▷ Yellow deposits around your eyes or on your skin
▷ White rings around the eyes
▷ Blood cholesterol of more than 5mmol/L
▷ Angina or leg pain (caused by narrowed arteries)

 ## PREVENTION

There are several lifestyle factors that affect your risk of developing high blood cholesterol. In particular, you should do the following.

- Eat a healthy balanced diet with lots of fruit and vegetables.
- Restrict your intake of saturated fat. This is found in red meat, meat pies, cream, hard cheese, butter and pastries.
- Exercise regularly, as lack of exercise increases LDL cholesterol levels and decreases HDL cholesterol. Aim for 30 minutes of moderate-intensity exercise five times a week.
- Lose weight if you are overweight. Obesity increases the risk of high LDL cholesterol and low HDL cholesterol.
- Avoid excessive alcohol consumption – men should have no more than 21 units each week and women no more than 14.
- Don't smoke. Smoking reduces your level of HDL cholesterol.

 ## Did you know?

Low-density lipoprotein (LDL) is 'bad cholesterol' because it builds up in your arteries. High-density lipoprotein (HDL) is 'good cholesterol' because it helps to get rid of excess LDL cholesterol.

CONVENTIONAL REMEDIES

Treatment for high cholesterol begins with making some important lifestyle changes: eat less saturated fat, lose weight, exercise more and quit smoking. You may also be offered medication, such as statins, niacin or ezetimibe, to lower your cholesterol, or aspirin to help prevent blood clots.

 ## NATURAL REMEDIES

You may like to try the following natural remedies to lower your cholesterol.

NUTRITIONAL MEDICINE Eating foods high in vitamin C may help to lower cholesterol. Add peppers, broccoli, kale, parsley, Brussels sprouts, kiwi fruit, strawberries and oranges to your diet.

ACUPUNCTURE This treatment focuses on re-balancing your body and improving blood flow in order to lower your cholesterol levels.

YOGA Yoga helps to reduce stress, which has been associated with high cholesterol. Deep breathing exercises, postures and meditation increase blood circulation, improve digestion and aid relaxation.

 ## HEALING FOODS

Some foods will have a positive effect on your blood cholesterol levels.

- Increase your level of HDL cholesterol by replacing saturated fat with healthier, unsaturated fat. This is found in oily fish, olive oil, avocados, nuts and seeds.
- Soluble fibre helps to remove cholesterol from the body. Good sources include psyllium, oat bran, beans, peas, potatoes and apples.
- Substituting some animal meat with soy protein, such as tofu, miso and tempeh, may help to lower blood cholesterol levels.

 ## HERBAL REMEDIES

The following remedies are helpful for protecting against high cholesterol.

HAWTHORN Take 150mg three times daily.

GARLIC Eat it fresh, or take a 1000mg odourless supplement one to four times a day.

OLIVE LEAF EXTRACT Take 500mg one to two times daily.

PSYLLIUM HUSK Take 1000mg three times a day.

 ## SEE YOUR DOCTOR

In addition to lifestyle factors, there are other things that can put you at greater risk of high cholesterol. You should see your doctor and get your cholesterol checked if:

- You have high blood pressure or diabetes
- You have heart disease or have had a stroke
- You have a family history of heart disease or stroke
- A member of your immediate family has familial hypercholesterolaemia (high cholesterol which runs in the family)
- You have kidney or liver disease, or an underactive thyroid gland.

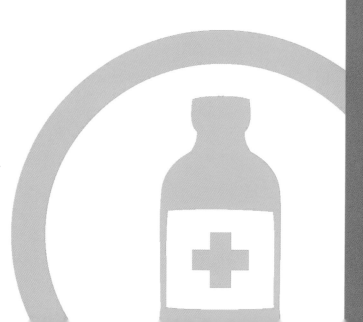

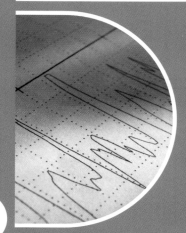

Palpitations

Palpitations (also known as arrhythmias) are variations in normal heartbeat rhythm, caused by a disruption of the electrical impulses that make the heart muscles contract. Normal heart rate is between 60 and 100 beats per minute when you are at rest, but sometimes your heart may beat faster or slower than usual or you may feel as though your heart skips a beat.

 SYMPTOMS

▷ Rapid heart beat
▷ Slow heart beat
▷ Your heart feels as though it skips a beat, or thumps suddenly
▷ Irregular heartbeat
▷ A fluttering sensation in your chest
▷ Sudden awareness of your heart beat

 PREVENTION

Depending on the type of palpitations you experience, they may be prevented easily with some simple lifestyle changes.

• Some medications can cause palpitations, such as beta-blockers, calcium channel blockers, and asthma and thyroid medications. You may need to discuss your medication with your doctor.

• Over-the-counter cold remedies can cause palpitations, but this is only likely if you have had heart problems in the past.

• Some substances, such as caffeine, tobacco and alcohol, and recreational drugs, including cocaine, amphetamines and marijuana, can stimulate the heart and cause palpitations, so avoid them.

• Manage your stress levels. Stress increases adrenaline, which can cause a rapid heartbeat and palpitations.

• Reduce your risk of heart disease by exercising regularly and eating a healthy diet.

 Did you know?

Most people experience extra heartbeats (ectopic beats) daily. An ectopic beat sometimes feels like a sudden thump in the chest, or as though your heart has missed a beat, but it is usually nothing to worry about.

CONVENTIONAL REMEDIES

Treatment for palpitations may be as simple as avoiding particular substances or situations that trigger them. Depending on the type of palpitations you have, your doctor may prescribe medicines for controlling your heart rhythm, such as beta-blockers to slow your heart rate, or anti-arrhythmic drugs. An injection of adenosine can also be given to normalise the heart rate. In some cases, surgery may be necessary to control the heart's rhythm, and a pacemaker may need to be fitted.

 NATURAL REMEDIES

Here are some natural ways of controlling your palpitations.

HERBAL REMEDIES Hawthorn contains flavonoids, which may help to control an irregular heartbeat. Try taking 150mg three times daily.

AROMATHERAPY Try adding a few drops of neroli, ylang ylang or lavender essential oils to bathwater to help calm palpitations.

NUTRITIONAL MEDICINE Include foods rich in magnesium in your diet, such as fish, spinach, nuts, and dairy products. Magnesium is a mineral that helps to regulate the heart's rhythm.

 HELPFUL THERAPIES

Practising yoga, tai chi or meditation regularly will help you to relax and reduce the frequency of palpitations caused by anxiety or stress. Try the following deep breathing exercise when you feel anxious or stressed:

1 Relax your shoulders and breathe in deeply through your nose for the count of two.

2 Then breathe out through your mouth for the count of 4. As you breathe, you should be able to feel your diaphragm (the muscle just below your breastbone) moving in and out.

 SEE YOUR DOCTOR

Although palpitations are very common and often harmless, sometimes they can be signs of an underlying medical condition, which is more serious. For example, they can be caused by an overactive thyroid gland, anaemia, high blood pressure or heart problems. See your doctor if your palpitations seem to last a long time and are worrying you.

Caution

Seek immediate medical attention if you:
- Have pain or pressure in your chest
- Feel extremely weak
- Feel dizzy or faint
- Have shortness of breath
- Feel nauseous while having palpitations.

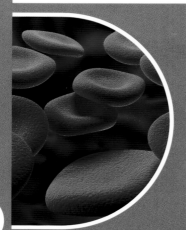

Anaemia

You have anaemia when you have too few red blood cells or too little haemoglobin (an oxygen-carrying protein) in your blood. This is most likely caused by an iron deficiency, but can also be due to a deficiency in vitamin B12 or folate. Anaemia is most likely to occur in pre-menopausal women, especially during pregnancy.

SYMPTOMS

▷ Tiredness and lack of energy
▷ Palpitations (rapid or irregular heart beat)
▷ Light headedness
▷ Pale skin
▷ Shortness of breath
▷ Feeling cold
▷ Headaches
▷ Changes in taste
▷ A sore or smooth tongue
▷ Sore corners of the mouth
▷ Itching
▷ Dry, peeling or spoon-shaped nails

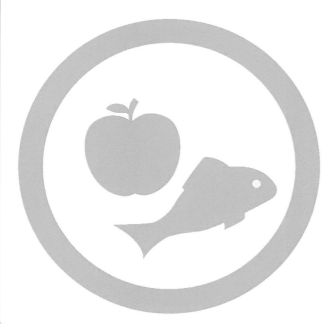

PREVENTION

Prevention involves making sure you eat a healthy balanced diet to get the nutrients you need, as well as addressing any other medical conditions that may be causing the anaemia.

- Ensure you get an adequate supply of iron, vitamin B12 and folate in your diet, especially if you are pregnant
- Women who experience heavy menstruation may need treatment to prevent anaemia
- Non-steroidal anti-inflammatory drugs such as ibuprofen and aspirin can cause gastrointestinal bleeding, which can lead to anaemia. It may be necessary to change medications
- Some people have underlying medical conditions that need attention. For example, stomach ulcers and Crohn's disease may cause blood loss, and coeliac disease can interfere with iron absorption.

CONVENTIONAL REMEDIES

As well as treating any underlying problems that may be making you anaemic, your doctor may prescribe iron supplements to address an iron deficiency and bring your iron levels back up to normal. Your red blood cell count and haemoglobin levels will be monitored carefully to ensure you are responding well to treatment. It may also be necessary to make dietary changes and take vitamin B12 or folate supplements.

NATURAL REMEDIES

Here are some natural treatments you might consider.

HERBAL REMEDIES Spirulina is a type of blue-green algae that may help to treat anaemia. Try taking one heaped 5ml teaspoon per day.

NUTRITIONAL MEDICINE Vitamin C helps your body to absorb iron from food. Good sources include broccoli, peppers, tomatoes, berries and citrus fruits.

HOMEOPATHIC REMEDIES Ferrum phosphoricum is a tissue salt that is used to treat iron deficiency. Try taking four tablets of Ferrum phosphoricum 6C twice daily until relief is obtained.

 ## HEALING FOODS

The following foods contain iron, vitamin B12 and folate, and they will help your body make enough red blood cells and haemoglobin.

IRON Found in dried fruits, such as apricots, raisins and prunes, green leafy vegetables, meat (especially liver), nuts, beans, pulses and blackstrap molasses. Some foods are fortified with iron, such as bread and breakfast cereals.

VITAMIN B12 Occurs naturally in meat, dairy products, eggs and fortified foods. If you follow a vegan diet, you should take a vitamin B12 supplement or eat fortified foods, as this vitamin is not found naturally in non-animal products.

FOLATE Found in many fruits and vegetables. Good sources include green leafy vegetables, beans, peas, oranges, bananas, yeast extract, liver and fortified foods.

 ## SEE YOUR DOCTOR

It is important that anaemia is investigated by your doctor as failure to do so may have other health consequences, such as an impaired immune system or heart and lung problems. Iron deficiency in pregnancy may increase the risk of low birth weight, premature birth and postnatal depression if it is left unchecked, whereas a folate deficiency can cause neural-tube defects, such as spina bifida, in a developing baby. So if you have the classic symptoms of anaemia (see opposite), check them out with your doctor without delay.

Caution

If you are taking medications, supplements, or if you are pregnant, consult your doctor before trying alternative remedies.

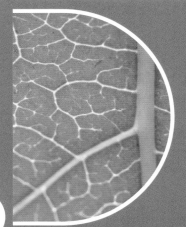

Varicose veins

Varicose veins are a common problem, most often occurring in the legs. Veins contain tiny valves which control the direction of blood flow, ensuring it flows upwards towards the heart. However, sometimes the valves become weaker, allowing blood to flow backwards and pool in the veins, causing swelling. While varicose veins don't usually cause health problems, they can become bothersome and unsightly.

 ## SYMPTOMS

▷ Lumpy, swollen, twisted blue or purple veins
▷ Aching, painful, heavy legs
▷ A throbbing or burning sensation
▷ Cramp in the legs
▷ Skin discolouration
▷ Ulceration
▷ Eczema-like rash (varicose eczema)

⊗ PREVENTION

A healthy lifestyle and good blood circulation may help to prevent varicose veins.

- Maintain a sensible weight. Obesity seems to increase the risk of varicose veins, as the extra weight puts pressure on the veins.
- Take regular exercise to keep your legs moving and improve blood circulation.
- Try to avoid standing or sitting for long periods of time as this can affect blood flow and make your varicose veins worse. Change your position often, and try to move about at least every 30 minutes.
- Don't smoke; this disrupts your body's circulation.

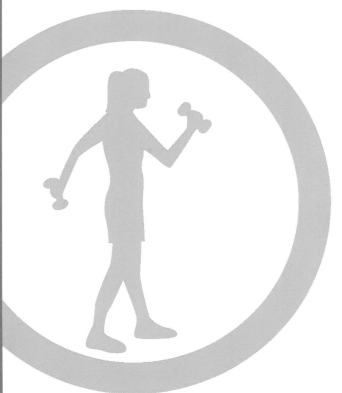

ⓘ Did you know?

Applied several times daily, witch hazel ointment may help soothe the swelling and bruising that are associated with varicose veins. This is due to its astringent properties.

CONVENTIONAL REMEDIES

Varicose veins don't usually require treatment and can be left alone if they are not giving you trouble. However, sometimes they can become uncomfortable or painful and require medical attention. Compression stockings can ease pain and discomfort; these apply pressure to the legs and encourage blood flow up towards the heart. Varicose veins can also be treated with sclerotherapy, which involves injecting the veins with a chemical to close them off. In some cases varicose veins may need to be removed with surgery.

 # NATURAL REMEDIES

There are a number of things you can try to help relieve symptoms of varicose veins.

HERBAL REMEDIES Horse chestnut (Aesculus hippocastanum) is helpful for treating chronic venous insufficiency. Take two 300mg tablets of horse chestnut extract (standardised to contain 20 per cent aescin) daily.

NUTRITIONAL MEDICINE Rutin is a bioflavonoid that may help to improve vein function and the symptoms associated with varicose veins. Try taking one 500mg rutin tablet daily.

YOGA Yoga postures will help improve circulation and encourage blood flow back to the heart. Try the shoulder stand for a few minutes each day to drain blood from your legs or, for a simpler option, lie with your body flat on the floor and your legs resting up against the wall.

 # HOMEOPATHIC REMEDIES

You can buy specially-prepared homeopathic remedies for varicose veins and circulatory disorders, or try the following.

Arnica montana 6C: Take one tablet three times daily for bruised, swollen legs that are very sore and feel better when you are lying down.

Hamamelis 6C: Take one tablet three times daily for large, sore, stinging, purple and bruised veins, and a tendency to experience bleeding haemorrhoids.

Pulsatilla 6C: Take one tablet three times daily for swollen, painful veins and heavy legs, which feel worse during warm temperatures.

 # SEE YOUR DOCTOR

If your varicose veins bother you, cause pain or keep you awake at night, see your doctor. This is especially important if:

- Your veins bleed
- You have excessive swelling
- Your skin changes colour
- You notice a rash or you develop ulcers.

 # IMMEDIATE RELIEF

To ease pain and discomfort when you are lying down, place some pillows under your legs to raise them above the level of your heart. When sitting, sit with your legs raised to help improve blood circulation, and don't sit with your legs crossed.

Restless legs

Restless legs is characterised by unpleasant sensations in the legs and the overwhelming urge to move them. Most people have mild symptoms, but they can be more severe, causing interrupted sleep and interfering with daily life.

 SYMPTOMS

▷ The need to move your legs when resting

▷ Aching, tingling, itching or pain in your legs

▷ Involuntary leg movements during the night

▷ Difficulty sleeping

 PREVENTION

Lifestyle changes may help to prevent symptoms and aid restful sleep.

- Exercise regularly.
- Avoid alcohol, caffeine and tobacco before going to bed.
- Do something relaxing before bed.
- Ensure your bed is comfortable and your bedroom is quiet and dark.
- Get up and go to bed at the same time each day.

 Did you know?

It is not clear what causes restless legs, but it is believed to be related to a low level of dopamine (a neurotransmitter) in the brain.

 CONVENTIONAL REMEDIES

If your symptoms are mild, simple lifestyle changes may be enough to provide relief. Dopamine agonists, such as ropinerol and pramipexole, which increase the level of dopamine in the brain, may be prescribed for more severe cases of restless legs.

 NATURAL REMEDIES

The following natural therapies may help relieve the symptoms of restless legs.

HERBAL REMEDIES Take 20 to 30 drops of butcher's broom extract in a little water up to three times daily to improve circulation.

NUTRITIONAL MEDICINE Restless legs may be associated with low iron levels. Good sources of iron include beef, chicken, beans, lentils and blackstrap molasses.

 SEE YOUR DOCTOR

If your symptoms are getting worse and disrupting your sleep and daily life, see your doctor. Restless legs can be due to an underlying health condition, such as kidney disease, diabetes or anaemia. It can also occur as a side effect of some medications, such as antidepressants.

Deep vein thrombosis

Deep vein thrombosis (DVT) is a blood clot in a deep vein, usually in the leg. The risk of developing this condition is increased by being immobile for a long time, such as during a long-haul flight or car journey, or a stay in hospital.

 ## SYMPTOMS

▷ Pain and swelling in the leg
▷ Heavy, aching leg
▷ Leg feels hot
▷ Skin changes colour

 ## PREVENTION

Here are some simple measures to help prevent DVT.

- Walk regularly to boost circulation in your legs.
- Obesity increases the risk of DVT, so lose weight if necessary.
- Eat a healthy diet.
- Stay well hydrated by drinking plenty of water.
- Don't drink alcohol.
- Don't smoke.
- Don't use sleeping pills while travelling.
- Wear special flight socks on long flights.

 ## CONVENTIONAL REMEDIES

DVT is treated with the anticoagulant drugs heparin and warfarin. These stop the blood clot getting bigger and help prevent further blood clots forming. Compression stockings may be worn to relieve pain and swelling and encourage blood circulation in the legs. After DVT it is important to keep mobile with gentle exercise.

 ## NATURAL REMEDIES

The following may help to prevent further clots.

NUTRITIONAL MEDICINE Vitamin E, Vitamin K and garlic have natural blood-thinning properties. (Seek medical advice if you are already taking anticoagulants.)

EXERCISE With your toes on the floor, raise and lower your heels 10 times. Then raise and lower your toes 10 times while keeping your heels on the floor. On long flights or car journeys, do these exercises at regular intervals to prevent blood pooling in the lower legs.

 ## SEE YOUR DOCTOR

If you think you may have DVT, see your doctor as soon as possible. If a blood clot is not treated, part of it may break off, travel to your lungs and block a blood vessel. This is a potentially life-threatening condition, known as a pulmonary embolism.

 ### Did you know?

If you have a family history of deep vein thrombosis, you have an increased risk of developing thrombosis yourself.

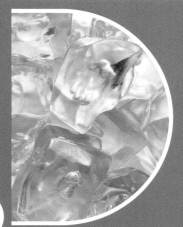

Chilblains

Chilblains are small, itchy lumps on the fingers, toes, ears or nose, which appear a few hours after prolonged exposure to cold. Although chilblains cause some discomfort, they usually go away on their own without further complications. Children, older people, and people with poor circulation are more likely to get chilblains.

118

 ## SYMPTOMS

▷ Small swellings on the skin
▷ Itching, burning skin
▷ Red or purple skin
▷ Sore and broken skin
▷ Blistering or ulceration of the skin

 ## PREVENTION

Here are some simple things you can do to protect yourself from the cold and help prevent chilblains.

- Keep warm. Wear gloves, socks, a hat and scarf, and other insulating clothing when you are outside in the cold.
- Warm your shoes and gloves on the radiator before you go outside.
- Make sure your home is warm, and free of draughts and damp.
- Wear socks in bed if you get cold feet.
- Don't wear tight-fitting shoes; this puts pressure on your feet and increases the risk of chilblains.
- Keep your hands and feet well-moisturised to prevent your skin from drying out.
- Have at least one hot meal a day in cold weather to warm up your body.
- Keep as active as possible to maintain good circulation.
- Don't smoke – nicotine contributes to poor circulation.

 ## Did you know?

In cold weather, the blood vessels in your fingers, toes and ears become narrower. When you go back into a warm environment, these blood vessels expand, which sometimes causes fluid to escape into nearby tissues. This leads to chilblains.

CONVENTIONAL REMEDIES

Always keep the parts of your body affected by chilblains warm. There are over-the-counter ointments that may relieve the symptoms of chilblains, and a mixture of friar's balsam and weak iodine (available from your pharmacist) can be painted over your chilblains. Antiseptic cream can be used on areas of cracked skin. A medication known as nifedipine, which dilates blood vessels, is sometimes prescribed for people who repeatedly suffer from chilblains.

 NATURAL REMEDIES

The following remedies may help provide some relief from chilblains.

NUTRITIONAL MEDICINE Use plenty of ginger, garlic, chilli and turmeric to add flavour when you are cooking. These foods are good for enhancing circulation.

AROMATHERAPY Add a few drops of peppermint, lavender, rosemary or eucalyptus essential oils to a carrier oil and massage into the affected areas.

ACUPUNCTURE This treatment may help to prevent chilblains by improving circulation to the hands and feet.

 HERBAL REMEDIES

The following herbs are thought to be helpful in improving general circulation.

- Take 30mg gingko biloba three to four times daily.
- Take 20 to 30 drops of hawthorn berry extract with water two to three times daily.
- Take 300g stinging nettle leaf powder each day.

 HOMEOPATHIC REMEDIES

You might like to try one of these remedies, depending on your symptoms.

Sulphur 30C: Take two tablets four times daily for chilblains that are inflamed.

Pulsatilla 30C: For painful chilblains, take two tablets four times daily.

Nux vomica 30C: For throbbing or pulsating chilblains, take two tablets three times daily.

 SEE YOUR DOCTOR

If you have cracked, broken or sore skin, see your doctor. Your skin may have become septic and need treating with antibiotics. Also, narrowing of the blood vessels may be a side-effect of some medications, such as beta-blockers. Speak to your doctor if you think your medication may be making you more susceptible to chilblains.

Caution

When you come in from the cold, never sit right next to a heater or place something hot directly on your skin. This increases the risk of chilblains. Warm yourself up slowly.

TOP 20
Conventional remedies

In case of accidents, minor aches, pains and common ailments, it's a good idea to keep some conventional medicines handy at home. Here are the top 20 remedies for your medicine cabinet with information on their uses. Always keep them in a safe place out of the way of children and pets.

1 SIMPLE ANALGESICS
- **Common names** paracetamol, Panadol, Tylenol
- **Used for** pain relief, headaches, fever
- !!! **Caution** Do not use if you have liver problems

2 NON-STEROIDAL ANTI-INFLAMMATORY DRUGS (NSAIDS)
- **Common names** ibuprofen, aspirin, naproxen
- **Used for** pain relief, especially where there is inflammation, swollen joints, sprains, arthritis
- !!! **Caution** do not use if you have asthma, IBS or stomach ulcers; do not give aspirin to children under 16

3 ANTIHISTAMINES
- **Available as** tablets, creams
- **Used for** hay fever, allergies, rashes, insect stings and bites, stinging nettles
- !!! **Caution** some may cause drowsiness

4 ANTACIDS
- **Common names** aluminium salts, Milk of Magnesia, Gaviscon, Alka-Seltzer
- **Used for** heartburn, indigestion and trapped wind
- !!! **Caution** check with your doctor before taking if you have a kidney disorder

5 ORAL REHYDRATION SALTS
- **Common names** Dioralyte
- **Available as** powder sachets
- **Used for** treating dehydration, diarrhoea, loose bowel movements, vomiting, and restoring body's natural balance of minerals and fluids

6 ANTIFUNGAL TREATMENTS
- **Common names** Clotrimazole, Micotin
- **Used for** relieving yeast infections, and treating oral thrush and fungal skin infections

7 HYDROCORTISONE 1% CREAM
- **Common names** hydrocortisone acetate
- **Used for** mild skin irritation, itching and mild eczema

8 CALAMINE
- **Available as** lotion or cream
- **Used for** itchy skin, rashes, sunburn

9 ANTI-DIARRHOEA TABLETS
- **Common names** Imodium, Arret, Diasorb
- **Used for** diarrhoea, food poisoning, gastroenteritis
- !!! **Caution** do not give to children under 12

10 SUNSCREENS AND SUNBLOCKS

- **Available as** lotions, creams, sprays
- **Used for** protecting skin against the sun's burning rays and minimizing risk of skin cancer. Choose one that offers UVA protection with an SPF of at least 15
- !!! **Caution** if sensitive to perfumes, opt for non-scented, hypoallergenic products

11 ANTISEPTIC

- **Common names** Dettol, Savlon, TCP
- **Available as** lotions, creams, sprays, wipes
- **Used for** cleaning cuts, grazes and wounds

12 THROAT LOZENGES AND SPRAYS

- **Common names** Benzocaine, Chloraseptic
- **Used for** relieving sore throats

13 EMOLLIENTS

- **Common names** E45, Dermal
- **Available as** creams, gels
- **Used for** relieving itching and moisturizing dry skin , eczema, dermatitis

14 PLASTERS

- **Used for** covering cuts and wounds

15 EYEWASH SOLUTION

- **Used for** washing grit and dirt out of eyes and treating eye injuries where tap water is not readily available

16 DECONGESTANTS

- **Available as** tablets or nasal sprays
- **Used for** relieving cold symptoms, such as blocked nose, and easing hay fever symptoms

17 MUSCLE PAIN RELIEF

- **Common names** Icy Hot, Deep Heat
- **Available as** sprays, gels, heat pads
- **Used for** muscular pains, and sprained joint pain

18 INSECT REPELLENTS

- **Available as** sprays, creams, gels, lotions, medicated towelettes
- **Used for** preventing insect bites and stings

19 INFANT SUSPENSION

- **Available as** flavoured liquids and sachets
- **Used for** relieving pain, teething pain, fever, cold symptoms in babies and young children
- !!! **Caution** contains paracetamol

20 COUGH MEDICINES

- **Types** suppressants for dry coughs; expectorants for chesty coughs with phlegm
- **Used for** relieving painful and irritating coughs

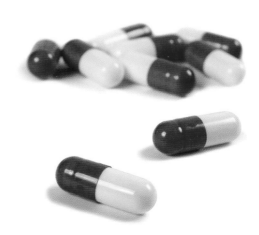

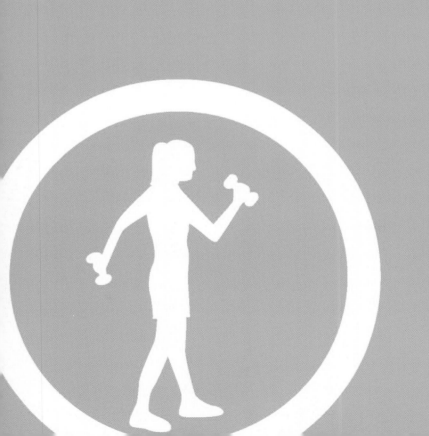

Respiratory problems

The respiratory system comprises the airways, breathing muscles and lungs, together with the arteries and veins that carry oxygen to and from the lungs. Its function is to supply oxygen, which is essential for the healthy and efficient functioning of all the body's cells, and to take away waste products, such as carbon dioxide.

When you inhale, air is breathed in through your nose and mouth and passes down the windpipe through the bronchi into your lungs. Inside the lungs are millions of tiny air sacs called alveoli where an exchange of gases takes place. The oxygen is passed into the bloodstream for distribution to the heart and thence to the rest of the body, while carbon dioxide is exhaled.

A properly functioning respiratory system is essential for good health, but diseases are becoming increasingly common in industrialised countries due to pollutants in the atmosphere, tobacco smoke and exhaust fumes. There is evidence that repeated exposure can increase the likelihood of developing respiratory problems, such as asthma, chronic bronchitis, emphysema and even lung cancer. Many minor common respiratory problems and disorders, such as coughing, runny nose and sore throat, are caused by infection, and these can be treated with conventional, traditional and natural remedies.

Your lifestyle and diet play an important role in building and maintaining healthy lungs. Regular exercise will make them strong and expand their capacity, while eating healthily helps your body to fight infections. However, the best protection you can give your lungs is not to smoke; if you are already a smoker, quit now before it is too late. Even second-hand smoke and passive smoking can affect your respiratory health, so get your partner or friends to give up cigarettes.

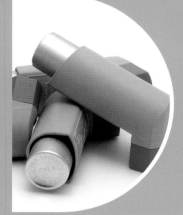

Asthma

The respiratory condition asthma affects around 5.4 million people in the UK alone. It causes the bronchi – the airways of the lungs – to become irritated, inflamed and swollen, which results in a narrowing of the airways. In many cases, asthma begins in childhood, but it can also develop at any point during life. Although there is no overall cure for this condition, there are many ways in which the symptoms can be managed and treated.

 SYMPTOMS

▷ Coughing
▷ Shortness of breath
▷ Wheezing
▷ A tight feeling in the chest

 PREVENTION

- Asthma can be triggered by common allergens, such as dust mites, pollen, smoke, animal fur or feathers, so reducing contact with these can help reduce the risk of an asthma attack. For dust mites, regularly cleaning your home is beneficial.
- Dust, fumes or chemical substances you come into contact with regularly (for instance, through your work environment) can also trigger asthma attacks. Being aware of this and trying to limit exposure wherever possible can help reduce the risk of an asthma attack or of asthma worsening.
- Regular exercise can improve lung capacity and strengthen your heart.

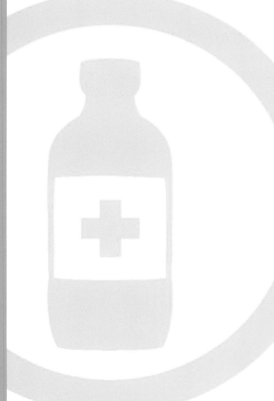 CONVENTIONAL REMEDIES

Asthma is controlled and managed using a variety of different methods, which are tailored to individual needs. Two types of inhalers, or puffers, which contain steroids and other medicines are usually prescribed. A reliever is used to treat the symptoms of asthma, and a preventer helps to prevent the symptoms. If you're prescribed a preventer, then it should be used every day, even when your asthma is fine. A reliever inhaler provides quick-acting relief if the symptoms of asthma flare up. You may also be given a spacer – a device that helps you to use your inhaler effectively. For bad asthma attacks, a course of steroid medicines may be prescribed.

NATURAL REMEDIES

There are various natural remedies you can try for easing different aspects of asthma.

NUTRITIONAL MEDICINE Foods containing the naturally occurring substance sulphite, used as a food preservative, can trigger asthma in some people. Watch your diet and cut down on sulphite foods, such as beer, wine, processed foods and shrimps. Sometimes food allergies can trigger asthma, so work with a nutritional therapist to try and identify and remove any potential allergens from your diet.

ALEXANDER TECHNIQUE Poor posture, especially hunching your shoulders and pushing the neck into the chest, can make the symptoms of asthma worse. Work with a qualified Alexander Technique practitioner to learn how to improve your posture and benefit your breathing.

YOGA Join a yoga class, as practising yoga, especially stretching postures and breathing techniques, can be beneficial.

AROMATHERAPY Put a few drops of eucalyptus essential oil onto a tissue and gently inhale it to help your breathing (steam inhalation isn't recommended for asthmatics).

HELPFUL THERAPIES The Buteyko Method, which involves learning breathing exercises and techniques to reduce over-breathing, is beneficial. Find a qualified practitioner to teach you.

OSTEOPATHY An osteopath may be able to use soft-tissue massage and manipulation techniques to relax the chest muscles and also to ease breathing problems.

 HERBAL REMEDIES

• If your asthma has been brought on by a cold or chest infection, then take one or two teaspoons of echinacea tincture with water two or three times a day for a week, or until the symptoms go.

• To ease the discomfort of a tight chest, take one teaspoon of cramp bark tincture with water three times a day, for up to a week.

 SEE YOUR DOCTOR

If you suspect that you may have asthma, see your doctor. Likewise, if you are asthmatic and your symptoms are getting worse or your medication is not working effectively.

Caution

• Don't abandon taking prescribed asthma medication.

• If you're having a severe asthma attack and are unable to breathe, dial 999 and request emergency medical treatment.

125

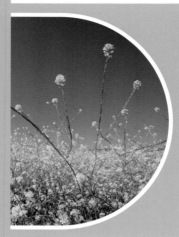

Hay fever

Hay fever is an allergic reaction to pollen, which is produced by seasonal grasses, occurring usually in the spring and summer. Like asthma, it is on the increase, and the symptoms listed below are common to other allergic reactions, including house dust mites, exhaust fumes and atmospheric pollution.

 SYMPTOMS

▷ Sore, swollen, itchy and stinging eyes
▷ Stuffed-up nose and sinuses
▷ Streaming nose
▷ Frequent bouts of violent sneezing
▷ Itching of the roof of the mouth
▷ Itching in the ears
▷ Mild form of asthma with tightness in the chest

 PREVENTION

As always, prevention is better than cure and the only real way to prevent hay fever is to avoid inhaling allergenic material. Although this is not practical, you could try the following measures.

• Keep the windows shut and avoid going outside early in the morning, late evening and just before and after thunderstorms when pollen counts are higher and more likely to trigger attacks.

• Don't open your car windows when you are travelling; if it's a hot day, turn on the air conditioning to stay cool. Make enquiries about getting a pollen filter fitted to your car.

• Some sufferers claim that wearing wraparound sunglasses to protect their eyes from pollen is also helpful.

• Smear some petroleum jelly around and just inside your nostrils to trap pollen and help prevent inhalation.

• You can take conventional anti-allergy medication before an attack (see below), or you can use a natural antihistamine, such as ginkgo biloba (up to 240mg daily) or nettle (500mg three times daily).

 Did you know?

Cutting back on your daily intake of dairy products may reduce mucus production and relieve hay fever symptoms. However, if you consume less milk, yoghurt and cheese, you must find other sources of calcium and other missing nutrients.

 Quick fix

You can quickly soothe sore, itchy eyes with a cool, damp flannel.

CONVENTIONAL REMEDIES

Antihistamines are commonly used to prevent allergic reactions. These are available as nose sprays, tablets and eye drops, or as syrups for young children. Although antihistamines are reasonably effective, they can cause drowsiness and other side effects. You can consult the packaging for details or ask the pharmacist or your doctor for advice.

Healing foods

Find a source of locally produced organic honey and have four 5ml teaspoons a day to help relieve hay fever symptoms. It is important that it is made by bees collecting the pollen from flowering plants in your area.

Herbal remedies

The usual remedies use cleansing and strengthening herbs for the respiratory tract.

- Take up to eight 200mg eyebright capsules to relieve symptoms.
- Bathe sore eyes with a soothing eyebright infusion or strained, sterilised marigold.

Homeopathic remedies

You can buy 'over-the-counter' homeopathic hay-fever tablets or try:

Allium cepa 6C: Take one tablet twice daily to relieve watering eyes and running, sore nose

Euphrasia 6C: Take one tablet twice daily to relieve watery, sore eyes and running nose with frequent sneezing

Sabadilla 6C: Take one tablet twice daily to relieve irritated eyes, blocked noise and violent sneezing.

NATURAL REMEDIES

You can experiment with a whole range of natural remedies to discover what works best for you. Here are some of the options you might consider.

ACUPRESSURE Points 41 and 47 may increase mucus drainage; points 50 and 51 may help stop bouts of sneezing.

AROMATHERAPY Place a drop of either basil or melissa oil in a handkerchief for instant relief from blocked sinuses and a stuffed-up nose.

NUTRITIONAL MEDICINE Eat more citrus fruit, berries and vegetables. They are good sources of Vitamin C and help protect mucus membranes. Oily fish and flax seed oil contain omega-3 fatty acids, which can counter inflammatory reactions triggered by pollen allergy.

SEE YOUR DOCTOR

If your symptoms do not diminish as a result of taking natural remedies or over-the-counter histamines, get professional help and consult your doctor.

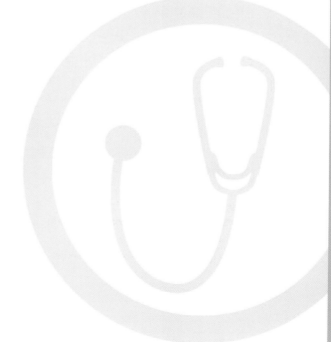

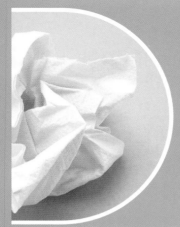

Common cold

Colds are viral infections of the upper respiratory tract and affect us all at some time or another. Although they are so common and highly contagious, there is no known cure. Colds are annoying and debilitating but most disappear within five days unless there are complications.

 ## SYMPTOMS

▷ Blocked nose
▷ Runny nose and sneezing
▷ Possible sore throat
▷ Possible fever
▷ Possible fever
▷ Tickly cough
▷ Headaches

 ## PREVENTION

Colds may be a sign that you are run down and need to boost your immune system. The best ways to prevent them include the following:

- Eat a healthy diet which contains vitamin C (citrus fruits, leafy green vegetables, tomatoes, peppers) and zinc (shellfish, meat, pumpkin seeds)
- Take a vitamin C supplement every day
- If possible, avoid crowded, over-heated places when cold viruses are circulating in winter
- Do not rub your eyes and nose after hand contact with cold sufferers
- Get outside and get plenty of fresh air and exercise
- Stay relaxed and calm and try not to get stressed or over-tired.

 ## CONVENTIONAL REMEDIES

There are so many over-the-counter cold and cough remedies but they can only relieve the symptoms at best, not cure your cold. These range from painkillers for headaches to decongestants. Antibiotics will not work unless there is a secondary bacterial infection.

 ### Did you know?

There are around 200 different cold viruses, which are transmitted by sneezing, coughing or hand-to-hand contact.

NATURAL REMEDIES

Most people have their own tried and tested home-made remedies for relieving the unpleasant symptoms of colds. These include the following:

- Squeeze the juice of a lemon into a cup of hot water and stir in one 5ml teaspoon honey. If wished, add some grated fresh ginger
- Drink lots of fluids to replace any lost through sneezing and sweating (if you have a fever)
- Gargle with saltwater
- Eat onions and garlic for their decongestant and antiseptic properties – make a French onion soup or just bake some whole in a little olive oil.

HERBAL REMEDIES Make a herb tea with some elderflower (for stuffed-up nose and catarrh), hyssop (for coughs) and peppermint (for reducing mucous). Taking echinacea and goldenseal drops every day in water helps to boost the immune system as well as relieving irritation of the mucous membranes.

 AROMATHERAPY

- Add 3 drops each lavender, eucalyptus and thyme oils to a bowl of boiling water and inhale the steam.
- Or sprinkle a couple of drops of eucalyptus, pine or lavender oil on to a handkerchief.
- Before going to bed, have a soothing bath and add a few drops of tea tree, eucalyptus, pine or lavender oil to the water.

 HOMEOPATHIC REMEDIES

These can be helpful in relieving cold symptoms.

Aconite 6C: Take one tablet every four hours at the beginning of a cold to relieve a stuffed-up nose and frequent sneezing.

Natrum muriaticum 6C: Take one tablet every three to four hours for a cold that starts with sneezing with white or clear discharge.

 SEE YOUR DOCTOR

Most colds do not necessitate a visit to the doctor and will clear up of their own accord in a few days. However, you should make an appointment if you experience any of the following symptoms:

- You have shortness of breath
- Your cough gets progressively worse and won't go away
- You have persistent fever for more than a week.
- You have a compromised immune system (for example, due to HIV) or chronic respiratory and/or heart disease.

 IMMEDIATE RELIEF

There is no quick fix for a cold but you can clear a blocked nose and make breathing easier by steam inhalation. Add some eucalyptus drops to a basin of boiling water, cover your head with a towel, bend over the steam and inhale deeply.

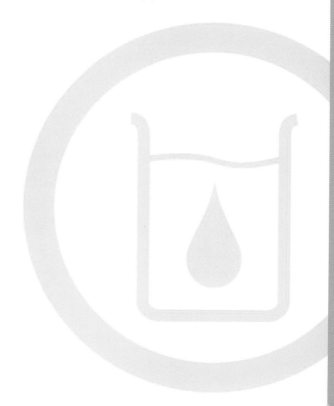

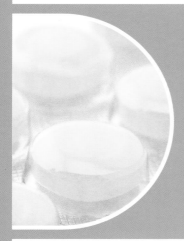

Coughs

Coughing is one of your body's natural defence mechanisms – a reflex action used by the respiratory system to clear the airways and remove or prevent infection. It may be caused by irritation of the throat or larynx, an increase in catarrh or saliva, or excess sputum, usually due to bacterial infection. Many coughs are just dry and irritating – a by-product of a cold – but they can be persistent and more serious.

 SYMPTOMS

▷ Dry tickly throat
▷ Dry, barking cough
▷ Deep, painful cough
▷ Clear or coloured mucous
▷ Possible sore throat

 PREVENTION

The best way to prevent unwanted coughs and respiratory problems is not to smoke and to avoid passive smoking situations. You can also:

- Exercise regularly to strengthen your lungs
- Try to avoid pollution, smog and traffic fumes or wear a face mask when you are cycling in heavy city traffic
- Wear a protective face mask when tackling any dusty housework and home improvements
- Do not sleep in air conditioning
- Put a humidifier in centrally heated rooms.

 CONVENTIONAL REMEDIES

You can choose from a wide array of cough mixtures and lozenges, which claim to soothe and loosen coughs. However, there is little evidence for their efficacy. Deep, painful and persistent coughing may be a symptom of a lower respiratory infection and might require antibiotics.

 Did you know?

Some people think that taking garlic capsules every day helps to prevent and relieve coughs. Garlic is decongestant and antibacterial.

NATURAL REMEDIES

For centuries, people have treated coughs with home-made medicines, herbs and nutritional remedies.

- Eat less dairy foods (milk, yoghurt, cheese) to reduce mucous formation.
- Try to eat some garlic, leeks and onions every day by adding them to soups, stews, bakes, etc.
- Apply a mustard pack to your chest.
- Slice some onions thinly into rings and layer them up in a bowl with brown sugar sprinkled between the layers. The following day, drain off the liquid and drink a teaspoonful at a time.
- Add freshly squeezed lemon juice and honey to hot water.
- Swallow one 5ml teaspoon honey, letting it trickle down your throat.

HERBAL REMEDIES Many herbs are traditionally used to treat coughs. You can make a herbal tea for chesty coughs with white horehound, thyme, coltsfoot, cowslip and peppermint, whereas marshmallow root can help ease dry coughs. You can also make herbal steam inhalations with eucalyptus and peppermint.

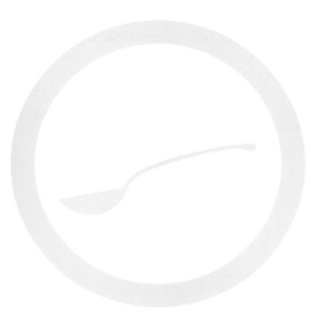

 AROMATHERAPY

- Add 3 drops of eucalyptus, cypress, thyme or sandalwood oil to steaming hot water and inhale deeply to soothe the airways.
- Mix eucalyptus, sandalwood or frankincense oils with a carrier oil and rub gently into the chest and throat, or heat the oil in a special burner and breathe in the fragrance.
- You can also use tea tree oil as a gargle – just add 2–3 drops to a cup of warm water and gargle three times a day.

 HOMEOPATHIC REMEDIES

The following remedies can be helpful in relieving cough symptoms. Choose the appropriate remedy for your symptoms.

Bryonia 6C: Take one tablet three times daily for dry, painful coughs.

Stannum 6C: Take one tablet three times daily for chesty coughs with greenish mucous.

 SEE YOUR DOCTOR

If your cough does not clear up and becomes progressively worse or you cough up blood-stained mucous, you must see your doctor. Coughs may be a sign of a more serious, underlying condition and this always needs checking out. If accompanied by a bacterial lung infection, you may be prescribed a course of antibiotics.

Quick fix

Sucking herbal cough lozenges may be soothing and bring instant relief in a coughing fit, although they will not cure your cough.

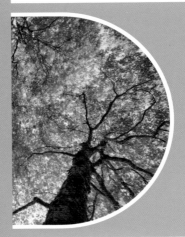

Bronchitis

Bronchitis affects the main airways of the lung (the bronchi). It causes inflammation and irritation, the production of more mucus than is normal and a hacking cough. It is common during the winter months, particularly after a cold, influenza or sore throat, but as well as infections, it can also be caused by environmental factors.

SYMPTOMS

▷ A bad, hacking cough
▷ Coughing up yellowy mucus
▷ Wheezing
▷ Breathlessness
▷ A sore throat
▷ Blocked nose and sinuses
▷ Headaches
▷ Chills or a fever
▷ General aches, pains and feeling unwell

PREVENTION

Good hygiene is beneficial, as bronchitis is often caused by a virus spread via coughing or sneezing. Wash your hands frequently or use anti-bacterial gel on them if you're in contact with people who have colds or flu.

- If you work in an environment where you could be exposed to breathing in irritating substances, protect your lungs by wearing a mask on your face.
- Damp or cold environments can also lead to bronchitis, so try to avoid such circumstances.
- If you're a smoker, then stop smoking, as the smoke can make you more likely to get bronchitis.
- If you have a low immune system, then try to eat a healthy balanced diet, so that your body gets a good dose of essential nutrients.

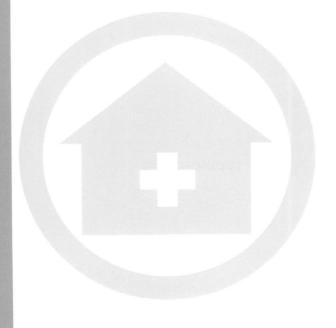

Did you know?

A humidifier can help keep the air in a room moist and aid your breathing. If you don't have one, you can create the same effect by simply placing a pot of water over a radiator.

CONVENTIONAL REMEDIES

Drinking plenty of fluids not only keeps you hydrated but also helps to thin the mucus and make it easier to cough up. Painkillers can be taken to ease any aches, pains or headaches. Over-the-counter cough medicines may provide some relief. It also helps to get plenty of rest and, where possible, have fresh air in a room. If your doctor thinks that you could have an increased risk of developing pneumonia, antibiotics may be prescribed.

 ## NATURAL REMEDIES

There are various natural remedies that may help ease the symptoms of bronchitis.

HERBAL REMEDIES Use expectorant herbs, such as elecampane and thyme, to encourage coughing and rid yourself of mucus. A herbalist can make up a tincture for you. Take echinacea, along with garlic, for their infection-fighting abilities, and try ginseng supplements to help reduce bronchial inflammation.

AROMATHERAPY Steam installation can provide much-needed relief for the congestion of bronchitis. Lean your head over a bowl of hot water to inhale. Add a drop of eucalyptus oil to clear your nasal passages, or lavender to relax your muscles and help your breathing. If you have no oils, then simply breathe in the steam. Inhale several times a day as required.

OSTEOPATHY An osteopath may be able to provide help for chronic bronchitis by working on the shoulder muscles, neck and back to ease any congestion and clear the air passages.

 ## NUTRITIONAL MEDICINE

- Include plenty of garlic in your diet, as it's good for your immune system.
- Avoid eating processed foods and dairy products whilst you have bronchitis, as they can encourage more mucus to form.
- Eat plenty of vitamin C – or take vitamin C supplements – as it can help thin the mucus.

 ## SEE YOUR DOCTOR

The symptoms of bronchitis are similar to those of pneumonia, which can be more serious. Don't try to self-diagnose – see your doctor, especially if your symptoms change. This is especially important if you have any other lung or heart conditions.

Helpful supplements

- Collodial Silver has natural antibiotic properties and can work with viruses and bacteria.
- Where bronchitis is triggered by an allergic reaction, such an environmental factor, taking the antioxidant supplement Quercetin can be beneficial.

133

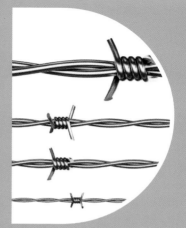

Sore throat

Most sore throats are due to minor bacterial or viral infections and they clear up after a few days. They are more common in winter, often accompanying the common cold or influenza, and are spread by airborne droplets, through coughing and sneezing, or by hand-to-hand contact. However, they can also be caused by allergies, such as hay fever, or irritation from smoking.

SYMPTOMS

▷ Throat feels sore with pain at back
▷ Difficulty swallowing
▷ Throat looks red
▷ Tonsils may be swollen and coated
▷ Possible swollen lymph nodes in neck
▷ May be fever, headache, pain in ears

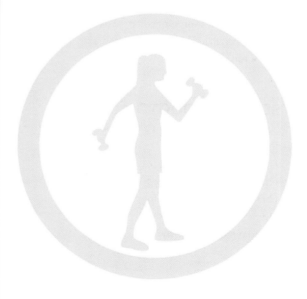

PREVENTION

Most sore throats are caused by viruses, so there are few preventive measures that you can take. However, you can reduce your chances of getting one and decrease the incidence and severity by:

- Eating a healthy diet
- Giving up smoking and avoiding smoky environments
- Drinking lots of fluids, especially water
- Wrapping up warmly in winter and wearing a scarf to protect your throat from cold
- Staying healthy, relaxed and stress-free to prevent becoming run-down and more susceptible to infections
- Not sharing towels, drinking or eating utensils with anyone who already has a sore throat.

ⓘ Did you know?

Most home remedies, especially honey, lemon and cider vinegar taken three times daily, are more effective in relieving sore throats than conventional over-the-counter preparations.

CONVENTIONAL REMEDIES

You can easily treat a sore throat yourself with over-the-counter painkillers, such as paracetamol, or by using a saltwater mouthwash and consuming plenty of fluids and soft foods. However, if the cause is bacterial rather than viral, your doctor may prescribe a course of antibiotics.

 ## NATURAL REMEDIES

The most common home-made remedy for a sore throat is to add the juice of a lemon and two 5ml teaspoons honey to a cup of hot water. Stir well to dissolve the honey and sip. Other remedies you can try include the following ones.

- Boost your immune system with raw fruit and fruit juice – drink plenty of citrus and pineapple juice.
- Take vitamin C and garlic capsules every day.
- Gargle with lemon juice and hot water or some cider vinegar and hot water.
- Swallow one 5ml teaspoon runny honey, letting it trickle down your throat.

AROMATHERAPY Add a few drops of tea tree or myrrh oil to a massage carrier oil or cream and gently massage them into your throat before wrapping a scarf around it to keep it warm.

 ## HERBAL REMEDIES

- You can gargle with echinacea, sage, thyme, rosemary or make them into a tea and sweeten with honey if wished.
- Marshmallow root or slippery elm tea will ease and soothe a sore throat.
- Make a sage infusion (see page 142) and after straining add one 5ml teaspoon each cider vinegar and honey. Use as a soothing gargle four times daily.
- In addition, try taking one 200mg capsule echinacea four times a day.

 ## HOMEOPATHIC REMEDIES

The following can be helpful in relieving a sore throat.

Belladonna 30C: Take one tablet four times daily for three days for sudden onset with red, dry painful throat and difficult swallowing.

Phytolacca 30C: Take one tablet four times daily for three days for intense dryness, burning in throat, pain in ears on swallowing and dark red tonsils.

 ## SEE YOUR DOCTOR

You should see the doctor if you experience the following symptoms:

- You have a temperature above 38°C (100.4°F)
- You have difficulty swallowing
- You have had a sore throat for more than two weeks
- You have a rash and/or vomiting.

 ## Quick fix

Suck antiseptic pastilles or natural herbal lozenges to ease a sore throat, or even some ice cubes, which are very soothing.

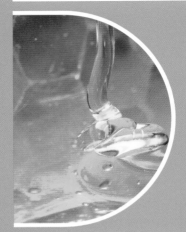

Tonsillitis

This is an inflammation of the tonsils, which is due to acute infection. The tonsils are lymph nodes on either side of the back of the mouth and their function is to protect against upper respiratory tract infections. If they become infected, they get inflamed and swollen with fluids and white blood cells, making swallowing painful and eating difficult.

 SYMPTOMS

▷ Sore throat
▷ Swollen, possibly coated, tonsils
▷ Difficulty swallowing
▷ Swollen lymph nodes in the neck
▷ Possible fever
▷ Headache and earache
▷ Breath smells unpleasant

 PREVENTION

Eating a healthy, varied diet, staying warm in cold weather and supporting the immune system with echinacea capsules (up to 600mg four times a day) will help keep you healthy and ward off respiratory and throat infections. In addition, you can:

• Avoid sharing utensils or towels with anyone who has a sore throat
• Wear a scarf in winter
• Boost your immune system with zinc and selenium – eat five Brazil nuts and a handful of pumpkin seeds every day
• Give up smoking.

 CONVENTIONAL REMEDIES

The usual treatment for tonsillitis is to drink plenty of fluids, take over-the-counter painkillers, such as paracetamol, and eat soft food. Gargling with saltwater or dissolved painkilling tablets may bring some relief as will sucking ice cubes or sore throat lozenges. If the cause is viral, you will have to rest and wait for the illness to run its course. However, if it caused by a bacterial infection, your doctor may prescribe a course of antibiotics.

 Did you know?

If you suffer from recurrent bouts of tonsillitis on a regular basis your doctor may even recommend an operation to remove your tonsils (a tonsillectomy).

NATURAL REMEDIES

Many of us practise natural medicine to treat tonsillitis and throat infections without even realising it. The traditional remedy is a soothing drink of hot water mixed with honey and freshly squeezed lemon juice.

NUTRITIONAL MEDICINE Because swallowing is painful, eat blended vegetable soups made with onions, leeks and garlic (antiseptic qualities), cabbage, peppers, broccoli and tomatoes (good sources of Vitamin C) and carrots and sweet potatoes (for beta-carotene content).

AROMATHERAPY Add a few drops of tea tree, thyme and lavender essential oils to a bowl of very hot water. Cover your head with a towel and bend over the bowl, inhaling the steam.

 # HERBAL REMEDIES

- Make a gargle by blending 4 tablespoons honey, 6 tablespoons lemon juice, 4 tablespoons apple cider vinegar, 1 crushed garlic clove and 1 teaspoon grated ginger.
- Alternatively, gargle with raspberry leaf tea or add a teaspoonful of chopped fresh sage leaves to a cup of boiling water, then cover and steep for 10 minutes, strain and use as a gargle when cool.

 # HEALING FOODS

- To soothe a painful, inflamed throat and tonsils, you can freeze pineapple juice in small containers and insert a wooden or plastic stick. Unmould and suck the ice lollies.
- Honey has natural antiseptic qualities, so swallow one 5ml teaspoonful four times a day.

 # HOMEOPATHIC REMEDIES

The medicine selected depends on the symptoms presented. However, if there is no response within 24 to 36 hours, you should consult your doctor.

Lachesis 30C: Take one tablet four times a day for three days to relieve swollen dark red or purple tonsils, which start on the left side and with pain shooting to the ear when swallowing

Phytolacca 30C: Take one tablet four times a day for three days to relieve dark red or purple tonsils with white pus, burning in the throat with pain worse on the right side.

 # SEE YOUR DOCTOR

You must call your doctor if you experience any of the following symptoms:

- Your sore throat persists for more than two weeks
- You have difficulty swallowing and cannot eat
- You have a fever above 38°C (100.4°F)
- You have a rash and/or vomiting
- You have an illness that lowers your immunity (such as HIV) or you are undergoing immuno-suppressive treatments, such as chemotherapy or steroids.

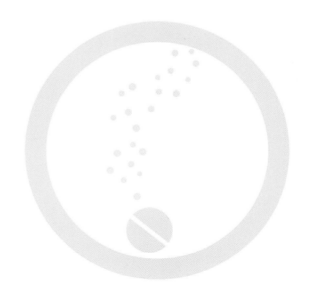

137

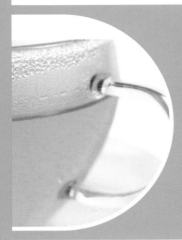

Sinusitis and congestion

When you can't breathe properly, you realise how much you take clear nasal passages for granted. Sinusitis occurs if the sinuses become infected or inflamed, causing large amounts of mucus to block them. Nasal congestion may also be due to allergies, or the after-effects of colds or flu.

SYMPTOMS

SINUSITIS

▷ Pain above eyebrows, in upper jaw, around eyes and nose
▷ Earache or even neck pain.
▷ A feeling of pressure in your face
▷ A blocked nose
▷ A headache
▷ Green or yellow mucus
▷ Mucus that drains from the back of your nose into your throat
▷ May cause a sore throat or cough
▷ Reduced sense of smell
▷ Fever

CONGESTION

▷ Being unable to breathe through your nose
▷ Headache
▷ Stuffy head
▷ Nasal discomfort
▷ Disturbed sleep

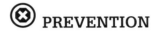 PREVENTION

• Chronic sinusitis is often linked to allergies, so identifying the potential allergens and doing your best to avoid them could prevent future bouts. Common allergens include dust, pollen, spicy foods and alcohol.

• Irritants, such as household chemical sprays or cleaning products, can trigger sinusitis, so avoiding these may help.

• Eating healthily and taking remedies such as echinacea to boost your immune system during the winter, when colds and flu are rife, may reduce your risk of sinusitis and congestion. Both are common after catching a cold.

Did you know?

Viral or bacterial infections are a common cause, but sinusitis can also be triggered by allergies, irritants or nasal polyps.

CONVENTIONAL REMEDIES

Painkillers can be used to help relieve the pain and bring down a fever, if you have one. Nasal decongestants may relieve the symptoms of a blocked nose. Some are available over-the-counter, but your doctor may also prescribe steroid nasal sprays. If your sinusitis could be caused by a bacterial infection, then antibiotics may be prescribed. For cases of chronic sinusitis that keep occurring and do not respond to treatment, surgery may be needed as a last resort. If nasal polyps are found to be blocking the nose, and causing recurring sinusitis, these may need to be surgically removed.

 NATURAL REMEDIES

The old-fashioned home remedies for dealing with sinus problems were to eat plenty of onions, leeks and garlic every day. If you don't like the flavour and smell of garlic, you can take it in capsule form.

NUTRITIONAL MEDICINE Dairy products are associated with the production of mucus, so it may be beneficial to cut down on the amount of dairy products you consume.

AROMATHERAPY Pop a drop of lavender, tea tree or eucalyptus essential oil into a base carrier oil, such as sweet almond oil, and gently massage it into your face. This can help ease the discomfort felt from sinusitis.

 ACUPRESSURE Pressing the acupoints on the large intestine meridian, which are located around the base of the nose, can help relieve the symptoms of sinusitis. Acupuncture can also help.

 HERBAL REMEDIES

- For chronic sinusitis, which may be due to an infection, take a daily echinacea capsule to boost your immune system and help fight the infection.
- Take pippali or long pepper supplements, or a tincture, to ease sinus headaches.

 HOMEOPATHIC REMEDIES

There are various homeopathic remedies that could help ease symptoms.

Kali Bich 6C, if you are experiencing a feeling of pressure around the bridge of your nose and have thick nasal mucus.

Sticta Pulmonaria 6C, for cases of chronic sinusitis and times when you don't have any mucus discharge.

 SEE YOUR DOCTOR

You can treat mild sinusitis yourself but if the condition is debilitating and very painful or persistent, see your doctor and get it checked out.

Quick fix

Put a few drops of eucalyptus essential oil in a bowl of steaming water. Lean over, covering your head with a towel, and inhale deeply for five to ten minutes. This should provide some relief from congestion. Repeat several times a day. Alternatively, add the oil to a warm bath.

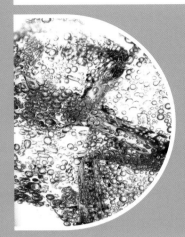

Hiccups

Hiccups are a reflex reaction, which occurs when your diaphragm suddenly contracts. As it contracts, the top of the windpipe closes immediately, causing the characteristic 'hic' noise. Short bouts of hiccups are relatively common and harmless and often have no apparent cause. Although cases of persistent hiccups lasting longer than 48 hours are quite rare, they can sometimes be caused by acid reflux, medication or an underlying disease.

 ## SYMPTOMS

▷ An involuntary 'hic' noise.
▷ Persistent hiccups can cause tiredness, exhaustion, disturbed sleep, embarrassment

 ## PREVENTION

Sometimes hiccups just occur – there doesn't seem to be any major reason why – but many other cases can be prevented.

- Overeating, eating a meal too quickly or suddenly having a very cold or extremely hot drink are all associated with bouts of hiccups, so avoiding these may reduce the risk.
- If you're prone to frequent hiccups, it may be worth avoiding fizzy, carbonated drinks, as these are linked to hiccups.
- Stress and over-excitement can bring on hiccups. If you're suffering from stress, find ways to relax.
- Smoking a lot or drinking alcohol are also known causes of hiccups, so give up smoking and drink less.

(i) Did you know?

The record for the longest running case of hiccups is held by Charles Osborne, an American who had hiccups for 68 years – from 1922 to 1990.

CONVENTIONAL REMEDIES

Whilst hiccups rarely need medical treatment, there are various self-help methods you can use to relieve the symptoms. Not everything works for everyone, but you could try the following.

- Hold your breath for a short period of time to stop hiccups – you may have to keep repeating this a number of times for it to work.
- Pull your knees up to your chest.
- Sip on some ice-cold water, suck an ice cube, bite on a lemon or drink a small amount of vinegar. All these can sometimes work – most likely due to the sudden shock to your system of tasting something cold, sour or strange!
- Lean forwards, with the aim of compressing your chest.
- If you're feeling athletic, do a headstand, as it could help get the diaphragm out of the spasm.

 # NATURAL REMEDIES

Try the following natural approaches to dealing with hiccups to find out what works for you.

HERBAL REMEDIES Slowly drinking spearmint or fennel tea, or sucking on a small piece of ginger, can help to stop hiccups.

NUTRITIONAL MEDICINE Some research suggests that a lack of magnesium may be linked to recurrent hiccups, so you could try taking magnesium supplements if you're susceptible to hiccups, or eat foods that are rich in magnesium, such as spinach or broccoli.

HYPNOTHERAPY If you are regularly prone to hiccups, or experience persistent hiccupping, then being hypnotised by a professional hypnotherapist could help ease your symptoms.

 # HELPFUL THERAPIES

The biochemic tissue salt, Mag Phos, has anti-spasmodic properties and can help relieve hiccup spasms. Take four 6C tablets when hiccups occur, or dissolve in hot water and sip every five to 15 minutes for the duration of the hiccup attack.

 # SEE YOUR DOCTOR

In cases where you experience persistent hiccups, for 48 hours or longer, your doctor may prescribe medication to bring the hiccups under control. The length of time you will need to take the medication will vary from weeks to months, depending on the severity of the hiccups.

 # IMMEDIATE RELIEF

The holistic therapy of yoga, which uses postural exercises, relaxation and breathing, can help relieve the spasm of hiccups. For instant relief, try lying on the floor with your arms at your side. Breathe in slowly and deeply, holding your breath for 10 seconds, before exhaling. Repeat 20 times.

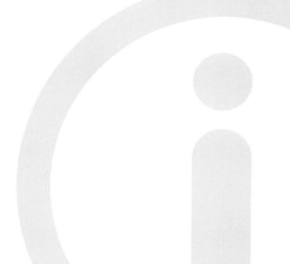

Using herbs at home

Using herbs in infusions (teas), decoctions, compresses and tinctures is simple when you know how. You can turn your kitchen into a pharmacy and make them yourself at home. It's easy, not expensive and does not take long to do – just follow the step-by-step instructions below.

HERBAL INFUSIONS

You can make an infusion (tea) from the dried or fresh leaves and flowers of plants. Drink them hot or cool, sweetened with a little honey to taste, if wished. Alternatively, they can be used as a gargle or mouthwash, or even added to the bath water.

1   Use one teaspoon of dried herbs or two teaspoons fresh herbs per cup of water.
2   Warm a ceramic, glass or stainless steel teapot (not an aluminium one) with hot water and then pour the water away.
3   Add the herbs and cover with water that is near boiling. Cover the pot and leave to steep for 10–15 minutes.
4   Strain the liquid, discarding the herbs, and drink or use as required.

HERBAL DECOCTIONS

These are similar to infusions but you can use the woody parts of the plant (stems, bark and roots) as well as the leaves and flowers. Instead of brewing, the herbs are simmered gently in the water until the liquid reduces.

1   Roughly chop or crush the herbs and place them in an enamel, stainless steel or glass saucepan – do not use an aluminium, copper or non-stick pan.
2   Cover the herbs with water – use 300ml ($^1/_2$ pint) for every teaspoon of herbs.
3   Bring to the boil, then reduce the heat and simmer gently for 10–15 minutes, until the liquid has reduced by one-third.
4   Strain immediately and drink or use while the decoction is still warm.

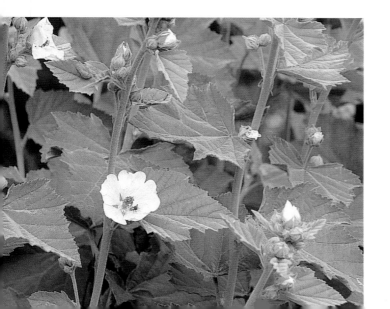
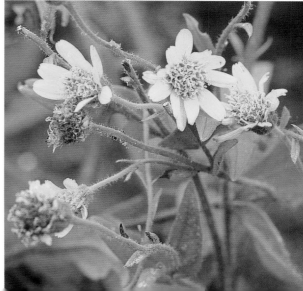

HERBAL COMPRESSES

These are very useful in reducing inflammation and speeding up healing. Herbal compresses are usually used hot for treating sprained muscles and aching joints, but you can also use cool ones for relieving feverish headaches.

1   Make a hot herbal infusion or decoction (see opposite).
2   Take a clean pad of cotton gauze or cloth and dip it into the hot liquid to soak it up.
3   Gently squeeze out any excess liquid and then apply the compress to the affected area.
4   When it starts to cool down, apply a fresh one.

HERBAL TINCTURES

These are similar to cold infusions but spirits are used instead of water, preserving the herbs and making them more concentrated. You can use alcohol, such as vodka or brandy, or apple-cider vinegar.

1   Chop the herbs or use dried ones. Place 225g (8 oz) fresh herbs or 115g (4oz) dried herbs in a large glass jar or container with a screwtop lid.
2   Add 600ml (1 pint) alcohol and cover the jar tightly.
3   Place the jar in a dark cupboard away from direct light and shake occasionally – at least three times a day – for two weeks.
4   Strain the liquid into dark-coloured bottles and stopper or seal securely. Store the bottles in a cool, dark place until required.

HERBAL POULTICES

These are commonly used to treat inflammation, skin irritations and itching, arthritis and aching joints, strained muscles and ligaments. They may also be used in first aid for treating wounds and drawing out pus.

1   Take some fresh herbs and chop finely – or use dried herbs. Mix to a pulp or paste with a little hot water.
2   Put the herbal paste on some clean cotton gauze or thin cloth and fold it over to enclose the herbs.
3   Apply the hot poultice to the affected area and cover with some clingfilm and a towel to retain the heat and moisture.
4   Replace the poultice as and when required.

HERBAL INHALATIONS

You can use a herbal infusion (tea) for these (see opposite). Use them for treating respiratory and chest infections, stuffed-up nose, catarrh and sinusitis.

1   Make some hot heat with the appropriate herbs.
2   Pour the hot, steaming tea into a basin and place on a table.
3   Put a large towel over your head and lean forwards over the basin, so your face is enclosed within the towel.
4   Breathe deeply and slowly, inhaling the steam, for a few minutes to clear your head and nasal passages.

143

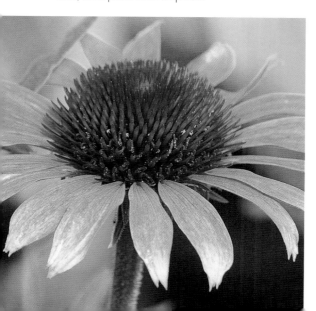

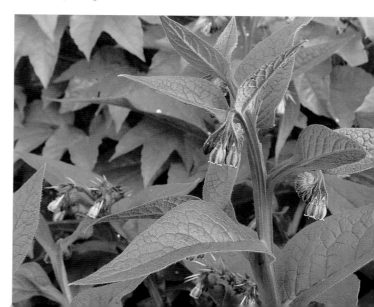

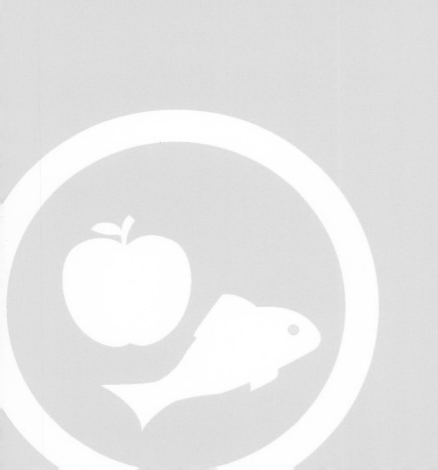

Immune system problems

The immune system is one of the defence mechanisms your body uses to protect it against micro-organisms that cause diseases. The key components of the system are the skin, mucus membranes, saliva, lymph nodes and vessels, spleen, adenoids, tonsils, thymus gland and white blood cells. These are all designed to either repel or prevent germs entering the body via the skin, mouth, nose and other openings, and to destroy any invasive viruses, bacteria, parasites and fungi that do cross these barriers.

To maintain optimum health and avoid infection or disease, you need to boost your natural immunity to germs and keep all these specialised defence mechanisms in efficient working order. In order to achieve this, your innate immunity and adaptive immunity must work together.

Your innate immune system consists of the key components (listed above) that you were born with. It attempts to repel invading disease-causing microbes and to fight any that breach its natural protective barriers. Your adaptive immunity is the one that you acquire from exposure throughout your life to different germs and diseases.

Signs of whether your immune system is functioning effectively include inflammation and swelling (blood flow to the infected area increases to fight the infection) and a raised temperature or swollen lymph nodes.

Eating a healthy diet that contains all the essential nutrients, taking regular exercise, getting enough sleep, managing stress, having good, supportive relationships with your family and friends, and avoiding exposure to toxic chemicals (in processed foods, cigarettes, alcohol, recreational drugs and environmental pollutants) can all help you to stay healthy, fight off infections and build a strong immune system.

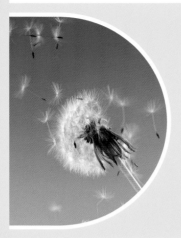

Allergies

An allergy is an adverse immune reaction to a substance or substances that are normally harmless. These substances are known as 'allergens'; they cause the immune system to over-react and produce a special type of antibody (IgE) to attack the invading material, while histamines are released which cause the symptoms of an allergic reaction. Common allergens include foods, pollens, spores, drugs, household chemicals, insects, animals and dust mites.

SYMPTOMS

Symptoms vary between sufferers, but some of the most common include the following:

▷ Sneezing and rhinitis (runny nose)
▷ Wheezing
▷ Excess catarrh
▷ Urticaria (hives)
▷ Coughing
▷ Swelling
▷ Itchy eyes, ears, lips, throat and palate (roof of mouth)
▷ Shortness of breath
▷ Sickness, vomiting and diarrhoea

PREVENTION

There is little that can be done to prevent allergies, apart from avoiding the allergens in question. The cause of allergies is unclear; however, they have been linked to overuse of antibiotics and other drugs, low intake of fruit and vegetables, and an imbalance in the bacteria in the gut, so taking steps to address these issues may help. There is also some evidence to suggest that breastfeeding can reduce allergies in susceptible children.

CONVENTIONAL REMEDIES

Allergies may be treated with antihistamines, nasal or topical steroids, and cromolyn sodium (which prevents the release of inflammatory chemicals). These can be used alone or in combination. Emergency treatment requires adrenaline, in the form of an injectible pen.

Did you know?

About 25 per cent of the UK population will suffer from an allergy at some point in their lives. Each year the numbers are increasing by five per cent, with as many as half of all those affected being children.

NATURAL REMEDIES

The traditional remedy is to take a little local honey in a cup of warm water with two tablespoons of apple cider vinegar to reduce the reaction to allergens. This is particularly useful during the hay fever season.

HERBAL REMEDIES Teas made from chamomile, elderflower, red clover and yarrow can reduce allergic reactions. Garlic has been traditionally used to boost immunity, either added to cooking or taken as capsules.

AROMATHERAPY Place a few drops of Roman chamomile in a vaporiser to treat an allergic reaction. Lavender oil, in a little light carrier oil, can be used in a gentle massage of the chest or the affected area to reduce spasm.

HEALING FOODS Foods that support your immune system include those that are high in vitamin C (fresh fruit and vegetables, in particular), zinc (eggs, nuts and seeds), vitamin A (fish and brightly coloured vegetables), and B vitamins (seafood, pulses, whole grains and nuts). You can take a vitamin C supplement (1000mg per day) to boost your body's defences.

 ## HOMEOPATHIC REMEDIES

Treatment will be undertaken on a constitutional basis (see page 202); however, the following remedies can address specific symptoms.

Urtica 30C will help with hives.

Pulsatilla 30C will help with thick catarrh and itching eyes.

Arsenicum 30C is for sneezing and itching eyes.

 ## SEE YOUR DOCTOR

Many allergies respond well to self-help and natural remedies but it is wise to see your doctor to get an accurate diagnosis. If you have a severe allergic reaction to any substance (anaphylactic shock), you must seek urgent medical advice. Symptoms can include swelling of the throat and mouth, difficulty swallowing or speaking, severe breathing difficulties, a drop in blood pressure and loss of consciousness.

Flower remedies

- During a sudden allergic reaction, offer Rescue Remedy or Emergency Essence.
- Beech is a basic essence for treating all allergies and conditions related to intolerance.
- Holly helps in cases of strong immune reactions, such as severe fits of sneezing, irritation or allergic shock.

Caution

Anaphylaxis (anaphylactic shock) is an extreme and severe allergic reaction. The whole body is affected, often within minutes of exposure to the allergen. This type of reaction is a medical emergency, and an ambulance must be called immediately.

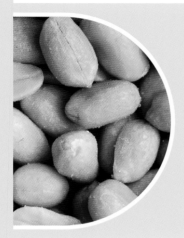

Food allergies

Food allergies occur when your immune system becomes confused, and instead of ignoring harmless food proteins that make their way into the bloodstream, it triggers a reaction that causes histamine to be released. This is the chemical that is responsible for such symptoms as hives, skin rashes and swelling. Anaphylaxis, or 'shock', is a severe, life-threatening reaction.

 SYMPTOMS

▷ A rash (particularly around the mouth)
▷ Tingling of the mouth and tongue
▷ Urticaria (hives)
▷ Swelling of lips or face
▷ Vomiting and diarrhoea
▷ Running nose
▷ Wheezing
▷ Eczema
▷ Tummy pain
▷ Headaches
▷ Breathing problems, pallor or loss of consciousness are anaphylactic reactions

 PREVENTION

The incidence of food allergies is increasing. The most common allergens (known as the 'big eight') are peanuts (and tree nuts), sesame seeds, soya, wheat, dairy produce, fish, shellfish and eggs. Exclusive breastfeeding for the first six months of a baby's life can reduce the incidence of food allergies significantly. Otherwise, avoiding the problem foods entirely is the best way to prevent attacks. There is some evidence that encouraging bowel health by eating a fibre-rich diet and taking probiotics can help to prevent allergies.

 CONVENTIONAL REMEDIES

Antihistamines are offered to deal with symptoms if an attack occurs or, in an emergency, adrenaline pens (EpiPens) can be used. Supplements may be prescribed to make up for shortfalls in your diet.

 ## Did you know?

Most serious food allergies begin in infancy or the preschool years, and are often outgrown. If you have a family history of food allergies or other allergic conditions, you are between 20 and 60 per cent more likely to suffer yourself.

NATURAL REMEDIES

There are many natural treatments that you can try, depending on your symptoms.

 HERBAL REMEDIES

- Horsetail tincture contains good levels of calcium, which is believed to be deficient in people who are suffering from food allergies.
- Stinging nettle (infusion or juice) can help reduce the allergic reaction, and supplement calcium.
- Agrimony tincture can ease bowel irritation and the recovery of damaged mucous membranes.
- To soothe gastric sensitivity and to heal mucous membranes, take goldenseal tincture three times a day in a little liquid.

 NUTRITIONAL MEDICINE

- Probiotics may be important in the control of food allergies because they improve digestion, helping the intestinal tract to control the absorption of food allergens; they also change the immune system response to food in the gut.
- A multivitamin and mineral tablet will ensure you get any nutrients that may be deficient; vitamins A, C and E are important for immune response.
- The nutrient quercitin (found in apples and onions) is rich in bioflavonoids and can reduce allergic reactions by reducing histamine release.
- Zinc is important for a healthy immune response. Take 35mg per day.
- Essential fatty acids (EFAs) have been shown to reduce inflammation and support the immune system. They are also responsible for general repair in the body, including the gut. Flaxseed oil, cold-water fish oils and borage oil can be taken in capsule form.

 HOMEOPATHIC REMEDIES

Constitutional treatment will be required to get to the root of the allergies, and also to encourage healing of the gut and a healthy immune response. Many sufferers will be offered bowel nosodes, to encourage bowel health.

Apis 30C can be used to treat hives.

Lycopodium 30C, for digestive complaints that follow eating suspect foods.

Aconite 30C can be taken at the first sign of an attack.

Arsenicum 30C is ideal for people who are highly sensitive to many foods, and respond by becoming ill, restless and exhausted, with breathing problems and digestive disorders.

 SEE YOUR DOCTOR

Breathing problems, pallor and loss of consciousness are anaphylactic reactions, and a medical emergency (see page 147). If you experience any of these, seek urgent medical help as they could be life-threatening.

Caution

Anaphylactic shock is a medical emergency and should be treated immediately. Do not delay. Call an ambulance.

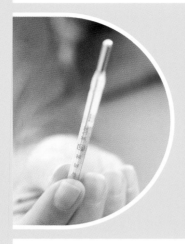

Fever

A fever is the body's reaction to an acute viral or bacterial infection. Raising the temperature helps to create an inhospitable environment for viral or bacterial invaders, and it also stimulates the production of disease-fighting white blood cells. Technically speaking, a fever is a body temperature above the normal of 37.0°C (98.6°F). In most cases, fevers are nothing to worry about unless they are accompanied by other symptoms.

 SYMPTOMS

▷ Chills
▷ Aching muscles
▷ Listlessness and fatigue
▷ Elevated body temperature
▷ Red cheeks
▷ Feeling hot and/or cold
▷ Shivering and shaking

 PREVENTION

A fever is actually a positive symptom, in that it provides evidence that your body is hard at work fighting off infection. There is nothing that can be done to prevent a fever, but you can keep yourself cool when it sets in, to prevent overheating.

 CONVENTIONAL REMEDIES

Paracetamol and aspirin are the two most common medications that are used to bring down a fever, with ibuprofen a close third. Note that children should not take aspirin as it can cause a rare condition known as Reye's syndrome.

 NATURAL REMEDIES

If you have a fever, you can try one of the following natural remedies.

FLOWER REMEDIES Rescue Remedy can be taken to ease any distress and calm you down. Chicory, Hornbeam and Cherry Plum are useful for all illnesses that may cause fever and, in particular, childhood illnesses.

HERBAL REMEDIES

- Yarrow and lime flowers are calming and cooling, and encourage sweating when you feel hot.
- Cinnamon, ginger and angelica can be used to produce heat when you are shivering.
- Hyssop, along with liquorice root and thyme, have traditionally been used to lower a high temperature.

AROMATHERAPY

- Tea tree encourages the body to sweat, while also helping to encourage the immune system to fight off invaders, such as bacteria and viruses.
- Lavender and peppermint are cooling oils, and help to soothe and bring down your temperature.
- Try sage, pine, rosemary and eucalyptus in a vaporiser in your room to support your immune system and open the airways.

HOMEOPATHIC REMEDIES

There are a number of homeopathic remedies that will be useful, according to the symptoms.

Belladonna 30C, for fever with a red, hot face and staring eyes.

Phytolacca 30C helps when there are painful ears and swollen glands, better on taking cool drinks.

Aconite 30C is ideal for a fever that comes on suddenly.

Ferrum phos 30C, for fever with a slow onset.

Gelsemium 30C can help when you feel drowsy and chilly, with aching limbs.

Merc sol 30C is suggested where there is yellow discharge with a fever.

SEE YOUR DOCTOR

If the fever lasts longer than a few days or your temperature is over 40°C (104°F), you should see your doctor to ascertain and treat the cause. Feverish babies under three months should always be seen by a doctor immediately; over three months, wait for 24 hours to see if it resolves.

Self-help

- Always drink plenty of fluids to prevent becoming dehydrated. Babies, in particular, can dehydrate quite quickly.
- Avoid eating heavy meals, which will divert the energy required for healing to your digestive system; instead, eat little and often. Fresh fruit and vegetable juices or vegetable soups contain immune-boosting vitamin C.
- Don't take fever-reducing medication for fevers under 38.9°C (102°F), unless suggested by your doctor. It's usually best to let your fever run its course, so your body can do the job of fighting infection.

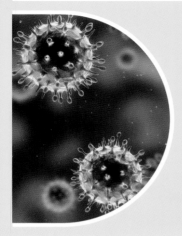

Influenza

Influenza is a viral disease of the upper respiratory tract, which is spread by the contaminated droplets other sufferers emit when they cough or sneeze. There are a number of different types of flu, some of which confer immunity once you overcome them, and others that mutate constantly, so your body cannot build up resistance.

 ## SYMPTOMS

▷ A high fever, possibly accompanied by shivering
▷ A sore throat
▷ Possibly a cough
▷ A running nose and sneezing
▷ Breathlessness
▷ Weakness
▷ Headache
▷ Stiff or aching joints and muscular pains
▷ Nausea and loss of appetite

 ## PREVENTION

• Always wash your hands after touching surfaces that others have touched, such as handrails on public transport.
• Anti-flu vaccines may work in the short-term for virulent, current strains, but, because the viruses constantly change, so too will the vaccines used against them.
• Boost your immune system by adopting a healthy diet and lifestyle.

 ## CONVENTIONAL REMEDIES

Conventional treatments for influenza consist of symptom-reducing drugs, such as paracetamol, cough suppressants, decongestants, pain-relievers and occasionally antihistamines. Antibiotics should never be offered for flu, as they have no effect on viruses. In severe cases, antiviral medication may be offered.

NATURAL REMEDIES

Barley water is the traditional natural remedy for relieving high fever – particularly when the cause of the fever is infection and inflammation. It also works to increase levels of immune-boosting B vitamins, and to keep you hydrated.

SELF-HELP Get plenty of rest, and aim to stay in bed for at least 48 hours. Don't push yourself; give your body time to fight off the infection and recover. Drink plenty of fluids, including vitamin C-rich fresh fruit and vegetable juices.

 HERBAL REMEDIES

- Fenugreek seeds crushed in a lemon and honey hot drink will help to bring down fever and soothe aching limbs.
- Echinacea is an immune stimulant that appears to activate your infection-fighting capacity when taken at the onset of a cold or flu; you can take it in tincture form.
- Ginger contains almost a dozen antiviral compounds; it helps to reduce pain and fever, suppresses coughing, and it has a mildly sedative effect to encourage rest. Grate some fresh root ginger into a hot honey and lemon drink, or look for tincture or tablet forms.

Flower remedies

- Crab Apple promotes purification of your blood, and helps you get strong enough to fight off infection.
- Olive is for overwhelming fatigue.
- Walnut can help to strengthen your immune system against invaders.
- Rescue Remedy or Emergency Essence can both help to soothe and calm you, promoting restful, restorative sleep.

 AROMATHERAPY

- Use a eucalyptus or peppermint essential oil inhalation to unblock sinuses and your chest.
- Add one to two drops of tea tree and geranium oils to a few tablespoons of a light carrier oil, and massage into your chest and head, to reduce symptoms and fight infection.
- Oils that act to bring down fever include chamomile, melissa and tea tree.

 HOMEOPATHIC REMEDIES

Choose remedies according to your symptoms.

Gelsemium 30C, when muscular weakness, aching and heaviness are the most predominant symptoms.

Rhus tox 30C, when there is aching in the joints rather than the muscles, and if you are restless and can't find a comfortable position.

Bryonia 30C, for a bad headache, and dry cough; if you feel intensely irritable and just want to lie still.

Eupatorium perfoliatum 30C, for very intense aching in the back and limbs with shivering chills.

Belladonna 30C, for a high fever, with red cheeks and staring eyes.

SEE YOUR DOCTOR

Most cases of flu get better of their own accord without medical intervention. However, if you suffer from asthma, chronic bronchitis or heart disease, have difficulty breathing or a cough that gets persistently worse you should see your doctor. Secondary chest infections and pneumonia can be complications.

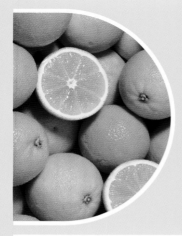

Glandular fever

Glandular fever is caused by the Epstein-Barr virus (a herpes virus), which multiplies in the white blood cells, harming the immune system's efficiency. Glandular fever is usually transmitted via saliva, hence its nickname of the 'kissing disease'. While symptoms may last for only six weeks, recovery is slow, and fatigue and low energy levels may linger for months. Most adults have been exposed to this virus by the age of 18 years and are immune.

SYMPTOMS

▷ Fever
▷ Fatigue
▷ Enlarged lymph nodes in the neck
▷ Inflamed throat and tonsils
▷ Little energy
▷ Sometimes a mild rash of small, slightly raised red spots

PREVENTION

Taking steps to boost your immune system will make it more likely that you will resist the infection and develop antibodies instead. However, there is nothing that can be done to prevent glandular fever apart from avoiding close contact with sufferers.

CONVENTIONAL REMEDIES

Almost all cases resolve within about four to six weeks without any drug treatment. Bed rest and plenty of fluid are normally suggested. In rare cases, corticosteroid drugs are required to reduce severe inflammation, particularly if your tonsils are swollen.

NATURAL REMEDIES

There are numerous natural remedies that may help to alleviate the symptoms and aid recovery.
FLOWER REMEDIES Olive will be helpful if you feel exhausted on all levels. Mustard is ideal for any depression, and Gorse will help with feelings of hopelessness.

HERBAL REMEDIES

- Herbs to promote healing include cleavers, echinacea and nettles, all of which stimulate immune activity as well as fighting infection.
- Infusions of yarrow and elderflower will help to control fever, and induce sweating.
- Liquorice supports the adrenal glands, which are under pressure in this illness, and also has some antibacterial and antiviral properties, which can help to prevent secondary infections.
- Tonic herbs, such as astragalus and ginseng, may help your recovery.

AROMATHERAPY

- Eucalyptus, lavender, rosemary and tea tree oils encourage the immune activity and fight the virus.
- Black pepper oil stimulates the spleen, which is involved in the production of new blood cells.
- Thyme oil is a powerful stimulant and is widely used to combat fatigue and lethargy. It can also stimulate a sluggish appetite.

HOMEOPATHIC REMEDIES

Constitutional homeopathic treatment is recommended, but the following remedies may be useful, taken up to six times daily, for two days.

Belladonna 30C, for sudden high fever, with red face and agitation.

Mercurius 30C, for tender glands and smelly sweat.

Calcarea 30C, for chilliness, sweating, a sour taste and fatigue.

Cistus 30C, for chilly feeling, with painful neck and glands, exacerbated by cold air and mental exertion.

Baryta carb 30C, for swollen glands – this remedy is particularly useful for children.

 ## NUTRITIONAL MEDICINE

EVENING PRIMROSE OIL has a beneficial effect on the immune system and encourages healing.

ROYAL JELLY will help fight feelings of fatigue and depression, and stimulate the immune system.

MAGNESIUM deficiency is common in many cases of glandular fever, and can be the result of a stressful lifestyle that caused you to become rundown. Take 300mg per day.

VITAMIN C stimulates the production of the white blood cells that produce antibodies against glandular fever. It is also an anti-inflammatory that helps to relieve a sore throat and aching muscles. Take 1000mg daily, or eat citrus fruit and plenty of green vegetables.

ZINC stops the Epstein Barr virus from replicating and entering your cells, and is also a powerful anti-inflammatory. Take 40mg daily.

 ## SEE YOUR DOCTOR

If you suspect that you may have glandular fever, see your doctor. A blood test will confirm whether you have the disease.

Caution

Glandular fever represents a relatively profound attack on the immune system, and you will need to work on building it back up again, probably for several months.

155

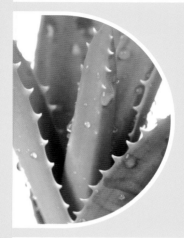

Chickenpox

Chickenpox is a very contagious viral infection, caused by the herpes-zoster virus, and it appears most commonly in childhood. It is characterised by spots, which fill with fluid to become little blisters. Eventually the spots dry up and form scabs, which may cause scars. The spots are very itchy, but scratching should be discouraged to prevent any infection. The incubation period is from 10 to 14 days, and sufferers are contagious from just before the spots appear.

 SYMPTOMS

▷ Headache
▷ Fever
▷ General malaise
▷ Spots, usually starting on the trunk and spreading to most parts of the body, including the mouth, anus, vagina and ears

 CONVENTIONAL REMEDIES

Your doctor may suggest calamine lotion to ease the itching, and paracetamol or ibuprofen to relieve symptoms and reduce the body temperature. In most cases, children will recover within about 10 days. In severe cases, antiviral medication may be offered. There is a vaccine against chickenpox but its use is questionable because it is normally a mild illness.

 NATURAL REMEDIES

There are many traditional remedies for chickenpox. For example, a witch hazel compress can be applied directly to the spots, or a little added to your bath, to ease discomfort. You can also add bicarbonate of soda to a bath to ease itching. Tie a handful of oatmeal in a muslin cloth or an old stocking, and hang it under the running tap when you fill the bath. Not only will this soothe the itching, but it will also encourage healing of the skin. Try dabbing some Vitamin E oil on the spots when they begin to dry up, to help prevent scarring.

 ## Did you know?

One bout of chickenpox normally gives lifetime immunity against the illness, but the virus that causes chickenpox (varicella-zoster) can lie dormant for years, then resurface as shingles (see page 158) in adults.

HERBAL REMEDIES

- Infusions of nettle are ideal for treating chickenpox as nettle is a strengthening herb that will help to heal the skin.
- Aloe vera gel, dabbed on the spots, can cool and help to promote healing.
- Calendula cream can be applied to the spots to soothe and encourage healing, as well as to prevent scarring. A handful of calendula flowers can also be added to a bath.
- Echinacea can help to support the immune system and reduce the duration of the illness.

 AROMATHERAPY

- A few drops of Roman chamomile can be used in the bath to soothe.
- Essential oil of lavender can be dabbed directly on spots to ease the itching and to encourage healing. Lavender also has an antibacterial action, which will help prevent a secondary infection.

 HOMEOPATHIC REMEDIES

Homeopathic remedies can be effective. Try the following, depending on the symptoms presented.

Variolinum 30C can be taken once in cases where there is an epidemic of chickenpox, before your child acquires the illness, and symptoms should be less severe.

Rhus tox 30C can be taken for a few days after contact with an infected child, and then again as soon as the first spots appear.

Aconite 30C is useful in the early stages of the illness.

Belladonna 30C is useful for fever.

 SEE YOUR DOCTOR

When fever lasts for more than a couple of days, or there is an obvious chest infection accompanying the rash, see your doctor. Very rarely, chickenpox pneumonia can occur as a secondary infection.

157

Flower remedies

- Chicory, Hornbeam and Cherry Plum can help relieve some of the discomfort.
- Impatiens can ease irritability.
- Crab Apple may be diluted and applied directly to the spots to encourage healing.
- Olive is useful for convalescence.

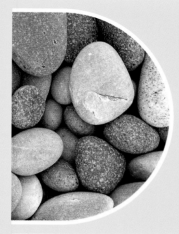

Shingles

Shingles is an extremely painful disease caused by the herpes zoster virus (also the chickenpox virus). Following an attack of chickenpox the virus remains dormant in the body. Many years later, a drop in the efficiency of the immune system may cause reactivation of the virus – this time in the form of shingles, causing acute inflammation in the ganglia (a mass of nerve cells) near the spinal cord.

 SYMPTOMS

▷ The first sign of shingles is sensitivity in the affected area, then pain
▷ Pain can be itching, tingling, throbbing, aching or stabbing
▷ There may be fever and nausea
▷ A rash of small blisters develops on the fourth or fifth day, usually on one side of the body and in a linear pattern
▷ These turn yellow within a few days, form scabs, then drop off, sometimes leaving scars.
▷ In some cases there may be persistent pain for months or years (post-herpetic pain)

 PREVENTION

Shingles tends to strike when you are run down, so ensure that you get plenty of rest, eat well, take some exercise and reduce your stress levels.

• Avoid direct contact with anyone else who has shingles.
• Boost your immune system by increasing your intake of vitamins and minerals (in particular, vitamins A, B and C, and the mineral zinc).
• Take a course of probiotics, the healthy digestive bacteria that can help to ward off infection.

 CONVENTIONAL REMEDIES

Antiviral drugs, such as acyclovir, are offered to reduce the severity of the active stage. Analgesic drugs, including capsaicin creams, may be offered if the pain is severe. If you develop, or are at an increased risk of, post-herpetic neuralgia, you may be prescribed medication, such as amitriptyline, which is usually used as an antidepressant but also acts on your nerves and can help to control pain.

 Did you know?

Shingles can be passed on by direct contact with fluid from the blisters, until they eventually dry up and crust over. This can also cause chickenpox in people who haven't had it before, but shingles isn't triggered by contact with someone who has chickenpox.

NATURAL REMEDIES

You can try some of the following natural remedies for treating shingles.

HERBAL REMEDIES Oats, St John's wort and vervain have a direct impact on the health of your nerves. Make an infusion of any of these and sip throughout the day. Ginseng encourages overall health and restores nervous stability, as well as combatting the effects of stress.

AROMATHERAPY Chamomile, eucalyptus, melissa, lavender and tea tree are all useful antiviral oils, which can be used in the bath, in a massage, or applied as a compress. Lavender, applied neat to painful areas, can soothe and encourage healing.

 # HOMEOPATHIC REMEDIES

The following remedies can be taken once every two hours for up to 10 doses.

Arsenicum 30C, for burning pains worse between midnight and 2 am, with skin eruptions and a restless, chilly and anxious state.

Lachesis 30C, when the left-hand side of the body is affected with swelling.

Rhus tox 30C, for red, blistered and itching skin – better for movement and warmth.

Fanunculus 30C, for nerve pains and itching, which are worse for movement and eating.

 # NUTRITIONAL MEDICINE

- Eat plenty of vitamin B-rich foods, such as whole-grain cereals, nuts, seeds and yeast extract, which aid the nervous system.
- High-dose vitamin C supplementation has been shown to reduce pain as well as help to dry up and heal the blisters. Take the highest dose you can without triggering diarrhoea, starting with 1000mg per day.
- Supplementation with Vitamin E is now known to reduce the long-term symptoms associated with shingles. Take 600iu per day, broken into three doses, with food. Vitamin E oil, applied directly to the sores, will encourage healing.

 # SEE YOUR DOCTOR

Shingles is very painful and it can cause serious complications and permanent damage if it affects your eyes. Always see your doctor for an accurate diagnosis, medical advice and treatment.

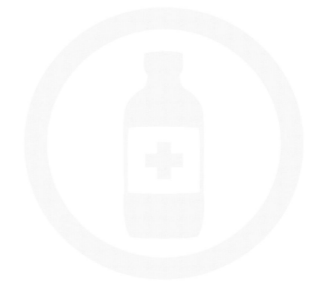

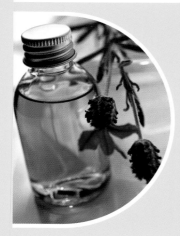

German measles

German measles (rubella) is a viral infection characterised by a mild rash and swollen lymph glands (usually in the back of the neck or behind the ears), and is most common in children. The incubation period is 14 to 21 days, and the disease can be spread from seven days before the rash appears, although it is most contagious once the rash is present. The condition only lasts three to five days.

 SYMPTOMS

▷ Mild fever
▷ Swollen, tender lymph nodes
▷ An itchy rash that appears first on the face and spreads downwards – usually beginning with pinprick pink or pale red dots that join together to form evenly coloured patches
▷ Headaches
▷ Loss of appetite
▷ Mild conjunctivitis
▷ A runny nose
▷ A sore throat

 PREVENTION

The main line of defence is the rubella vaccine, which is normally given to children at 12 to 15 months as part of the MMR vaccine. A second dose is offered between the ages of four and six years of age. Apart from this, it's difficult not to acquire this very contagious disease once you have been in contact with a sufferer, although cases are less common since immunisation against the disease began.

 CONVENTIONAL REMEDIES

Your doctor may suggest paracetamol to bring down any fever and reduce discomfort. Don't give aspirin to children, as it can cause a rare condition called Reye's syndrome. Creams and ointments can be prescribed if the rash is very itchy; these include calamine lotion and mild steroid preparations.

NATURAL REMEDIES

The following natural treatments may help to ease the symptoms of German measles.

AROMATHERAPY A few drops of lavender oil on the bedclothes, or on a hanky near the bed, eases symptoms and is very calming. For a build-up of phlegm, a few drops of tea tree or eucalyptus oil in a vaporiser will encourage easier breathing.

FLOWER REMEDIES Rescue Remedy will ease distress, and help to calm. Chicory, Hornbeam and Cherry Plum are indicated for childhood illnesses.

NUTRITIONAL MEDICINE Eat plenty of raw fruits and vegetables to cleanse the system. Increase your intake of foods containing vitamin C and zinc, to aid the action of the immune system. Acidophilus should be taken during and after any illness, to encourage the growth of healthy bacteria in the gut.

 HERBAL REMEDIES

- Hot yarrow tea, cooled and drunk several times daily, will relieve symptoms.
- An infusion of elderflower combined with peppermint will help to cool a fever and calm you – and your child.
- Very high fever can be treated with an infusion of catmint, taken as required.

Self-help

Frequent, tepid baths will relieve any itchiness and bring down a fever. Add some Epsom salts or bicarbonate of soda to the water.

 HOMEOPATHIC REMEDIES

Homeopathic remedies are useful in all cases of rubella. Choose the appropriate one for you.

Pulsatilla 30C, when there is thick yellow discharge from the nose and hot, red eyes.

Belladonna 30C, for fever, a bright red rash and hot face.

Phytolacca 30C, for painful ears and swollen glands, better on taking cool drinks.

Aconite 30C if there is a high fever and not too much mucus.

Merc sol 30C where there is yellow discharge from the nose and a fever.

 SEE YOUR DOCTOR

Rubella is a 'notifiable disease', so you should contact your doctor if you suspect it. The symptoms in small children may be mild, but if a pregnant woman comes into contact with the condition, there is a serious risk of miscarriage and birth defects.

Caution

If you are pregnant and are unsure of your immune status, ask your doctor.

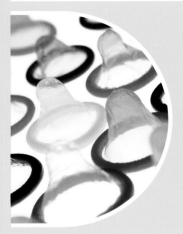

Herpes simplex

Herpes simplex (HSV) is a virus of which there are two main strains. Oral herpes (HSV-1) causes cold sores around the lips or nose; genital herpes (HSV-2) affects the genitals, buttocks or anal area. HSV-2 is usually, but not always, sexually transmitted. HSV-1 is transmitted by contact with infected saliva, and it is possible to carry the virus without experiencing any symptoms whatsoever.

 ## SYMPTOMS

▷ Blisters or ulcers, usually on the mouth, lips, gums or genitals
▷ Enlarged lymph nodes in the neck or groin area (although usually only at the time of the initial infection)
▷ Fever (during the first episode)
▷ Fever blisters
▷ Genital lesions, which burn or tingle
▷ Mouth ulcers

 ## PREVENTION

Once you have the herpes-simplex virus, you will carry it for life, but you can prevent attacks by:

- Eating a healthy diet, with plenty of fresh fruit (especially citrus fruit which are rich in vitamin C and bioflavonoids) and vegetables, whole-grain cereals and good-quality proteins to boost your immune system
- Not kissing anyone who has a cold sore or sharing towels and face cloths with them
- Applying sunblock to lips to protect them from sunshine and cold winds
- Using a condom to reduce the risk of catching or spreading herpes.

 ## CONVENTIONAL REMEDIES

Some cases are mild and may not need treatment. If cold sores are particularly troublesome, your doctor may prescribe idoxuridine paint or the antiviral drug acyclovir (in tablet or cream form), or another antiviral agent. Genital herpes can be treated with antiviral medication, such as famciclovir, acyclovir and valacyclovir. Topical antibiotic ointments also may be applied to prevent secondary bacterial infections.

 ## Did you know?

Most people with genital herpes have five to eight outbreaks per year, but not everyone has recurrent symptoms; over time, the number of outbreaks usually decreases. Oral herpes can recur monthly or only once or twice a year. You may be able to anticipate an outbreak if you notice a tingling sensation, (a prodrome).

NATURAL REMEDIES

At the first sign of cold sores appearing round the mouth, rub the area with a cut slice of lemon. To relieve blisters and other symptoms, try the following.

AROMATHERAPY Bergamot, eucalyptus and tea tree oils will help to treat the blisters, and should be applied at the first sign of a sore. Lavender oil will help to heal blisters as they begin to erupt, and can be used until they heal.

 HOMEOPATHIC REMEDIES

Homeopathy can prevent recurring cold sores, but constitutional treatment will be required. The following remedies may help, depending on the symptoms.

HSV-1

Natrum mur 30C, for deep cracks in the lower lip, dry mouth and puffy burning sores.

Rhus tox 30C, for mouth and chin sores, and ulcers at the corner of the mouth.

Sempervivum 30C, for ulcers in the mouth, and bleeding gums; worse at night.

Capsicum 30C, for cracks at the corners of the mouth, pale lips, rash on chin, blisters on tongue and bad breath.

HSV-2

Vaccinotoxinum 30C, taken when the infection shows its first signs

Apis mel 30C, which will prevent the blisters from appearing (stop if blisters do appear).

Rhus tox 30C, when you feel a stinging sensation.

Arsenicum 30C, for small blisters that burn.

 HERBAL REMEDIES

- St John's wort tincture applied at the first sign of tingling should stop a cold sore from appearing.
- Apply calendula tincture or ointment to blisters to ease pain.
- Echinacea or goldenseal can help to combat the infection and boost your immune system.
- Lemon balm tea can be effective, as it has considerable antiviral activity against herpes simplex.

 SEE YOUR DOCTOR

If you suffer from recurrent attacks of cold sores around your mouth or nose, you should see your doctor. If you experience any of the other symptoms that are listed opposite, especially in the genital area, make an urgent appointment. You may need a course of antiviral drugs.

Caution

The virus can be dangerous in newborn babies, or in people with a weakened immune system. HSV is believed to be more contagious when blisters are present, but it can be transmitted without active lesions.

Eat your way to health

The saying 'You are what you eat' is very true – eating too much of the wrong foods can play a significant role in a variety of health conditions. If you are keen to eat more healthily, then here are the five main nutritional components that make up a healthy, well-balanced diet.

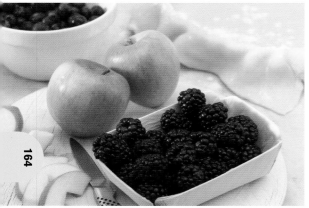

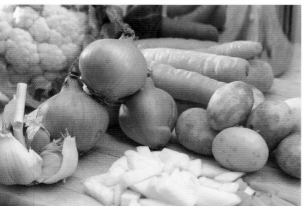

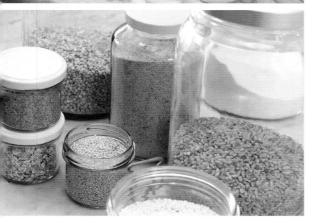

FRUITS AND VEGETABLES

Fruits and vegetables are an important source of many essential vitamins and minerals. Ideally, you should aim to eat at least five portions of fruits and vegetables each day.

These five portions are easily achieved, especially if you spread them out throughout the day. One portion is equivalent to one apple, one banana, three heaped tablespoons of vegetables or a slice of melon. As well as fresh fruit and vegetables, you can include dried, canned or frozen options, plus one glass of fruit or vegetable juice.

STARCHY FOODS

About one-third of your daily diet should be made up of starchy foods (carbohydrates), such as bread, potatoes, pasta and cereals. They are a good source of essential nutrients, plus they provide you with energy and 'fuel' for your body.

Wholemeal bread and whole-grain cereals, such as brown ice or wholewheat pasta, contain more fibre than their white counterparts, so, ideally, you should eat them regularly.

SUGAR AND FAT

Although your body needs some fat, foods containing sugar and fat should be eaten in limited quantities. Where possible, opt for low-fat or reduced-sugar foods, and choose fats that are rich in monounsaturated fatty acids, such as olive oil, rather than saturated ones like butter.

MEAT, EGGS, FISH AND PULSES

The third important food group to include in your healthy diet is protein, which comes in the form of meat, fish, eggs or pulses. Meat is packed full of vitamins and minerals, including iron and zinc, and it's a good source of vitamin B12. Fish has lots of vitamins and minerals, too, and oily fish, such as fresh salmon, tuna, kippers, sardines, herring or mackerel, is particularly good for your health. Aim to eat three to five servings of protein daily. For ultimate health, avoid fatty cuts of meat and opt for lean varieties instead or trim the fat off before you cook it (and remove the skin from chicken). Ideally, include two portions of fish in your diet each week, one of which should be an oily fish.

Note For vegetarians and other non-meat eaters, good sources of protein include eggs, tofu, pulses and beans.

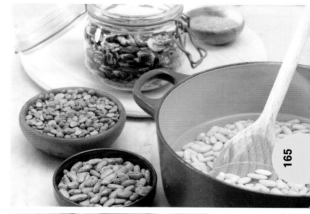

DAIRY PRODUCTS AND MILK

Dairy products and milk are important nutritional elements and are good sources of protein and calcium, which is good for your bones. Aim to have 600ml (1 pint) skimmed or semi-skimmed milk each day – drinking six to eight cups of tea or coffee with milk in is equivalent to at least one-third of this. Eating a small pot of yoghurt or a matchbox-sized piece of cheese provides you with the same amount of calcium as 200ml (⅓ pint) milk.

Note Many cheeses and yoghurts are high in fat, so opt for lower-fat, healthier versions instead.

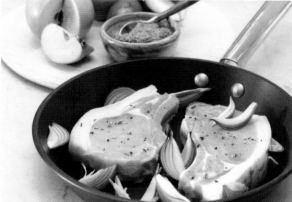

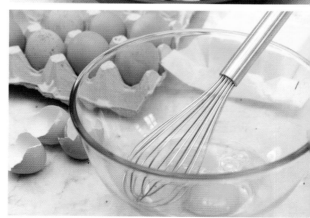

165

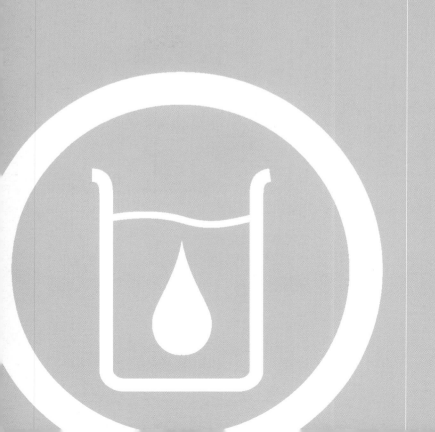

Digestive problems

In the digestive tract, which extends from the mouth to the anus, food is digested and processed, and waste products are eliminated. The nutrients in the food you eat (protein, fats, carbohydrates, vitamins and minerals) are absorbed into the bloodstream and carried around the body to the cells.

Digestion begins when you start chewing the food in your mouth. It passes down the oesophagus into your stomach, where it is churned and partially digested with gastric juices to a semi-liquid consistency. It passes into the small intestine where the nutrients are broken down into molecules and pass into the blood vessels and lymphatic system. The undigested residues enter the large intestine, where water and minerals are absorbed back into the body and the liquid digestive products are turned into semi-solid waste. The waste (faeces) passes into the rectum for storage and is subsequently expelled through the anus.

It is a complicated process and a variety of digestive problems can occur, ranging from relatively harmless ones like indigestion and constipation to far more serious conditions, such as inflammatory bowel disease. The system has its own built-in defence mechanisms, however, and can react rapidly against irritants, such as contaminated food (food poisoning or gastroenteritis) or alcohol, through vomiting and/or diarrhoea.

To stay fit and healthy, you need to look after your digestive system, which means eating plenty of fibre-rich whole-grain cereals, fruit and vegetables to provide the bulk to carry away body waste and keep stools soft. Good personal hygiene, eating regular meals and a variety of nutritious foods will all help to prevent many common digestive problems.

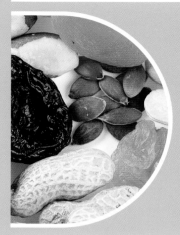

Constipation

Most doctors define constipation as having a bowel movement less than twice a week, although some say that a movement every four or five days is adequate. However, constipation is not so much about regularity as stools. Do you have to strain to pass stools more than a quarter of the time? Do you feel a sense of incomplete emptying after a bowel movement? And, most importantly, are your stools hard? If so, you are likely to be suffering from constipation.

 ## SYMPTOMS

▷ Straining on the toilet
▷ Wind
▷ Bloating
▷ Stomach/abdominal pain and cramps
▷ Lethargy
▷ Headaches

 ## PREVENTION

- The single most effective way to prevent constipation is to ensure that your diet is rich in fibre; this means eating plenty of fresh fruit and vegetables, whole-grain cereals, and fewer refined convenience foods.
- Also important is water to bulk up the fibre and encourage healthy evacuation – drink at least six large glasses a day.
- Some foods, particularly milk and milk products, tend to delay things in the large intestine, causing constipation. Try abstaining from dairy produce for two weeks to see if it makes any difference.
- Regular exercise will help to stimulate bowel movements.

 ## CONVENTIONAL REMEDIES

You can buy over-the-counter laxatives in your local pharmacy. Apart from adopting a high-fibre, high-fluid regime, laxatives and suppositories are the usual conventional treatments for constipation. Natural or vegetable laxatives are available.

NATURAL REMEDIES

Treatment is generally based on the cause of your constipation, but the follow natural remedies should be useful for treating symptoms.

HERBAL REMEDIES Laxative herbs can be drunk as herbal infusions up to three times daily; these include liquorice, marshmallow root and senna. Aloe vera is also quite a powerful laxative. Take just one teaspoon of gel a day, or drink a small glass of aloe vera juice three times daily.

 AROMATHERAPY

- Massage a drop of marjoram or fennel oil, which has been diluted in grapeseed oil, into the abdomen, to relieve constipation.
- Rosemary and mandarin (as well as any other citrus oils) stimulate peristalsis, which is the rhythmic movement along the digestive tract. Use in a warm abdominal massage, or add five drops of each to your evening bath.

 NUTRITIONAL MEDICINE

- Acidophilus supplements will encourage the health of the intestines, and make bowel movements more normal.
- Eat dried apricots and figs as snacks, and add seeds and bulking agents, such as bran and psyllium husks, to your breakfast cereal.
- Prunes are a classic laxative remedy; soak them overnight and eat them for breakfast with a little probiotic yoghurt.

 HOMEOPATHIC REMEDIES

In homeopathy, constipation is regarded as a constitutional problem, but the following remedies can help with occasional symptoms.

Lycopodium 30C, when there is flatulence but no need to open bowels for long periods of time. Hard stools, passed with pain.

Nux vomica 30C, for constipation that alternates with diarrhoea.

Opium 30C, when there is no desire to pass a stool.

Silicea 30C, when there is a burning sensation after a bowel movement.

Causticum 30C, for a stitch-like pain accompanying a bowel movement.

Bryonia 30C, for large, hard, dry stools, with congestion in the abdomen causing distension, and a burning feeling in the rectum.

Alumina 30C, for no desire to open the bowels until the rectum is full; stool may be covered in mucus.

 SEE YOUR DOCTOR

If laxatives are not having any effect, or you are suffering from abdominal pain, weight loss, blood in your stools or pencil-thin bowel movements, you should see your doctor to ensure that there is not an obstruction or another problem. There are many possible causes of constipation, some of which are minor and others that are more serious. Always consult your doctor immediately if a child under three is constipated.

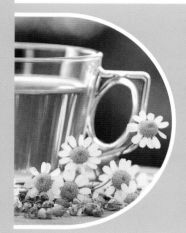

Diarrhoea

Diarrhoea, defined as the profuse evacuation of watery stools at least three times a day, may be accompanied by vomiting and abdominal pain and is usually due to a viral or bacterial infection, parasites, or toxins in the bowel, when it is known as gastroenteritis. It can also be caused by a long-term condition, such as IBS or Crohn's Disease (see pages 178–181), and may be an indication of food allergy (see pages 148–149).

 ## SYMPTOMS

▷ Urgent need to have a bowel movement
▷ Liquid stool, at least three times per day
▷ Sometimes cramping or abdominal pain
▷ Sometimes nausea and/or vomiting
▷ May be loss of appetite

 ## PREVENTION

Basic personal hygiene can help to prevent diarrhoea.

- Pay close attention to hand-washing, especially after going to the lavatory, touching pets and gardening.
- Always make sure that you wash your hands with soap and water before and after touching food, especially raw meat or poultry.
- Good food hygiene and refrigeration of food can also help to prevent diarrhoea.

 ## CONVENTIONAL REMEDIES

Medical advice is usually to eat more carbohydrates and to take plenty of fluids for 24 to 48 hours. Anti-diarrhoeal drugs, such as loperamide, can relieve symptoms by slowing down the movement of bowel contents, and sometimes by increasing water absorption from the gut. An electrolyte mixture (rehydration fluid) may be suggested if there is any dehydration.

NATURAL REMEDIES

Natural treatments will address the symptoms, and encourage normal, healthy bowel movements.

AROMATHERAPY Massage your abdomen with a few drops of antiseptic and relaxing oils, such as chamomile, lavender and neroli, to ease diarrhoea; this is particularly helpful if diarrhoea is linked to anxiety. If an infection is suspected, use eucalyptus or tea tree oil instead. Fennel and ginger oils (one drop of each) can be added to a warmed carrier oil, such as grapeseed, to deal with any abdominal pain or cramping.

HERBAL REMEDIES

- Peppermint and blackberry leaf tea act as astringents to the gut, and can help to ease the condition.
- An infusion of meadowsweet provides a gentle treatment for diarrhoea as it tones the lining of the small intestine.
- Chamomile, drunk as an infusion, may reduce intestinal cramping and ease the irritation and inflammation associated with diarrhoea.
- Calendula ointment can be applied to a sore bottom to soothe and heal.

Good kitchen hygiene

To minimise the risk of diarrhoea and food poisoning, always:

- Use separate chopping boards for raw meat, poultry, fish and vegetables
- Cover raw meat and poultry and keep them separate from other foods in the fridge
- Wash knives and kitchen utensils carefully
- Always wash your hands with soap and warm water after handling food, especially raw meat and poultry.

 ## NUTRITIONAL MEDICINE

- Taking a probiotic, such as acidophilus, during and after an attack can help to build up healthy bacteria in your gut.
- Increasing your fibre intake during an attack of non-infectious diarrhoea is now known to alleviate diarrhoea by making stools more solid. Try taking psyllium seed, or eating whole-grain cereals.
- Avoid dairy products for the duration of the attack, as they promote mucus in the gut, which can allow pathogens to proliferate.
- Eat plenty of apples, which contain the soluble fibre pectin, which helps to bulk out stools, and also heal the gut.

 ## HOMEOPATHIC REMEDIES

Chronic diarrhoea should be treated constitutionally, but acute attacks may be treated with one of the following remedies.

Aconite 30C, for diarrhoea that comes on suddenly, with a distended abdomen

Pulsatilla 30C, for diarrhoea that is worse at night, and made worse by rich foods.

Colocynth 30C, for diarrhoea accompanied by griping pains, with yellowish, thin and copious stools.

Argentum nit 30C, for diarrhoea caused by anxiety, characterised by belching and cravings for sweet and salty food.

 ## SEE YOUR DOCTOR

Call your doctor urgently if a baby or child with diarrhoea shows symptoms of dehydration, including a sunken fontanelle (the soft spot on top of the head), unresponsiveness, drowsiness, prolonged crying, glazed eyes or a very dry mouth. For adults, if diarrhoea contains blood, lasts longer than five days or occurs after foreign travel, see your doctor.

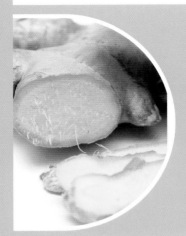

Nausea & vomiting

Nausea and vomiting can be symptoms of gastroenteritis, inner-ear infection, pregnancy, motion sickness, food poisoning, migraine, over-eating (especially the wrong kinds of foods), heat exhaustion, and medication, as well as many other health problems. A constant feeling of nausea with no vomiting but with a headache and abdominal pain may also be stress- or anxiety-related.

 ## SYMPTOMS

Nausea and vomiting are symptoms rather than ailments in their own right, but they are characterised by the following:

▷ Feelings of sickness
▷ Sometimes dizziness
▷ Emptying of stomach contents
▷ Retching

 ## PREVENTION

Careful hygiene (hand washing after dealing with pets, going to the lavatory or preparing food) is important, and avoiding towel-sharing can also help to prevent infections from being passed on. In reality, however, the cause of the nausea and vomiting must be addressed to prevent them occurring.

 ## CONVENTIONAL REMEDIES

A fluid-only diet is usually recommended for 24 hours, with fluid replacement solutions offered in the event of dehydration. A variety of anti-nausea medications (antiemetics) can be prescribed, although many of these are not appropriate for children and pregnant women or while breastfeeding.

 ## Did you know?

In children, vomiting can be the result of coughs or colds (due to excess mucus) or a raised temperature.

NATURAL REMEDIES

Treatment should be offered according to the cause of the nausea and vomiting, but the following natural remedies may be useful.

AROMATHERAPY The essential oils of peppermint or lavender can be used in a vaporiser and inhaled to alleviate nausea and vomiting. Similarly, thyme or tea tree can be used for their antiseptic properties. Massage the tummy and chest with a few drops of lavender or chamomile in a light carrier oil to calm and reduce any spasm.

FLOWER REMEDIES Rescue Remedy or Emergency Essence will be useful for prolonged or distressing vomiting; it will help to reduce panic and calm the mind and body. Holly or Beech may help if the vomiting is linked to fearfulness, stress and emotional problems.

 ## HERBAL REMEDIES

- Make a cup of very weak blackcurrant or chamomile tea and drink lukewarm, in small sips. This will help to soothe the digestive tract.
- Chewing a little fresh or candied ginger will help to settle the stomach, and is particularly useful for motion sickness or pregnancy-related nausea.
- Echinacea, peppermint and thyme can be drunk as infusions or added to a footbath when there is infection at the root of the illness.

 ## HOMEOPATHIC REMEDIES

These can be very effective. If the condition is chronic, constitutional treatment is indicated. There are remedies that will help for acute attacks.

Arsenicum 30C is the best one to try first, when nausea and vomiting are accompanied by diarrhoea, and symptoms seem to be worse between midnight and 2am.

Nux vomica 30C, when nausea is made better by vomiting, and may be caused by overindulgence (after a party, for example).

Tabacum 30C, for nausea and vomiting relieved by uncovering the abdomen. This is a good one for travel sickness.

Phosphorus 30C, for cravings for cold water, which is then vomited, and burning pains in the stomach.

Pulsatilla 30C, for vomiting after rich fatty food, with tearfulness.

Arnica 30C, when vomiting follows a head injury.

Aconite 30C, when vomiting and severe pain last for more than an hour, and are not relieved by vomiting.

 ## SEE YOUR DOCTOR

Any case of vomiting that continues for longer than 24 hours, or occurs in a child who is under the age of three months, should be seen by a doctor. Children dehydrate very quickly, and if there is floppiness, a sunken fontanelle (the soft spot on top of the head) in a baby, or fewer wet nappies, make sure that you see your doctor urgently. Blood in the vomit should also always be investigated.

 ## Quick fix

For immediate relief for nausea, try wearing an acupressure wristband. They are sold in most pharmacies for treating motion sickness.

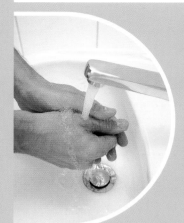

Gastroenteritis & food poisoning

Gastroenteritis is an infection of the digestive tract, caused either by a virus, such as the norovirus, or by bacteria, as in food poisoning. It is highly infectious, but most people only suffer mild symptoms, lasting a few days.

 SYMPTOMS

▷ Nausea and vomiting
▷ Diarrhoea
▷ Abdominal pain
▷ Headaches
▷ High temperature
▷ Possible dehydration

 PREVENTION

- Wash your hands after going to the lavatory, and after touching any surfaces in public places.
- Avoid direct contact with the body fluids of a person with gastroenteritis: use separate towels, don't share cups or plates, and make sure the toilet is cleaned thoroughly after each bout of vomiting or diarrhoea they suffer.
- To avoid food poisoning, practise good food hygiene rules.
- Prepare and store raw and cooked foods separately.
- Make sure food is thoroughly cooked through, especially poultry, pork and eggs.
- Don't eat foods that are past their 'use by' date.
- Wash your hands before preparing food and after contact with raw meat and poultry.

 Did you know?

You can ease back into eating again when you start to get your appetite back with the BRAT diet. Eat the following foods.

- **B**ananas – ripe ones
- **R**ice – must be plain, boiled
- **A**pples – raw ones
- **T**oast – preferably dry whole wheat without butter.

 CONVENTIONAL REMEDIES

Sufferers of mild to moderate cases of gastroenteritis should stay at home and make sure they get plenty of fluids. Rehydrating salts, available over-the-counter, are recommended for vulnerable groups, such as the elderly, or after prolonged bouts of gastroenteritis. For severe cases, your doctor might prescribe loperamide to reduce diarrhoea, or metaclopramide for vomiting. Antibiotics may sometimes be prescribed to prevent secondary infections in the most vulnerable groups.

NATURAL REMEDIES

There are many treatments to soothe the digestive tract and restore normal function. Natural remedies focus on helping your digestive system to recover normal function after an attack of gastroenteritis or food poisoning.

NUTRITIONAL MEDICINE Eat small, easily digested meals, including plain, non-fatty foods, such as clear soups, dry toast, boiled rice and bananas. Avoid smoking, alcohol, caffeine-containing drinks, and spicy or fatty foods.

AROMATHERAPY Massage a few drops of chamomile and geranium essential oils, blended with a light carrier oil, into the abdomen to bring relief from discomfort. Use a blend of basil, oregano and lavender in the bath.

 # HERBAL REMEDIES

- Take a course of probiotics after any kind of stomach upset, to restore the balance of healthy bacteria in the gut. Choose ones that supply a billion units of acidophilus per dose.
- Garlic tablets and manuka honey have an antibacterial effect, which could help in cases of bacterial infection.
- Powdered ginger added to a hot drink can help to ease nausea, and has an anti-inflammatory effect on the gut.
- Slippery elm powder mixed with hot water will help to soothe the digestive lining after an infection.

 # HOMEOPATHIC REMEDIES

Homeopathic remedies can be taken hourly, as required. As always, choose the appropriate remedy for the symptoms presented.

Arsenicum 30C, for burning pains in the abdomen and great thirst.

Pulsatilla 30C, for symptoms worse at night, and tearfulness.

Baptisia 30C, if a salmonella infection is suspected – stools dark, bloody and smelly, nearly liquid.

Phosphorus 30C, for a burning sensation when stools are passed, with vomiting and cravings for cold water, which is then vomited.

Sulphur 30C, for burning diarrhoea that is worse around 5am, with a red and itchy anus.

 # SEE YOUR DOCTOR

If your symptoms last longer than three days, contact your doctor. If there is blood in your stools or vomit, seek medical advice straight away. You should also get help if you suffer any symptoms of dehydration, such as an inability to pass urine, dry mouth and eyes that appear sunken. Gastroenteritis can be dangerous in the elderly, the very young, or those who are suffering from other health problems that weaken the system, so a close eye should be kept on them.

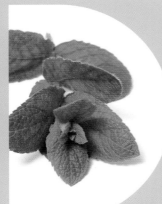

Indigestion & heartburn

Indigestion, or dyspepsia, is a burning pain in the upper abdomen caused by a reflux of stomach acid irritating the lining of the oesophagus. Heartburn has the same cause but tends to be felt just behind the breastbone.

 SYMPTOMS

▷ A burning pain in the throat, chest and/or stomach that is worse when you are lying down
▷ Sour acidic taste in the mouth
▷ A sore throat

 PREVENTION

- Don't smoke, as the chemicals in cigarette smoke irritate the digestive lining.
- Keep your weight down.
- Avoid foods that bring on indigestion, such as rich, spicy, fatty dishes, chocolate, pastry, acidic fruit juices, alcohol, and caffeine-containing drinks.
- Eat small meals and don't stuff yourself full.
- Wear loose clothing, without tight waistbands.
- Don't eat too late at night; always make sure that at least three hours elapse after a meal before you go to bed.
- Raising the head of the bed with wooden blocks can help to prevent acid reflux.

 CONVENTIONAL REMEDIES

Antacids, which are available over-the-counter in pharmacies, neutralise stomach acids and ease symptoms, but you shouldn't take them longterm or exceed the stated dosage. For severe, recurrent indigestion, your doctor might prescribe protein pump inhibitors (PPIs) or H2-receptor antagonists (such as cimetidine) that inhibit the production of stomach acid. Prokinetic drugs are for particularly severe symptoms, and they work by speeding up the rate at which the stomach empties.

 Did you know?

Acid reflux is a common problem that affects many people and it is seldom serious, but in the long-term it may lead to the lining of the gut becoming damaged.

NATURAL REMEDIES

There are lots of ways to lessen the effects of acid reflux. The traditional remedy to ease heartburn and indigestion is two or three teaspoons of apple cider vinegar in a glass of water before meals. The vinegar lowers the acidity of stomach acids but allows them to digest food efficiently.

HELPFUL THERAPIES Both acupressure and reflexology may be helpful in relieving indigestion.

NUTRITIONAL MEDICINE Baking soda is a natural antacid and you can mix a little with water in a glass for instant relief.

 ## HERBAL REMEDIES

- Liquorice powder containing a substance called glycyrrhizin is effective at soothing indigestion. Don't take it if you have any other health problems, though, as there can be interactions.
- Aloe vera juice has anti-inflammatory, pain-killing properties.
- Peppermint tea can relieve mild indigestion when sipped after a meal.
- Marshmallow root tea can coat and soothe the lining of the oesophagus.

 ## AROMATHERAPY

- Neroli, peppermint and chamomile oils have a healing and soothing effect on the digestive system; use in the bath or mixed with a carrier oil for a light massage of the abdominal area.
- Chamomile and lavender oils can be used in the same way for relief of cramping and wind. Inhaling peppermint oil from a vaporiser can help with flatulence.
- Heartburn can be relieved by massaging your abdomen with a few drops of neroli or chamomile in a warm carrier oil, such as grapeseed.

 ## FLOWER REMEDIES

- Impatiens is ideal if you tend to do everything too quickly, and pay the consequences later.
- Olive will help with fatigue caused by overindulgence.
- Oak is good for persistent indigestion caused by an inability to change poor lifestyle habits.

 ## HOMEOPATHIC REMEDIES

For relief of symptoms, try one of the following.

Nux vomica 30C, for heartburn, discomfort and flatulence, especially after a heavy meal or overindulgence.

Carbo veg 30C can help if you have a full, heavy feeling, and feel sleepy after eating.

Lycopodium 30C relieves tiredness and bloating after eating, and helps when you have a burning in your throat.

 ## SEE YOUR DOCTOR

If you are suffering recurrent bouts of indigestion, if it is particularly painful, or if it suddenly feels worse than it has felt before, see your doctor.

Caution

Taking aspirin or NSAIDs, such as ibuprofen, to relieve the pain of indigestion will only make it worse.

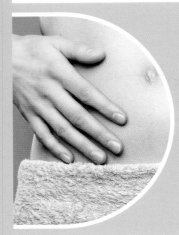

Inflammatory bowel diseases

Crohn's disease and ulcerative colitis are both chronic relapsing/remitting conditions in which inflammation of the lining of the bowel causes uncomfortable and potentially dangerous symptoms.

 ## SYMPTOMS

▷ Diarrhoea, with blood and/or mucus in the stools
▷ Abdominal cramps, especially after eating
▷ Relapsing and remitting episodes
▷ Fever and joint pain
▷ Weight loss
▷ Vitamin and mineral deficiencies
▷ Fatigue

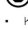 ## PREVENTION

- Keep a food diary and note down which foods make your symptoms worse, so you can avoid them. One study found that the commonly implicated foods were wheat, milk, yeast, corn, egg, potato, rye, tea, coffee, apples, mushrooms, oats and chocolate.
- Eating six small meals rather than three large ones a day can help. Focus on high-vitamin, low-sugar foods.
- If you are a smoker, giving up can ease the symptoms of Crohn's disease.

 ## CONVENTIONAL REMEDIES

Mild to moderate cases of Crohn's disease and ulcerative colitis may be treated with aminosalicylates, which reduce inflammation. If the symptoms are more severe, however, steroids such as budesonide and prednisolone may be given during active episodes, but there are potential dangers if they are used long-term. Immune system suppressants, such as azathioprine, may be prescribed during a non-active phase to try and prevent relapses.

 ## Did you know?

No one is entirely sure about the causes of Crohn's disease and ulcerative colitis, but it seems that there may be a genetic element as well as some environmental triggers.

NATURAL REMEDIES

Before taking any natural treatments alongside the conventional ones, discuss them with your specialist to avoid interactions.

NUTRITIONAL MEDICINE Several studies have indicated that fish oils ease symptoms and prevent relapses, so it's well worth taking daily fish oil capsules. Zinc, selenium, vitamin B12 and folic acid deficiencies are common, so take a good multivitamin and mineral supplement to replace all these.

FLOWER REMEDIES Try Rescue Remedy or Emergency Essence when you experience any pain or discomfort. Blend the Bach flower remedies Impatiens, Willow, Agrimony and Wild Oat with a little water, and sip throughout the day to encourage healing and deal with symptoms.

 HERBAL REMEDIES

- Probiotic supplements with healthy digestive bacteria are useful.
- Some people swear by drinking a small glass (100ml) of aloe vera juice three times a day.
- Liquorice root powder containing glycyrrhizin can have a soothing effect on the bowel.
- Garlic powder tablets can help to deal with any fungal growth in the digestive system.
- Slippery elm powder can be mixed with a little warm water to soothe and heal inflammation of the gut.

 AROMATHERAPY

- A blend of lavender and peppermint can be massaged into the abdomen or added to the bath to relieve conditions associated with stress, and also relax any spasms.
- A few drops of juniper or cedarwood oil added to the bath have an antispasmodic, sedative and tonic effect.
- Essential oil of basil can help to reduce symptoms, used in the bath or simply inhaled from a vaporiser when you feel discomfort.

 HOMEOPATHIC REMEDIES

Treatment should be constitutional, but the following remedies may be useful.

Arg nit 30C, if you are anxious and suffer from flatulence and diarrhoea.

China 30C, for painless diarrhoea accompanied by a swollen abdomen and flatulence; worse after milk, gluten or fruit.

Ignatia 30C, if your bowels are particularly sensitive during periods of emotional distress.

Podophyllum 30C, for abdominal pain that is better for heat and when lying down; often explosive diarrhoea.

 SEE YOUR DOCTOR

Always consult your doctor if there is blood in your stools, if you have recurrent diarrhoea or abdominal pain, or if you lose weight for no obvious reason.

Reduce stress

Take steps to reduce the stress levels in your life. Identify the main stressors and try to deal with them by changing your daily routines, or taking up some form of relaxation therapy, such as yoga or meditation.

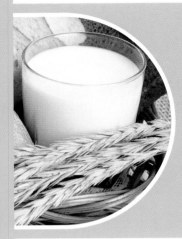

Irritable bowel syndrome

About one-third of the population are affected by irritable bowel syndrome (IBS) at some point in their lives, but only half of them will consider it severe enough to consult their doctor. It's a chronic condition, but, fortunately, plenty can be done to relieve it and to prevent recurrence.

 ## SYMPTOMS

The following should last for at least six months before a diagnosis of IBS is confirmed:
▷ Abdominal pain that is relieved by defecation
▷ Bloating
▷ Constipation or diarrhoea

You may also have at least two of the following:
▷ Needing to strain to pass stools
▷ Feeling the bowel movement is incomplete
▷ Having to rush to the lavatory for a bowel movement
▷ Fewer than three bowel movements a week
▷ More than three bowel movements a day
▷ Excess wind

 ## PREVENTION

• Keep a food diary and find out which foods improve symptoms and which make them worse.
• Eat small, regular meals and chew your food properly.
• Drink eight large glasses of water a day, and cut down on tea, coffee, alcohol and fizzy drinks.
• Get 30 minutes of exercise five days a week to stimulate the normal functioning of your digestive system.
• Stress make the symptoms of IBS worse, so try to relax and reduce the amount of stress in your life.

 ## CONVENTIONAL REMEDIES

Your doctor will probably recommend making lifestyle changes before prescribing drugs, but antispasmodic medicines, such as mebeverine and peppermint oil, can help. Bulk-forming laxatives might be prescribed for constipation, and loperamide may be offered for IBS-related diarrhoea.

NATURAL REMEDIES

There are different types of IBS so it's worth seeing a therapist for an individual diagnosis, but the following natural remedies could help.

FLOWER REMEDIES Impatiens will help with attacks that come on as a result of stress or overindulgence.

 ## NUTRITIONAL MEDICINE

- Some IBS symptoms are caused by the action of gut bacteria on fibre, and it's worth trying a very low-fibre diet for a while, then gradually reintroducing foods that contain fibre until you find a level you can tolerate.
- A gluten-free diet is helpful to many sufferers.
- Other possible irritants can include dairy products, eggs, yeast, onions, potatoes and chocolate. Exclude them all, then reintroduce one at a time to see which, if any, cause symptoms.
- Many sufferers report that symptoms are eased by taking probiotics.

 ## HERBAL REMEDIES

- Cynara artichoke supplements seem to be very effective at reducing pain and bloating, and results can be seen within 10 days.
- Agrimony and hops can be blended into an infusion and drunk before meals to regulate digestion and ease discomfort.
- Wild yam and cramp bark can be taken in either capsule or tincture form to ease painful spasms and cramps.

 ## HOMEOPATHIC REMEDIES

Constitutional treatment will be necessary, but the following remedies should help in the shortterm.

Arg nit 30C, for digestive upsets accompanied by nervousness, bloating, nausea and greenish diarrhoea.

Asafoetida 30C, for a feeling of constriction in the digestive tract, and a bloated abdomen, but inability to pass wind.

Colcynthis 30C, for cutting pains and cramping that are worse before diarrhoea.

Lycopodium 30C, for chronic digestive discomfort and bowel problems, with bloating and a feeling of fullness that comes on early in a meal.

Podophyllum 30C, for abdominal pain and cramping followed by watery, offensive diarrhoea.

 ## SEE YOUR DOCTOR

If any change in your bowel habits lasts longer than six weeks, or if there is blood in your stools, consult your doctor. You should also seek medical advice if you have a family history of bowel cancer, or if you are over 60 years old.

Pilates

This is an exercise system that works to strengthen the abdominal and pelvic muscles. If you are prone to constipation, Pilates can help you to push more effectively.

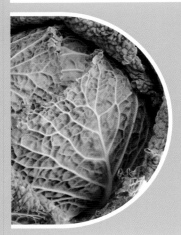

Peptic ulcers

A peptic ulcer is an area of damage to the lining of either the stomach or the wall of the small bowel, caused when the layer of mucus that normally protects them from stomach acids is compromised. The most common cause is a bacteria called Helicobacter pylori but NSAIDs (non-steroidal anti-inflammatory drugs), such as aspirin, naproxen and ibuprofen, taken over long periods of time, can also be a factor. They also tend to run in families.

 SYMPTOMS

▷ Acute abdominal pain, usually just below the breastbone
▷ Burning pain extending into the back
▷ Pain that is worse immediately after eating
▷ Heartburn
▷ A bitter taste in your mouth
▷ Nausea or vomiting
▷ Regurgitating food

 PREVENTION

• Avoid food and drink that exacerbate symptoms, including spicy foods and alcohol.
• Smoking is a known cause of ulcers, so giving up can help to prevent them.
• Alcohol can cause peptic ulcers, so only drink in moderation.
• Avoid NSAIDs – ask your pharmacist for advice on the other options.
• Drink a large glass of water before each meal to dilute stomach acids.
• Stress caused by injury or trauma is another cause of peptic ulcers. You may not be able to prevent these happening but you can take steps to manage the stress effectively.

 CONVENTIONAL REMEDIES

The two types of medication offered for the treatment of ulcers include proton pump inhibitors (PPIs) and H2-blockers, both of which are designed to reduce the production of acid in your stomach. If the *Helicobacter pylori* bacteria is diagnosed, you will also be offered antibiotics.

 Did you know?

Stress seems to play an important role and if you have peptic ulcers you should reassess your life to introduce more relaxation and try to eliminate any stressful situations and relationships. You could even sign up for a stress management course.

NATURAL REMEDIES

Most natural treatments are designed to heal the gut and ease symptoms.

AROMATHERAPY A lovely oil known as Althea soothes mucous membranes, and relieves gastritis and peptic ulcers. Use a few drops in abdominal massage, or in the bath.

 HERBAL REMEDIES

- Antibacterial herbs, such as echinacea, red clover and thyme, can be drunk daily as an infusion to combat any bacteria present.
- Manuka honey heals and strengthens the stomach lining and kills harmful bacteria.
- Slippery elm encourages the health of the mucous membranes, and can be taken in capsule, tincture or infusion form. Meadowsweet has a similar effect.
- An infusion of chamomile can help to relieve the pain, particularly if it is sipped just after meals.
- Powdered liquorice containing glycyrrhizin can help to heal peptic ulcers by increasing the production of the mucus that lines the stomach.

 NUTRITIONAL MEDICINE

- Increase your intake of EFAs (essential fatty acids), which are natural anti-inflammatories, and protect the lining of the entire gastro-intestinal tract. Fish oil or flaxseed supplements may be useful.
- Fresh cabbage juice and raw cabbage can strengthen the lining of the stomach.

- A diet rich in dietary fibre (psyllium or flax seeds) can help to protect the gut.
- Zinc is crucial to the health of your stomach lining, so eat plenty of whole grains, shellfish and pumpkin seeds or take supplements of 50mg per day.
- Vitamin C will promote healing of ulcers – take 1000mg per day, and increase your intake of vitamin C-rich foods.

HOMEOPATHIC REMEDIES

Arg nit 30C is ideal for ulcers with gnawing pain and belching.

Arsenicum 30C is indicated for ulcers with a burning feeling that is worse for food and drink.

Hydrastis 30C may be appropriate if the symptoms include gastritis and abdominal pain.

Graphics 30C, for burning and constricting pains that are often better for eating, but may later cause vomiting.

Nux vomica 30C may help if symptoms are worse after heavy meals, alcohol and stimulants such as coffee or tobacco.

SEE YOUR DOCTOR

See your doctor if you have difficulty swallowing food, have lost weight, notice blood in your vomit or faeces, or experience sudden, extreme abdominal pain.

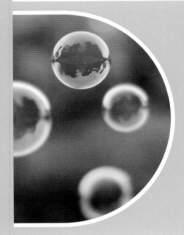

Wind

Every human being passes wind, but some people do so in excessive quantities. Bowel gases come from the air that we swallow while eating, from fizzy drinks, and from the digestion of foods in the intestine. If the digestive system is not working efficiently and foods decompose in the gut, wind can have a sulphurous smell and there may be abdominal bloating as well.

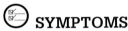 **SYMPTOMS**

▷ Frequent passing of wind
▷ Foul-smelling wind
▷ Embarrassing intestinal noises
▷ Bloating

 PREVENTION

- Avoid gas-producing foods, such as beans, lentils, cauliflower, cabbage, broccoli and cucumber, as well as fizzy drinks.
- Slimming products that contain sugar substitutes, such as sorbitol and fructose, can also cause flatulence, as can fruit juices.
- Eat small meals of easily digestible foods, such as potatoes, rice, yoghurt and bananas.
- Eat slowly and chew each mouthful thoroughly.
- Keep a food diary to see which foods exacerbate symptoms.
- Get plenty of exercise, which will help your digestive system to work more efficiently.
- Avoid chewing gum and smoking, both of which cause you to swallow air.

 CONVENTIONAL REMEDIES

Charcoal tablets, available over-the-counter, absorb abdominal gases effectively, but cannot be taken with any other medication. You can also buy a charcoal pad to wear in your underwear to absorb bad smells. A supplement called alpha-galascitosidase can improve the way in which you digest carbohydrates.

NATURAL REMEDIES

Excess wind can be a symptom of irritable bowel syndrome (see pages 180–181), so the remedies listed there may help – or you can try the following.

TRADITIONAL REMEDIES Try drinking the juice of a lemon in a glass of water with a half teaspoon of bicarbonate of soda to quieten a noisy digestive system.

NUTRITIONAL MEDICINE Some people are lactose-intolerant and don't have the correct enzymes to break down milk products. Try avoiding them for a few weeks to see if your symptoms improve. You could also try excluding wheat- and gluten-containing products to see if this makes a difference.

 HERBAL REMEDIES

- Drink peppermint tea after a meal or take peppermint oil capsules to aid digestion.
- Probiotics should help. Choose one that contains a billion units of acidophilus per dose.
- There are lots of herbs you can use in your cooking that have an anti-flatulent effect. Basil, dill, turmeric, rosemary, coriander, cloves, cardamom, fennel seeds, caraway seeds and anise are all good.
- Chamomile tea can relieve spasms and discomfort associated with wind.

 AROMATHERAPY

- Marjoram, ginger and fennel will help your body to disperse wind, and calm any associated pain. Add a few drops of each to a light carrier oil and massage into your abdomen.
- Massaging your abdomen with a drop of fennel oil in a light carrier oil can help to release trapped wind and encourage healthy digestion.

 HOMEOPATHIC REMEDIES

Choose the appropriate remedy for the symptoms.

Carbo veg 30C, for feelings of heaviness, sleepiness and belching after meals, with offensive-smelling flatulence.

Lycopodium 30C, for a bloated, rumbling abdomen, and when passing wind eases abdominal discomfort.

Colocynthis 30C, for cutting, cramping pain in the tummy that is relieved by bending double.

Chamomilla 30C, for searing pains caused by wind; you'll feel worse for warmth.

Ipecac 30C, for pains that feel like a hand clutching your intestines, with pains moving from left to right.

 SEE YOUR DOCTOR

If you have abdominal pain and bloating that won't clear up after a few weeks; if you have blood in your stools; or if you keep getting persistent diarrhoea or constipation, consult your doctor.

 IMMEDIATE RELIEF

To relieve trapped wind, kneel on the floor, then lean forwards, so that your forehead touches the floor, with your arms straight forward, palms face down.

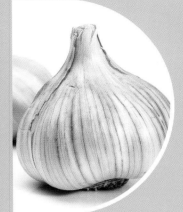

Intestinal worms

Infestations of worms in the digestive system are quite common, particularly in young children, who usually contract them at school. Worms can sometimes be seen around the anus or in the faeces, and they inflame the area of the bowel or rectum where they attach themselves. The most common worms in our climate are threadworms.

 SYMPTOMS

▷ Diarrhoea
▷ Bad breath
▷ Dark circles under the eyes
▷ Restlessness at night
▷ Anaemia
▷ Itching around the anus
▷ Loss of weight, fever and irritability are symptoms of round worms
▷ Anaemia and nutritional disorders can be caused by hookworms

 PREVENTION

• Encourage children to wash their hand regularly, particularly after going to the lavatory, dealing with pets or handling food.
• Avoid scratching the anus area.
• Worms thrive on sugar, so keep this to a minimum in your diet.
• Changing the bedclothes regularly and washing them at a high temperature can prevent the spread of worms.

 CONVENTIONAL REMEDIES

Over-the-counter preparations are available to stun or kill worms, which are then excreted in the faeces. These are called anthelmintic drugs, and they will be chosen according to the type of worm present. Only one or two doses are normally required. Laxatives may sometimes be offered to aid the expulsion of worms living in the intestines.

Did you know?

Round worms are the largest found in the human body, and the ones most likely to cause problems; tapeworms are usually picked up from undercooked, infected meat; and giardia lamblia and hookworms are picked up from countries where water and sanitary conditions are substandard.

NATURAL REMEDIES

Some natural treatments depend on the type of worm present but the following remedies will all help to rid you of an infestation.

FLOWER REMEDIES Rescue Remedy is good for discomfort or distress. Rub into the pulse points, and around the anus to relieve itching. Crab Apple is excellent if you feel unclean or polluted.

AROMATHERAPY Rub a drop each of eucalyptus, lavender and tea tree oil into a bland ointment, such as petroleum jelly or chickweed. Rub around the anus to prevent itching, and to prevent eggs from being laid. This is particularly helpful at night.

HERBAL REMEDIES

- A teaspoon each of cayenne pepper and senna can be combined in a cup of live yoghurt and taken by the teaspoon before meals. The former stuns the worms and the latter encourages their expulsion.
- Wormwood tea will stun the worms, but should only be taken under the supervision of a registered herbalist.
- Garlic is toxic to worms. Crush and add it to a tablespoon of honey and take before meals, followed by a tincture of laxative herbs such as liquorice and dandelion root to aid expulsion.

 NUTRITIONAL MEDICINE

- Acidophilus tablets should be taken for several weeks to improve the health of the bowel.
- Carrots, turnips and apples are traditional remedies used to clear worms. Grate them together and take three times daily.
- Ripe pumpkin seeds are useful in the treatment of intestinal worms, especially tapeworms. One tablespoon of the seeds should be peeled and crushed, and then infused in 250ml of boiling water and drunk. This will kill the parasites and help to expel the worms.

HOMEOPATHIC REMEDIES

Select the appropriate remedy for your symptoms.

Cina 30C may alter the balance of the body, so that you expel threadworms naturally.

Teucrium 30C, for an itchy bottom and nose, worse in the evening and with restless sleep.

Santoninum 30C, when all else fails.

 SEE YOUR DOCTOR

Conventional treatment is always necessary for any roundworm or tapeworm infestations. See your doctor if treatment is not effective after two courses, or if you begin to lose weight.

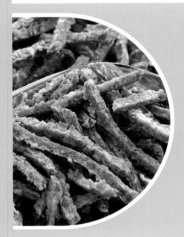

Haemorrhoids

Haemorrhoids, which are also commonly known as piles, are enlarged and swollen blood vessels in or around the lower rectum and anus. They are caused by increased pressure on the blood vessels in the area, as a result of being overweight, lifting heavy objects, pregnancy, constipation or prolonged diarrhoea, or simply ageing.

188

 ## SYMPTOMS

▷ Bleeding when passing stools
▷ An itchy feeling around the anus
▷ Intense pain, particularly when passing a stool
▷ Bright-red bleeding after passing a stool
▷ Discharge of mucus when passing a stool
▷ Straining and feeling as though bowels are still full after a movement

 ## PREVENTION

• Include plenty of fibre in your diet, to ensure that bowel movements are efficient and you don't strain.
• Avoid lifting heavy articles, and try to maintain a healthy weight.
• Drink plenty of water to keep stools soft.

 ## CONVENTIONAL REMEDIES

You can choose from a number of over-the-counter preparations that act as anti-inflammatories and help to reduce pain and itching. Creams containing corticosteroids can be prescribed to reduce the inflammation. If pain is intense, analgesic ointments can be prescribed. Long-term haemorrhoids may be addressed by 'banding', in which a very tight elastic band is placed around the base of the haemorrhoid. There are a number of other options available, including surgery.

NATURAL REMEDIES

There are lots of remedies that can help with symptoms and encourage healing.

TRADITIONAL REMEDIES Witch hazel and/or lemon juice can be applied neat to haemorrhoids, to reduce swelling and bleeding.

AROMATHERAPY A warm bath with 10 drops of bergamot (or a compress, with a few drops of this oil) will help to reduce pain, and act as an antiseptic. Myrrh oil is cooling and anti-inflammatory; use in the same way.

 HERBAL REMEDIES

- Calendula cream or ointment will encourage healing and relieve itching.
- Horse chestnut relieves swelling and inflammation, and helps to strengthen vein walls. Take in tea or capsule form, or apply externally as a compress.
- Butcher's broom contains anti-inflammatory and vein-constricting properties, and has traditionally been used for the treatment of haemorrhoids and varicose veins. Take in tea or capsule form.
- A strong, warm infusion of yarrow can be applied to the affected area to soothe and heal.
- Aloe vera gel is soothing for burning and pain.

 NUTRITIONAL MEDICINE

- Increasing your fibre intake is the most important step you can take. Try psyllium, ground flax seeds or ispaghula husks.
- Bioflavonoids stabilise and strengthen blood vessel walls and decrease inflammation. They have been found to reduce anal discomfort, pain and discharge during an acute attack of haemorrhoids. Boost your intake of bioflavonoids by eating more citrus fruit, grapes, berries and whole grains, or take a 500mg supplement per day.

 HOMEOPATHIC REMEDIES

Treatment should be constitutional, but the following remedies will help.

Hamamelis 30C can be taken two or three times daily to treat the cause of haemorrhoids.

Aloe 30C, for haemorrhoids that are swollen and protrude like a bunch of grapes, and soothed by cold compresses.

Calc fluor 30C, for haemorrhoids with bleeding and itching, or sore internal piles.

Nux vomica 30C, for itching, painful haemorrhoids, with a constricted feeling in the rectum and chronic constipation.

Pulsatilla 30C, for itching, uncomfortable haemorrhoids that are likely to protrude.

 SEE YOUR DOCTOR

Always see your doctor if you experience profuse bleeding, or if the haemorrhoids become hard and dark in colour (which means that a clot may have formed within them).

 IMMEDIATE RELIEF

Apply some ice, never directly to the skin but wrapped in a clean towel, for a local anaesthetic effect. This helps to relieve the irritation as well as the pain.

TOP 20
Super-healing foods

The everyday foods you eat can help to keep you healthy and prevent or treat some common medical problems.

1 HONEY

Nutrients B vitamins, minerals (depending on plant sources), antioxidants

Good for sore throats, coughs and colds; healing wounds; hay fever

Caution don't give honey to children under 12 months as it can cause infant botulism

2 GINGER

Nutrients Vitamins A and B2 (riboflavin), iron, phosphorus, potassium

Good for nausea, food poisoning, motion sickness; vertigo; respiratory ailments; menstrual pain; lowering blood cholesterol

3 GARLIC

Nutrients Vitamins A, B, C, calcium, potassium, iron, selenium

Good for fighting infection; relieving colds, bronchitis, congestion; fungal infections; protecting against food poisoning; lowering cholesterol and high blood pressure; asthma; diarrhoea and indigestion

4 ONIONS

Nutrients Vitamin C, potassium

Good for chest infections; lowering blood pressure; diabetes; preventing cancer

5 CARROTS

Nutrients Vitamin A (beta-carotene), B and C, iron, fibre

Good for eye health, healthy skin; gum disease; asthma and respiratory problems; protecting against cancer

6 BROCCOLI

Nutrients Vitamins C and K, calcium, potassium, fibre

Good for protecting against cancer and infections; improving cognitive function

7 WATERCRESS

Nutrients Vitamins A and C, folic acid, calcium, iron, potassium, lutein

Good for protecting against cancer; urinary infections; good eye health and reducing risk of cataracts and age-related macular degeneration

8 AVOCADOES

Nutrients Vitamins B2 (riboflavin) and E, fibre

Good for healthy skin and treating skin problems; fighting stress; good digestion; boosting immune system; lowering cholesterol levels

9 TOMATOES

Nutrients Vitamins A, C, iron, antioxidant lycopene, folic acid

Good for preventing cancer (especially prostate); chronic fatigue syndrome; aiding memory and fighting dementia

10 APPLES

Nutrients Vitamins B, C and E, fibre, potassium, antioxidants

Good for fibre helps digestion; food poisoning; lowering blood pressure and cholesterol

11 BANANA

Nutrients Vitamin B6, potassium, zinc, fibre

Good for digestive ailments, constipation, diarrhoea; convalescing after illness; relieving muscular cramping

12 CITRUS FRUITS (LEMONS, LIMES, ORANGES, PINK GRAPEFRUIT)

Nutrients Vitamin C and bioflavonoids, folic acid (oranges)

Good for boosting body's natural immunity; treating coughs, colds, flu, sore throats; arthritis; lowering cholesterol; protecting against heart disease and cancer; gum disease

13 BERRIES

Nutrients Vitamin C, antioxidants

Good for fighting infection; preventing heart disease and cancer; urinary tract infections (cranberries and blueberries); respiratory tract infections; improving short-term memory loss (blueberries)

14 SEEDS (PUMPKIN, SUNFLOWER, FLAX SEEDS)

Nutrients Vitamin E, zinc

Good for heal;thy nervous system; good digestion; reducing risk of dementia and enhancing memory and thinking skills

15 NUTS

Nutrients protein, B vitamins, Vitamin E, zinc, selenium, magnesium, iron, healthy oils, folic acid

Good for healthy nervous system, fatigue and stress; lowering cholesterol; preventing memory loss

16 WHOLE GRAINS

Nutrients protein, B vitamins, vitamin E, folic acid, fibre, zinc

Good for constipation; protecting against bowel disease, heart disease, cancer, diabetes; high blood pressure

17 OATS

Nutrients protein, Vitamins B6 and E, magnesium, fibre

Good for treating constipation; lowering cholesterol and blood pressure; protecting against colon cancer

18 BEANS AND LEGUMES (LENTILS, DRIED PEAS)

Nutrients protein, B vitamins, fibre, calcium, iron, magnesium, zinc

Good for constipation; protecting against cancer, bowel and heart disease

19 LIVE YOGHURT

Nutrients protein, Vitamins A and D, calcium

Good for stomach ailments, food poisoning, constipation; fighting fungal infections; boosting the immune system

20 OILY FISH

Nutrients protein, Vitamins A, B12 and D, Omega-3 fatty acids, iodine

Good for a healthy heart and preventing heart disease; healthy nervous system; protecting against memory loss and Alzheimer's disease

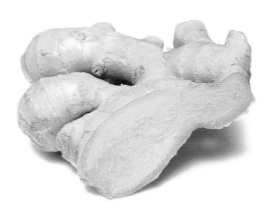

Urinary problems

The urinary system performs some important functions in the body: filtering the blood, expelling waste products and excess water, and maintaining the correct balance of blood flow and pressure, and fluids and minerals. It is composed of the bladder, kidneys, two ureters and the urethra (the tube through which urine passes leaving the body).

The kidneys purify the blood by filtering out waste products and toxins. While the cleaned blood returns to the heart, the filtered liquid is turned into urine to be channelled through the ureters into the bladder where it is stored before being expelled by the body through the urethra.

Most of the time, your waterworks will function efficiently and well, but the urinary tract is susceptible to infection, especially in women, due to its location near the anus and vagina. If bacteria enter the urethra, other parts of the system, such as the bladder and kidneys, can become infected, too, if the problem is left untreated. Difficulty in passing urine, pain when you urinate, or an increase in the volume of urine can be symptoms of more serious disorders and will warrant medical investigation.

Drinking plenty of fluids, especially cranberry juice, eating a high-fibre diet, good personal hygiene and going to the toilet promptly when you feel the need to urinate (at least once every three hours during the day) can all help to prevent urinary tract infections and keep your system flushed out and healthy.

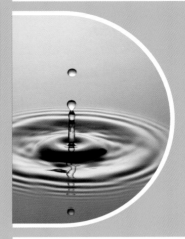

Incontinence

Incontinence is an involuntary loss of bladder control, leading to the unplanned leakage of urine. It can be embarrassing and awkward, especially with stress incontinence, as it can occur when coughing, sneezing or making sudden movements. Stress incontinence becomes more common as people get older, especially in women, with about one in five over-40s experiencing it.

 ## SYMPTOMS

▷ A sudden release of urine – from a few drops to your whole bladder

▷ A sudden urge to urinate (known as urge incontinence and caused by an overactive bladder)

 ## PREVENTION

One of the common causes of stress incontinence is weakened pelvic floor muscles. The muscles get weaker after having children and after menopause. Regularly practising pelvic floor exercises, especially after childbirth and as you get older, can help to reduce the chance of incontinence and accidental leakages. Pelvic floor exerciser gadgets are available, or you can simply learn to do the exercises yourself.

NOTE If you're not sure which your pelvic floor muscles are, try stopping the stream of urine when you are urinating. The muscles you use are the ones you want to strengthen.

PELVIC FLOOR EXERCISE

1 Sit or stand with your knees apart and tighten your pelvic floor muscles. Hold whilst counting to five, then relax. Repeat five times.

2 Tighten your muscles again, but this time only for a few seconds, before releasing. Repeat this faster muscle action for up to five minutes. Aim to do the exercises for five minutes every day, gradually increasing the amount of time you hold your muscles.

 ## Did you know?

This is not solely a women's problem; men can suffer from incontinence, too, especially when prostate problems are an issue.

CONVENTIONAL REMEDIES

Various types of incontinence pads are available, to save some of the embarrassment of an unexpected leakage. Strengthening the pelvic floor muscles is commonly recommended for anyone suffering from stress incontinence, as is losing weight if you're overweight. In some cases, medication may be prescribed (such as Duloxetine), in addition to exercises. For anyone who is severely affected, surgery may be required.

Electrical stimulation, involving the use of a specially designed electrical device, is sometimes used to help the pelvic floor muscles become stronger. If a urine or kidney infection is suspected to be the cause of urge incontinence, then antibiotics may be prescribed.

 NATURAL REMEDIES

The following natural remedies may be helpful in treating and relieving incontinence.

AROMATHERAPY The essential oil cypress has astringent and relaxing properties. Mix a few drops with a base carrier oil, such as sweet almond oil, and gently massage into your lower abdomen.

HOMEOPATHIC REMEDIES Take Causticum 6C to help symptoms of involuntary incontinence as a result of sneezing, coughing or laughing. Pulsatilla 6C or Ferrum Phos 6C may help incontinence that occurs when lying down in bed.

NUTRITIONAL MEDICINE Simple dietary amendments may help to reduce the symptoms of incontinence. Cut back on caffeine, as it has diuretic properties, avoid drinking fizzy, carbonated drinks and eat less tomato-based foods, as they could irritate the bladder.

HELPFUL THERAPIES Biofeedback, a method that encourages people to learn to improve their health by gaining control over bodily functions, may offer some help with incontinence. Find a local therapist and see if it works for you.

 HERBAL REMEDIES

Some herbs may help sufferers of incontinence. You can try the following remedies.

- Gingko supplements or tincture can help a weak bladder and incontinence.
- Try taking varuna to help improve muscle tone and bladder control.
- Take healing horsetail tincture to help the urinary system.
- For men with incontinence linked to prostrate problems, take the herb saw palmetto. Supplements are available and should be taken as directed on the packaging.

 SEE YOUR DOCTOR

Many people are too embarrassed to seek medical help, but if your symptoms are severe or interfering with your daily life, see your doctor.

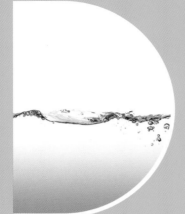

Water retention

Water or fluid retention can affect anyone, but it's particularly common in women around the time of a menstrual period or during pregnancy, and it can get worse as you get older. Even though it may be caused by underlying heart or kidney diseases, water retention is seldom linked to other health problems and, although a nuisance when it happens, it is not a serious concern.

 ## SYMPTOMS

▷ Swelling of the feet and ankles
▷ Swelling around the abdomen
▷ Swelling in the hands
▷ Swelling in the face
▷ You may weigh more in the evening than in the morning
▷ The need to loosen clothing or shoes

 ## PREVENTION

- If you are prone to water retention, especially around your ankles and legs, it can be useful to wear support stockings to try and prevent fluid build-up occurring. This is especially pertinent if you tend to sit down for long periods or spend a lot of time travelling in cars or planes.

- Putting your legs up in a raised position – for example, propped up on a footstool or on a couple of cushions – can help to prevent the swelling recurring.

- Leading a healthy lifestyle, including eating a varied, well-balanced diet and taking regular exercise, can help to prevent water retention.

- Maintain a healthy weight for your height and build. People who are overweight are at more risk of fluid retention.

- Avoid standing still for long periods of time, as this can trigger water retention.

 ## Did you know?

Water retention can sometimes be caused by not drinking enough, so make sure you drink six to eight glasses of water a day to keep your body fully hydrated.

CONVENTIONAL REMEDIES

Diuretics or water tablets are often prescribed to relieve water retention. They work by increasing the amount of urine the kidneys produce, making you need to go to the lavatory more often. Sometimes the tablets can cause side-effects, such as feeling dizzy when you stand up. If water retention occurs during pregnancy, do not take diuretic tablets – consult your doctor for advice. If you are overweight, your doctor may suggest losing weight, as this can help reduce water retention, too. Support or compression stockings may be advised, especially if your job involves a lot of standing around or travelling.

 ## NATURAL REMEDIES

The following natural therapies and remedies may help to relieve the condition.

NUTRITIONAL MEDICINE If you eat a lot of salt, or regularly add salt to your meals, then cutting down on salt consumption can have a positive effect on reducing fluid retention. Include more naturally potassium-rich foods in your diet. They can help reduce the salt levels in your body and relieve areas of swelling. Bananas are a good option, as are tomatoes.

AROMATHERAPY Add a few drops of soothing lavender or rosemary essential oil to a carrier oil, such as sweet almond, and gently massage the area affected by water retention. Repeat daily as necessary.

 ## HERBAL REMEDIES

- Dandelion is one of nature's best diuretics, so try drinking dandelion tea or using a tincture.
- Another diuretic herb available in tincture format is corn silk. One ml tincture should be diluted in 5ml water three times a day. A professional herbalist will be able to mix you up a special blend for the ultimate diuretic remedy.

 ## SEE YOUR DOCTOR

If you have persistent swelling around the abdomen or in your feet and ankles, possibly accompanied by breathlessness or fatigue, see your doctor. Fluid retention can sometimes be linked to underlying kidney or heart conditions, and some further tests and investigations may be required.

 ## IMMEDIATE RELIEF

You can ease the discomfort of swollen feet or ankles by making up a warm, soothing foot bath and then soaking your feet in the water with a few drops of rosemary essential oil added.

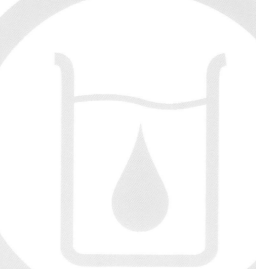

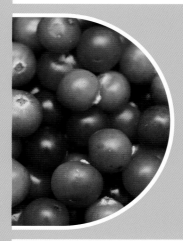

Cystitis

This bladder condition occurs due to infections or irritations of the bladder, or lower urinary tract. It is more common in women than men – up to 40 per cent of women will get cystitis at some point in their life – and it can trigger a range of uncomfortable symptoms. One of the main causes is bacteria, such as E. coli, which gets in the urethra from other areas of your skin and travels up into your bladder.

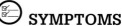 ## SYMPTOMS

▷ Frequent urination
▷ Pain or burning when urinating
▷ Feeling like you need to keep urinating, but not being able to
▷ Blood in urine
▷ Cloudy or dark coloured urine
▷ Feeling unwell as a whole
▷ Pain or discomfort in your lower back or lower abdomen

 ## PREVENTION

There are various ways in which cystitis can be prevented, particularly if you are prone to it.

- Wear cotton underwear and loose clothing.
- Try to empty your bladder before and after having sex.
- Drink more fluid, particularly water, every day.
- Empty your bladder frequently, or at least once every three hours, rather than hanging on.
- Avoid using scented products in the bath, such as bubble bath, as it may cause irritation.
- Avoid spermicidal products – speak to your doctor about alternatives.
- Reduce any stress in your life and eat a healthy diet that is rich in vitamin C – a poor diet and stress can both lower your immunity to infections.

CONVENTIONAL REMEDIES

Over-the-counter painkillers can be used to help relieve the pain of cystitis. If you have an infection, your doctor may prescribe a course of antibiotics for three to six days. If cystitis occurs repeatedly, further investigations may be required.

 ## NATURAL REMEDIES

Various natural remedies can help ease the symptoms and discomfort of cystitis. Here are some options.

HERBAL REMEDIES The herb bachu has natural antiseptic and diuretic properties and can help soothe the pain and burning feeling that cystitis produces. Corn silk is another diuretic and yarrow is a urinary antiseptic. Take individually, or choose a tincture that combines all three (a herbalist can make this up for you). The usual dosage is 1ml tincture diluted in 5ml water three times a day.

NUTRITIONAL MEDICINE Boost your immune system by taking vitamin C or echinacea.

 ## HOMEOPATHIC REMEDIES

Cantharis 6C or Sarsapilla 6C can be taken for burning pain when urinating.

Merc cor 6C, for when urination is painful and you have blood in your urine.

 ## SEE YOUR DOCTOR

Always see a doctor if you have any of the following:

- Your symptoms persist and don't improve within two to three days
- You have blood in your urine
- You have a high temperature, feel nauseous and are being sick
- You have severe abdominal or lower back pain
- You're diabetic, pregnant or over 65
- You have, or have had, any other kidney related problems, such as kidney stones.

 ## IMMEDIATE RELIEF

You can take regular warm baths to help ease the pain and discomfort of cystitis, avoiding the use of any scented bath products.

Healing drinks

- Drink a pint of pure unsweetened cranberry juice daily during an attack of cystitis. The juice contains an acid that helps acidify the urine and prevent bacteria from sticking to the bladder lining. If you don't like the taste, then opt for cranberry tablets containing 200mg of cranberry extract instead.
- Marshmallow root also has a similar effect, by increasing levels of acid in urine and reducing the growth of bacteria. Brew a pot of marshmallow root tea and drink two to three cups daily.

 ## Quick fix

Pop half a teaspoon of bicarbonate of soda in a glass of water and drink it. This can help make your urine less acidic.

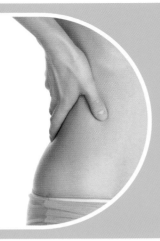

Kidney stones

Kidney stones are solid masses that form in the kidney from substances found in the urine, such as calcium and acid. They can remain in the kidney, or travel through the urinary tract – small stones may pass out without causing much discomfort and you may not even know you have them. However, if a stone becomes large, moves into the ureter and gets stuck, it can cause severe pain, infection and, in some instances, damage to the kidneys.

 SYMPTOMS

▷ Pain or aching on one or both sides of your back
▷ Spasms of severe pain
▷ Blood in the urine
▷ Cloudy urine
▷ Burning feeling when you urinate
▷ Fever or chills
▷ Vomiting

PREVENTION

About 50 per cent of people who have had kidney stones develop more within the next 10 years. Once you have had one or more stones and know what type you are susceptible to, there are practical steps you can take to reduce your risk of further kidney stones.

- If you've had a uric acid stone, then cutting down on the amount of meat you eat can help, as when meat breaks down it makes uric acid.
- If you've had a calcium oxalate kidney stone, then it helps to cut down on foods that are high in oxalate, such as spinach, rhubarb, coffee and chocolate.
- Drinking lots of water – between two and three litres daily – can help reduce the levels of the substances that form kidney stones and flush them through your system.
- Keep active, take regular exercise and aim to eat a healthy, balanced diet.

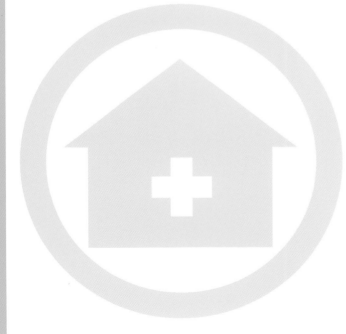

CONVENTIONAL REMEDIES

Drinking a lot of water and just being active can sometimes be enough to flush a small stone through the body. Painkillers can be taken to help with the pain. If there's a kidney infection alongside the stones, then antibiotics may be required. For large stones that are not passed through naturally, a treatment called extracorporeal shock wave lithotripsy is used under local anaesthetic to break down the kidney stones. If stones get stuck in the ureter or are very large, surgery may be required to remove them.

NATURAL REMEDIES

There are some helpful self-help home remedies for you to try. Swap your usual teabags for a pot of dandelion or nettle tea. They both act as natural diuretics, helping your kidneys to function well. Use two 15ml tablespoons dried leaves, or you can buy them as teabags. Ideally, drink two to three cups of dandelion or nettle tea daily.

HERBAL REMEDIES Use herbs with diuretic properties to increase and dilute your urine, such as herbal tinctures of gravel root, stone root or parsley piert. To ease an inflamed urinary system, you can take a tincture of marshmallow and couch grass. Just dilute 1ml tincture in 5ml water three times a day.

 NUTRITIONAL MEDICINE Take vitamin B6, vitamin K and magnesium supplements, as they may help reduce the crystallisation process that causes kidney stones to form. Take vitamin A and the amino acid lysine, to lower levels of calcium excretion.

 ## HEALING FOODS

- Eat plenty of cranberries, or drink cranberry juice, to help any associated infection.
- Include bran in your diet, as it can reduce the absorption of calcium and lower levels of calcium in the urine.

SEE YOUR DOCTOR

If you are experiencing severe pain in the kidney region and any other symptoms of kidney stones, don't self-diagnose or try and treat it yourself – always see a doctor for a professional diagnosis and treatment.

201

Caution

Natural remedies can be helpful for future kidney stone prevention and for helping ease any further symptoms, but they should not be used as a first port of call.

TOP 20
Homeopathic remedies

Homeopathy is a holistic treatment, which is based on the principle that 'like cures like'. Diluted natural substances are used to stimulate the body's natural defences. The remedy used will depend on the ailment and symptoms, but treatment should always be on a constitutional basis, taking into account the patient's personality, emotional attributes, personal likes and dislikes, and physical features. It is better to consult a qualified homeopathic practitioner rather than self-diagnose.

1 ARGENTUM NITRICUM

Constitutional features cheerful and outgoing when well; anxious when unwell

Used for nervous disorders, anxiety, chronic fatigue syndrome, depression; and digestive problems, including indigestion and irritable bowel syndrome

2 ARSENICUM ALBUM

Constitutional features restless and anxious with desire for order and tidiness

Used for digestive problems, food poisoning, diarrhoea, vomiting, peptic ulcers; and skin ailments, e.g. eczema and psoriasis; conjunctivitis; sore throat; and dandruff

3 BELLADONNA

Constitutional features lively and sensitive but prone to sudden-onset illness

Used for fever, headaches, neuralgia; arthritis; tonsillitis, earache; German measles; abdominal pain with nausea and vomiting

4 BRYONIA ALBA

Constitutional features for people in business working hard, who may feel angry or disappointed

Used for acute illnesses; rheumatism, arthritis, sciatica and backache; headache; diarrhoea, indigestion and gastritis

5 CHAMOMILLA

Constitutional features constitutional medicine, for hypersensitive people

Used for toothache, teething and earache; arthritis; painful periods; withdrawal symptoms after giving up caffeine, alcohol or smoking

6 HEPAR SULPHURIS

Constitutional features mentally and physically sensitive

Used for skin conditions, acne, boils, abscesses; sore throat, coughs, bronchitis; neuralgia

7 IGNATIA

Constitutional features for idealists, romantics, grief and disappointment

Used for digestive problems, diarrhoea, stomach cramps; headaches; coughs

8 IPECACUANHA

Constitutional features constitutional medicine

Used for asthma; coughs; morning sickness, nausea and vomiting

9 LACHESIS

Constitutional features intense, competitive, talkative, prone to jealousy

Used for depression; menopause; asthma; back pain, sciatica; neuralgia

10 MERCURIUS SOLUBILIS

Constitutional features calm, reserved, susceptible to temperature changes

Used for arthritis; colds, sore throat, tonsillitis, ear infections; mouth ulcers; colitis

11 NATRUM MURIATICUM

Constitutional features constitutional medicine, for sensitive people with suppressed emotions

Used for back pain; colds; headache, premenstrual tension; mouth ulcers, cold sores; eczema, psoriasis; irritable bowel syndrome; asthma

12 NUX VOMICA

Constitutional features ambitious workaholics, impatient, competitive

Used for stress, fatigue; sleep problems, insomnia; headache; asthma, hay fever; irritable bowel syndrome, peptic ulcers, colic

13 PHOSPHORUS

Constitutional features enthusiasm for life, empathy for other people, fear of being alone

Used for respiratory problems, bronchitis, coughs; digestive disorders, peptic ulcers, gastroenteritis; angina; nose bleeds

14 PULSATILLA

Constitutional features emotional, timid, or symptoms due to hormonal changes and pregnancy

Used for asthma, hay fever; arthritis, diarrhoea, constipation, irritable bowel syndrome; pregnancy sickness; period problems, postnatal depression; conjunctivitis; ear infections

15 RHUS TOXICODENDRON

Constitutional features cheerful and lively when well; depressed and agitated when ill

Used for rheumatism, arthritis, sprains, neck pain and stiffness; influenza; shingles, chicken pox; eczema

16 SABINA

Constitutional features do not feel cold but intolerant of heat

Used for heavy periods, nosebleeds; arthritis, gout; back pain

17 SANGUINARIA

Constitutional features regularly recurring conditions, such as migraine

Used for allergies, asthma, hay fever; migraine, menopausal hot flushes; shoulder pain

18 SEPIA

Constitutional features exhausted, feeling drained and dull

Used for headaches; backache; constipation; fatigue, depression, premenstrual syndrome; cystitis, nausea in pregnancy

19 SILICA

Constitutional features delicate, lacking stamina, sensitive, poor self-esteem

Used for abscesses, skin infections; headaches

20 SULPHUR

Constitutional features intellectual, self-confident, self-absorbed

Used for arthritis; acne, eczema, abscesses; conjunctivitis; diarrhoea; tonsillitis; migraine; dandruff

203

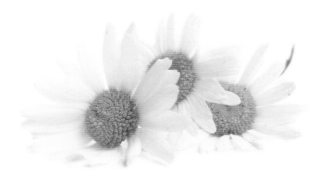

Emotional and nervous disorders

We lead such busy, stressful lives that emotional disorders and psychological illnesses are relatively common and can profoundly affect our quality of life. Our emotional health is shaped by our experiences, relationships and body image. People who feel valued and comfortable about themselves, who can manage stress, can forge strong, close relationships with family and friends, can adapt to changes in their lives, and recover rapidly from setbacks tend to be psychologically healthy and less likely to suffer from emotional and nervous disorders.

Some health problems, such as headaches and migraines, are not indicative of your emotional health, but fatigue, anxiety and insomnia may be a temporary reaction to a difficult stressful situation or symptomatic of deeper psychological disorders. Some health conditions, such as chronic fatigue syndrome (ME), are still controversial and experts are divided as to whether they are physical or entirely psychological illnesses.

You cannot eliminate stress, difficult situations and trauma from your life, but you can take positive action to enable you to cope with them, to manage your condition, and to adapt accordingly. As with other aspects of your health, good nutrition and regular exercise have an important role to play. Natural remedies and therapies, including yoga, meditation, relaxation, massage, aromatherapy, herbal medicine and homeopathy, are also helpful. In addition, depending on the problem and its severity, there are many conventional treatments, such as medication, counselling, cognitive behavioural therapy and self-help groups.

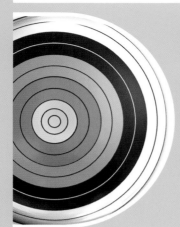

Headache

Most people experience the head and neck pain associated with a headache at some point. Headaches can be brought on by a variety of factors, including tiredness, hunger, stress, bad posture, sunlight, vision problems, or certain foods and drinks. They can vary according to the severity of the symptoms and the frequency with which they occur.

 ## SYMPTOMS

▷ Mild to moderate pain on both sides of your head
▷ Pressure around your head
▷ Tightened neck muscles
▷ Pressure behind your eyes

 ## PREVENTION

In order to prevent headaches, it helps to understand what is causing them, so that you can make the appropriate lifestyle changes.

• Note how often you get headaches, how severe they are and how long they last. This will help you identify what triggers them. For example, you may find you get headaches when you are hungry, anxious, driving, or after working at a computer screen for long periods.
• Try to manage your stress levels. Stress is a frequent cause of tension headaches.
• Take regular exercise. Aim for 30 minutes of moderate physical activity five days a week. This helps to reduce stress and the likelihood of getting a stress-related headache.
• Are you using painkillers frequently? You may get withdrawal headaches when you are not taking them. Either stop taking the painkillers altogether, or try to wean yourself off them gradually.

 ## Did you know?

There are many different types of headache, including tension-type headache, cluster headache, migraine, hypnic headache, primary thunderclap headache as well as medication-overuse headache. Tension-type headache is the most common.

CONVENTIONAL REMEDIES

Try to identify the cause of your headaches and eliminate it. Over-the-counter painkillers can be taken for most headaches, such as paracetamol, aspirin or ibuprofen. The antidepressant amitriptyline may be prescribed for frequent headaches; this helps to reduce the occurrence and duration of headaches. Cognitive behavioural therapy (a talking treatment) can help you to deal with stress.

 NATURAL REMEDIES

The following remedies may help to provide welcome pain relief from headaches.

ACUPUNCTURE This treatment stimulates the flow of energy through your body to relieve pain and reduce the frequency of headaches.

CHIROPRACTIC Relieves muscular tension in the head, neck and shoulders and corrects posture to stop the pain of headaches.

REFLEXOLOGY This works on the spinal reflex areas of the foot to reduce tension in the spine.

 HERBAL REMEDIES

- For tension headaches, drink rosemary or lime blossom tea.
- For fatigue headaches, sip chamomile tea.

 AROMATHERAPY

Try these essential oils for relief from headaches.

- Add a few drops of lavender, peppermint or bergamot essential oils to a carrier oil and massage into the back of your neck.
- Add eucalyptus, spearmint, sweet marjoram or basil essential oils to a vaporiser.
- Add several drops of peppermint, grapefruit or rosewood essential oils to a nice warm bath.

 HOMEOPATHIC REMEDIES

The homeopathic remedy you select will depend on the type of headache you have.

Belladonna 30C: Take two tablets three times daily for a throbbing, pulsating headache.

Nux vomica 30C: Take two tablets three times daily for a headache triggered by food or drink.

Arnica 30C: Take two tablets four times daily for a headache caused by trauma or injury.

 SEE YOUR DOCTOR

Although most headaches don't require medical attention, you should see your doctor if:

- You have frequent headaches (on more than 15 days of the month)
- Your headache comes on suddenly and is extremely painful
- You have a stiff neck, high temperature, a rash, nausea or vomiting
- You start having headaches after an accident or head injury
- You feel weak, numb, confused, or you have slurred speech
- You have disturbed vision.

 IMMEDIATE RELIEF

To bring instant relief, apply a hot flannel to your forehead or neck and hold it there for a few minutes.

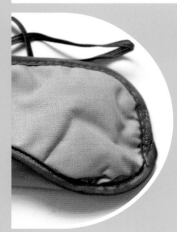

Migraine

Migraines are severe, throbbing headaches, which may last just a few hours or even several days. They can be triggered by a number of different factors, such as stress, dehydration, tiredness, smoking, chocolate, cheese, red wine or orange juice. Anyone can suffer from migraines, but they are more common among women than men.

 SYMPTOMS

▷ Intense pain on one side of the head, or at the front of the head
▷ Nausea or vomiting
▷ Visual disturbances, such as partial loss of vision or flashing lights
▷ Sensitivity to light, sound or smells
▷ Stomach ache
▷ Feeling hot or cold, or sweating

 PREVENTION

In order to prevent migraine attacks, it helps if you can identify the factors that trigger them, so that you can try to avoid them.

• Keep a diary of when your migraines occur, the symptoms you have, how long they last, and anything you ate beforehand.
• Eat regular meals. Fluctuating blood sugar levels caused by eating irregularly can trigger migraines.
• Avoid dehydration by getting plenty of fluids.
• Establish a regular sleeping pattern; try to go to bed and get up at the same time each day.
• Try to manage your stress levels.
• Taking regular exercise may help to prevent migraines.

 CONVENTIONAL REMEDIES

Many people find they are able to manage their migraines by keeping away from the things that cause them. In the event of a migraine attack, it helps to lie down in a quiet, dark room. Over-the-counter remedies, such as paracetamol, aspirin or ibuprofen, help to relieve symptoms. Triptan medicines work by constricting blood vessels in the brain. Your doctor may also prescribe anti-sickness medicines or non-steroidal anti-inflammatory drugs, and, in some cases, referral to a migraine clinic may be necessary.

 Did you know?

It is not clear what causes migraines. It is thought that blood vessels in the brain become narrower, temporarily restricting blood supply. When they widen again, this causes a severe headache.

NATURAL REMEDIES

Try the following natural remedies and therapies to reduce the severity of migraines.

NUTRITIONAL MEDICINE Migraines could be related to low levels of magnesium. Good food sources of this mineral include spinach, nuts, seeds and whole-grain cereals.

ACUPUNCTURE This may be effective in reducing the frequency of migraines by using needles to stimulate the flow of energy through the body.

AROMATHERAPY Add a few drops of rosemary essential oil to a bowl of steaming hot water. Cover your head with a towel, lean over the bowl and inhale the steam for 10 minutes.

 HERBAL REMEDIES

Taking the following herbs may help to relieve the symptoms of migraines.

- Take 380mg feverfew once or twice daily.
- Take 60mg butterbur two to four times a day.
- Take 530mg dong quai twice daily.

 HOMEOPATHIC REMEDIES

The remedy will depend on the type of pain:

Bryonia 30C: Take two tablets three times daily for sharp pain in the forehead or back of the head, which may be accompanied by either nausea or vomiting.

Natrum muriaticum 30C: Take two tablets four times daily for a beating pain in the head which is made better when lying down in a dark room.

Lachesis 6C: Take two tablets three times daily for migraine which is triggered by food or drink.

 SEE YOUR DOCTOR

You should see your doctor if:

- You have a sudden, severe headache for the first time, especially if you are over 50
- You can't seem to do anything to relieve your symptoms
- You are having frequent migraines (daily or weekly)
- You experience fever, vomiting or a rash
- You keep having stiffness, numbness or tingling on the same side of your body.

 Quick fix

For some migraine sufferers, drinking two or three glasses of cold tap water at the first signs of an oncoming migraine may be sufficient to prevent it.

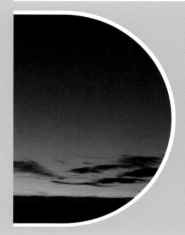

Fatigue

Fatigue is characterised by tiredness and exhaustion, which can have either a physical or an emotional cause. People may experience fatigue due to sleeping difficulties, stress, anxiety, being overweight or underweight, too little exercise or pregnancy. Sometimes fatigue can be so severe that it interferes with normal day-to-day life.

 SYMPTOMS

▷ Physical or mental tiredness
▷ Weakness and lack of energy
▷ Palpitations (irregular or rapid heart beat)
▷ Feeling faint
▷ Breathlessness
▷ Difficulty concentrating and making decisions
▷ Lack of motivation
▷ Depression

 PREVENTION

Lifestyle changes, such as having a good diet, taking more exercise and getting more sleep, should help to prevent fatigue.

- Eat plenty of fruit, vegetables and protein to maintain your energy levels. Don't skip meals as this will lead to fluctuating blood sugar levels and cause fatigue.
- Try to avoid sugary foods, such as cakes and biscuits. These will cause a surge in blood sugar levels, which will then drop quickly leaving you tired and irritable.
- Take regular exercise. Aim for 30 minutes of moderate-intensity physical activity five days a week, but don't exercise just before going to bed.
- Try to find ways to cope with stress, and learn how to relax.
- Go to bed and get up at the same time each day, and don't take naps during the day.
- Don't eat a heavy meal before going to bed.
- Avoid caffeine, alcohol and tobacco before you go to bed, and cut down on these substances in general.
- Try and do something relaxing before bedtime each night, such as taking a warm bath.

 Did you know?

Lack of physical activity can cause fatigue. If you don't exercise regularly, your level of fitness falls, so when you do need to be active, you get tired more easily.

CONVENTIONAL REMEDIES

People often find their fatigue improves by having a good rest, eating properly and exercising. If fatigue is caused by an underlying medical condition, such as anaemia or a thyroid disorder, appropriate treatment should relieve any associated tiredness.

 ## NATURAL REMEDIES

You may find the following natural remedies are useful for combating fatigue and making you feel more energetic.

NUTRITIONAL MEDICINE Make sure your diet contains adequate amounts of B vitamins, which are important for the release of energy from food. Good sources include meat, yeast extract, beans and bananas.

AROMATHERAPY For an energising, stimulating massage oil, try blending six drops of grapefruit and four drops of ginger essential oils with 30ml jojoba oil.

ACUPUNCTURE Thin needles are placed at specific locations on your body in order to unblock the flow of energy and relieve fatigue.

 ## HERBAL REMEDIES

You may like to try taking one of the following herbs to relieve fatigue and boost your energy.

- 1–2ml American ginseng extract three times daily.
- Four drops of gentian extract at least four times a day.
- 550mg ginger root twice daily.
- 1–4ml Kola nut extract three times a day.
- 500mg Siberian ginseng three times daily.

 ## EXERCISE

Deep breathing exercises may relieve fatigue by releasing tension and improving oxygen circulation.
1 Lie on your back and relax with your knees bent.
2 Place one hand on your chest and the other on your stomach.
3 Breathe in deeply through your nose and exhale through your mouth.
NOTE Breathe in from your abdomen – you should feel your stomach rise higher than your chest. Continue this breathing exercise for a few minutes.

 ## SEE YOUR DOCTOR

If you feel constantly tired and self-help measures don't seem to be working, see your doctor. Fatigue can be caused by other conditions, such as anaemia, asthma, thyroid problems, diabetes, malnutrition, infection or chronic fatigue syndrome.

Caution

Don't take high-energy fizzy commercial drinks to relieve your fatigue. They are full of sugar and, after a brief blood sugar surge, you will end up feeling even worse than you did before.

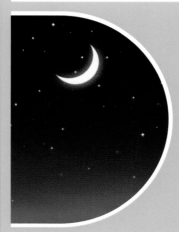

Insomnia

Most people will have trouble sleeping sometimes, but insomnia is a chronic sleep disorder, characterised by the frequent inability to fall asleep or stay asleep. This can go on for days, months or even years. There are, however, things you can do to help yourself get a good night's sleep and wake up feeling refreshed the following day.

 SYMPTOMS

▷ Difficulty getting to sleep
▷ Frequently waking in the night
▷ Waking early in the morning, and inability to get back to sleep
▷ Difficulty concentrating
▷ Irritability and tiredness

 PREVENTION

Simple changes to your evening routine can help you to sleep better. Prevention is better than cure, so try the following measures and see if they help.

- Don't take naps during the day.
- Ensure your bed is comfortable. Use thick curtains, blinds or an eye mask to block out light, and wear earplugs if noise disturbs you.
- Don't use the bedroom for activities unrelated to sleep, such as watching television, making phone calls or eating.
- Ensure that you always go to bed and get up at the same time every day.
- Write down any worries you may have before going to bed.
- Do something relaxing every night before you go to bed, such as taking a warm bath.
- Don't eat a heavy meal late in the evening.
- Avoid coffee, tea, alcohol or nicotine six hours before bed.
- Exercise regularly, but not within four hours of going to bed.
- Avoid checking the clock throughout the night. If you can't sleep, get up and do something else for a while.

 Did you know?

There is no 'normal' amount of sleep that is right for every individual. In general, most adults sleep for seven to nine hours each night, but older people tend to need less sleep, while children need a lot more.

CONVENTIONAL REMEDIES

Treatment for insomnia involves addressing the cause of the disorder, such as reducing caffeine and alcohol intake. Sleeping tablets, such as benzodiazepines, Z medicines or melatonin, help aid sleep but are only for short-term use. Cognitive behavioural therapy may be recommended to help change your sleeping habits and negative thoughts about your insomnia.

 ## NATURAL REMEDIES

There are many natural remedies you can try to help you sleep. Here are some options.

NUTRITIONAL MEDICINE Milk, eggs, turkey, chicken and fish are good sources of the amino acid tryptophan, which is thought to have a calming effect and help to induce sleep.

ACUPUNCTURE This treatment calms your nervous system, relieves stress and re-balances your energy, giving you a sense of deep relaxation.

REFLEXOLOGY Apply firm pressure to the top of the pad of your big toe, to clear your mind and body in preparation for sleep.

 ## HERBAL REMEDIES

To aid relaxation, try one of these popular remedies.

- Drink chamomile tea to soothe and calm you.
- Take one 450mg capsule of valerian root before bed to aid sleep.
- Take one to two 250mg Rhodiola rosea capsules daily to help relieve stress.

 ## AROMATHERAPY

Essential oils can calm and soothe and prepare you for a restful night's sleep.

- Place a drop of soothing lavender essential oil on a tissue, and put it under your pillow.
- Have a warm bath with a few added drops of marjoram, rose or roman chamomile essential oils to relax you before bed.
- Mix up to 15 drops of ylang ylang, sandalwood or clary sage essential oils (you can create your own combination) with 30ml jojoba oil and use it for a relaxing massage.

 ## SEE YOUR DOCTOR

Insomnia can sometimes have an underlying cause, such as a physical or psychological medical condition. If it is persistent and is affecting your physical and mental health, you should see your doctor. After the appropriate treatment, your insomnia may go away.

 ## Quick fix

Lettuce has been used as a soporific since ancient times. Eat a lettuce sandwich before going to bed. Alternatively, a hot, soothing milky drink may help to relax you.

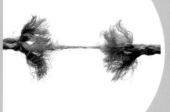

Stress

Stress is the mental or physical strain you experience when you are under pressure. This can be caused when you are faced with situations that you find difficult to handle. Common causes of stress include a wide range of factors, such as work pressures, money problems, relationship and family issues and bereavement.

 SYMPTOMS

▷ Anxiety, depression, frustration or tearfulness
▷ Loss of control
▷ Difficulty concentrating
▷ Behavioural changes
▷ Headaches and other aches and pains
▷ Difficulty sleeping and restlessness
▷ Changes in appetite
▷ Sweating
▷ Nervous twitching, or pins and needles
▷ Palpitations (rapid or irregular heart beat), breathlessness or dizziness
▷ Constipation or diarrhoea

 PREVENTION

Identifying the things that make you stressed and learning how to cope with them in a different way is the key to preventing symptoms of stress. You also need to look after your physical and mental health.

- Learn some relaxation techniques to calm you down and relieve muscle tension.
- Make an effort to do things you enjoy. See your friends, read a book, listen to music or do whatever makes you happy.
- Write down the things that are making you feel stressed; this can help you work out ways of organising and prioritising your responsibilities.
- Talk to someone about how you feel; this can give you a new perspective on the things that are troubling you.
- Eat a healthy, balanced diet with plenty of fruit and vegetables.
- Limit your alcohol and caffeine intake, and don't smoke.
- Exercise regularly.

 Did you know?

When under stress, your body releases chemicals, including cortisol, adrenaline and noradrenaline. These chemicals build up and produce the emotional and physical symptoms that we associate with stress.

CONVENTIONAL REMEDIES

Learning how to handle difficult situations, having a good work-life balance, and looking after your health are all important for managing stress effectively. Stress and anger management techniques, and talking therapies, such as cognitive behavioural therapy or counselling, can teach you how to deal with stress. Medication may be given to treat anxiety or depression, if these are symptoms of stress.

 # NATURAL REMEDIES

For natural relief from stress, you can try taking the following therapies.

NUTRITIONAL MEDICINE Vitamin C is an antioxidant that may help reduce the physical and psychological symptoms of stress. Good sources include red and green peppers, oranges and other citrus fruits, kiwi fruit, broccoli, strawberries and Brussels sprouts.

AROMATHERAPY Blend nine drops of bergamot, three drops of geranium and three drops of frankincense essential oils with 60ml jojoba oil. Add one-quarter of this blend to a nice warm bath.

REFLEXOLOGY Massage the ball of your foot to help you relax, and gently tug your toes to release tension in your head and shoulders.

 # HERBAL REMEDIES

- Take 500mg Korean ginseng three times daily to help your body cope with the effects of stress.
- Green tea may help to reduce levels of stress hormones and promote relaxation.
- Take 450mg Valerian root daily to reduce tension, anxiety and irritability and aid restful sleep.

 # HOMEOPATHIC REMEDIES

The following remedies may help to relieve the symptoms of stress.

Aconite 6C: Take two tablets four times daily for anxiety, restlessness and trouble sleeping.

Arsenicum 6C: Take two tablets four times daily for worry with an upset stomach.

Phosphorus 6C: Take two tablets three times daily for anxiety and nervousness.

 # SEE YOUR DOCTOR

If you are having difficulty dealing with stress, see your doctor. Stress is a common problem, and they will be able to help you cope. It may also be necessary to run some tests to check that your symptoms are not due to another underlying medical condition.

 # IMMEDIATE RELIEF

If you are in a traumatic situation, an emergency or you are feeling very stressed, take some Bach Rescue Remedy to calm you down.

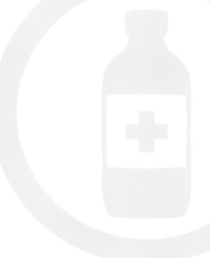

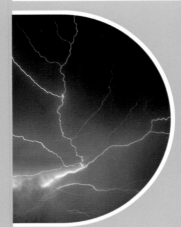

Neuralgia

Neuralgia is extreme nerve pain in the face or other parts of the body. Pain in the face may come on suddenly and last for a few seconds or minutes at a time, or pain in the body may last for days or even months. Neuralgia can be a very difficult condition to live with – even smiling or the lightest touch of a breeze can cause pain.

 SYMPTOMS

▷ Tingling, numbness
▷ Stabbing, shooting, shock-like pains in the face
▷ Pain in the mouth, teeth and gums
▷ A burning, aching sensation
▷ Throbbing pains in the body
▷ Intense itching

 PREVENTION

To prevent pain from neuralgia, it helps to avoid the things that trigger an attack or make the pain worse.

• Wind and draughts can trigger pain, so avoid sitting near open windows or air conditioning. When outside in breezy weather, protect your face with a scarf.
• Avoid very hot or cold drinks that can trigger pain. Drinking through a straw can help prevent liquid from causing pain in your mouth.
• Rough, synthetic or tight clothing can aggravate your skin and cause pain. Try wearing loose clothing made from natural fibres, such as cotton.

 CONVENTIONAL REMEDIES

For trigeminal neuralgia, anticonvulsants, such as carbamazepine, are prescribed to numb pain and help settle nerve impulses. If these are ineffective, surgery may be recommended to release pressure on the trigeminal nerve. Other options include stereotactic radiosurgery, or injections to numb the pain. Postherpetic neuralgia is treated with painkillers, such as paracetamol or codeine, or tricyclic antidepressants to reduce sensitivity to pain. Topical creams containing capsaicin (made from hot peppers), or lidocaine patches containing local anaesthetic may help to relieve pain.

 Did you know?

Trigeminal neuralgia is thought to be caused by blood vessels pressing on the trigeminal nerve, which runs through the face. Postherpetic neuralgia may be a result of nerve damage caused by shingles infection, and can occur in different parts of the body.

216

NATURAL REMEDIES

The following natural remedies may be helpful.

NUTRITIONAL MEDICINE Eat more foods that are rich in B vitamins, such as brewer's yeast, beans, pulses and dairy products. These provide support for the nervous system.

AROMATHERAPY Place a few drops of calming lavender or chamomile essential oils in a carrier oil and massage into painful areas.

ELECTRO-ACUPUNCTURE This is similar to traditional acupuncture, but a low-frequency electric current (1Hz) is passed down the needles.

 HOMEOPATHIC REMEDIES

Treatment depends on the type of pain you have.

Kali phosphate 6C: Take four tablets three times daily for pain that is relieved by cold.

Belladonna 30C: Take two tablets three times daily for pain that suddenly comes and goes.

Magnesium phosphate 6C: Take four tablets three times daily for pain that is relieved with warmth.

 HERBAL REMEDIES

The following remedies may provide some relief.

- Take 1 or 2ml passion flower tincture up to three times daily, to soothe and calm your central nervous system.
- Take one 150g capsule of St Johns wort three times daily to reduce inflammation, or 1ml of extract in water up to three times a day.
- Take 15 to 30 drops of wood betony two to three times daily; this has a calming, sedative effect.

 SEE YOUR DOCTOR

If you suspect that you have neuralgia, see your doctor. Facial pain can also be caused by dental problems and sinus infection; these need to be ruled out before it can be ascertained whether or not neuralgia is responsible.

 IMMEDIATE RELIEF

If your neuralgia is not aggravated by cold temperatures, you can place gel-filled cold packs in the freezer and hold them against painful areas to numb the pain.

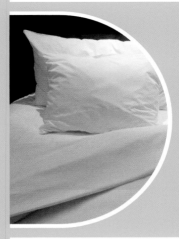

Chronic fatigue syndrome (ME)

Chronic fatigue syndrome is long-term general weakness and muscle pain. Many people have symptoms that come and go, but for others, the condition is so debilitating and serious that they have to spend much of their time in bed, and they may even end up wheelchair-bound.

 SYMPTOMS

▷ Generally feeling unwell
▷ Physical and mental exhaustion
▷ Muscle aches and pains
▷ Poor memory and difficulty concentrating
▷ Difficulty moving
▷ Headaches
▷ Sleeping difficulties
▷ Sensitivity to light and sound
▷ Depression
▷ Painful lymph nodes
▷ Stomach problems
▷ Sore throat
▷ Dizziness and nausea
▷ Palpitations (rapid or irregular heart beat)

 PREVENTION

There are positive things that you can do to help prevent the severity of the symptoms associated with chronic fatigue syndrome.

- Learn to manage your stress levels, and make time for relaxation.
- Eat a healthy balanced diet with plenty of fruit and vegetables. Be sure to include foods that release energy slowly, such as oats, whole-grain cereals, beans and pulses.
- People with chronic fatigue syndrome are often sensitive to substances such as alcohol and caffeine, and certain foods, so try to avoid these.
- Keep a diary, so you can track how your energy levels change from day to day. This will help you to pace yourself better.
- Improve your quality of sleep by relaxing before bed each night. Go to bed and get up at the same time each day and try to avoid taking naps during the day.

 Did you know?

It is not clear what causes chronic fatigue syndrome. It may be triggered by viral infections, such as glandular fever, a genetic predisposition, stress, depression or trauma.

CONVENTIONAL REMEDIES

It is important for people to ensure they get the right balance of physical activity and rest that is suitable for them. Painkillers or antidepressants may be prescribed to relieve symptoms. Cognitive behavioural therapy is a talking treatment that helps people to cope with the effects of chronic fatigue syndrome. Supervised, graded exercise therapy aims to increase physical activity slowly, and tailors exercise duration and intensity to your own limits.

 NATURAL REMEDIES

You may find the following natural remedies helpful, depending on your symptoms.

NUTRITIONAL MEDICINE Take 100mg Coenzyme Q10 per day for healthy cell function and energy production.

AROMATHERAPY Add 12 drops of rosemary and 18 drops of bergamot essential oils to a spray bottle containing 90ml distilled water. Use as a reviving, energising air freshener.

ACUPUNCTURE This stimulates your body's energy to relieve fatigue, boost your immune system and help you sleep better. See a qualified practitioner.

 HERBAL REMEDIES

- Take 500mg Korean ginseng three times daily to help increase stamina, relieve stress, boost immune function and improve concentration.
- Mix 1ml echinacea extract in a little water two to five times daily to boost your immune system and reduce the risk of infection.
- Take 470mg astragalus three to six times daily to strengthen your immune system and reduce inflammation.

 HOMEOPATHIC REMEDIES

The following remedies may help relieve symptoms. Take whichever is appropriate for you.

Arsenicum 6C: Take two tablets four times daily when feeling cold and weak.

Gelsemium 6C: Take two tablets four times daily when feeling physically tired with heavy, aching muscles.

Pulsatilla 6C: Take two tablets four times daily for aches and pains and when feeling emotional.

 SEE YOUR DOCTOR

If you suspect that you have chronic fatigue syndrome, you should see your doctor, who will be able to help you manage your condition. It may be necessary to conduct some tests to rule out other conditions that have similar symptoms to chronic fatigue syndrome, such as kidney disease, anaemia or thyroid problems.

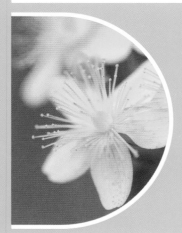

Depression

Depression is a mental illness that is characterised by feelings of sadness and hopelessness lasting for more than two weeks. Depression interferes with everyday life, preventing people from getting on with the things they would normally do. Symptoms can be psychological, social or physical, and can affect anyone at any age.

 SYMPTOMS

▷ Feeling low, with negative thoughts about the future
▷ Little interest in doing things you used to enjoy
▷ Anxiety and low self-esteem
▷ Inability to concentrate
▷ Trouble making decisions
▷ Irritability
▷ Unable to cope with normal things
▷ Feelings of guilt
▷ Trouble sleeping
▷ Tiredness and lack of energy
▷ Aches and pains
▷ Lack of appetite and weight loss (but sometimes weight gain)
▷ Loss of libido
▷ Social inactivity, work and home life problems
▷ Thoughts of self-harm

 PREVENTION

A healthy lifestyle is important for preventing depression. The following can be helpful.

- Eat a balanced diet with plenty of fresh fruit and vegetables. Try to avoid sugar highs and lows, caused by foods such as cakes, biscuits and chocolate.
- Exercise regularly. Exercise will help you feel better about yourself and get you out of the house.
- Don't drink excessively. Men should drink no more than 21 units of alcohol per week, and women no more than 14.
- Avoid drugs such as cannabis and cocaine; these are likely to make you feel worse.
- If you smoke heavily, try to cut down or, better still, stop altogether.
- Make an effort with social relationships – with friends, family and work colleagues.
- Keep up with your interests and hobbies.
- Learn how to deal with stress and relax.

 Did you know?

People with a family history of depression have an increased risk of experiencing depression themselves. Depression can also be triggered by life events, such as bereavement or loss of employment.

CONVENTIONAL REMEDIES

For mild depression, self-help measures, such as self-help books, an exercise programme or local-support groups, may be all you need to recover. If depression is more severe, there are antidepressants, such as SSRIs (selective serotonin reuptake inhibitors), which alter levels of chemicals in the brain, to improve mood. Psychological treatments, such as cognitive behavioural therapy, interpersonal therapy or counselling, may also be recommended.

 ## NATURAL REMEDIES

You may like to try the following treatments alongside conventional remedies.

NUTRITIONAL MEDICINE A lack of omega-3 fatty acids in the diet (found in cold-water fish, flax seeds and walnuts) may contribute to symptoms of depression. If your diet is lacking, consider taking an omega-3 supplement.

ACUPUNCTURE This treatment frees up the body's energy, increases the production of 'feel good' chemicals in the brain, and promotes relaxation.

AROMATHERAPY Aromatherapy massage with essential oils, such as orange, sandalwood or lavender, can help aid relaxation and relieve symptoms of depression.

 ## HERBAL REMEDIES

Here are some herbal remedies that you might find useful in treating depression.

- St John's wort may be as effective as antidepressants. Take 300mg three times daily. **NOTE** St John's wort can interfere with other medications, so check with your doctor if necessary.
- Try taking 60mg of ginkgo biloba daily to relieve symptoms.

 ## EXERCISE

Research shows that exercise is an effective way of treating depression and boosting self-esteem. It is thought to work by increasing levels of serotonin (a neurotransmitter in the brain) and endorphins (the body's natural painkillers). Try doing 30 minutes of physical activity, such as running, brisk walking, or aerobics three to five times a week. You may need to work up to this, depending on your fitness level. Also consider other types of exercise, such as weight training, yoga or tai chi.

 ## SEE YOUR DOCTOR

In severe cases of depression, early diagnosis is very important. If you are feeling depressed and the symptoms persist and do not improve as time passes, you should see your doctor or seek professional advice and counselling.

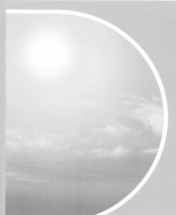

Seasonal affective disorder

Seasonal affective disorder (SAD) is a type of depression experienced by people during the winter. Symptoms occur repeatedly at the same time each year, and improve over spring and summer. As with other types of depression, SAD affects normal daily life and can be quite debilitating.

 SYMPTOMS

▷ Feeling low and unhappy
▷ Irritability and tearfulness
▷ Stress, anxiety and low self-esteem
▷ Lack of motivation
▷ Little interest in things you used to enjoy
▷ Difficulty concentrating and making decisions
▷ Lack of energy
▷ Spending more time sleeping
▷ Feelings of guilt
▷ Increased appetite (especially for carbohydrates) and weight gain

 PREVENTION

You can help prevent symptoms of SAD by getting as much exposure to natural light as possible. You may also benefit from some lifestyle changes.

• Try and get outside for a short walk each day, whatever the weather.

• Make sure your indoor environment is as bright as possible, and try to sit near a window.

• Exercise regularly, outside if possible. Exercise increases the level of serotonin (the 'feel good' hormone) in the brain. Aim for 30 minutes of moderate to vigorous physical activity five times a week.

• Eat a healthy, well-balanced diet with plenty of fresh fruit and vegetables. Eating properly can have a profound effect on your mood.

• Try to reduce your stress levels, and learn how to relax.

 ## Did you know?

It is not clear what causes SAD, but it is thought to be related to a lack of sunlight during the winter months. Reduced sunlight decreases the production of serotonin, a chemical in the brain, which is found to be low in people with depression.

CONVENTIONAL REMEDIES

Antidepressants, such as selective serotonin reuptake inhibitors (SSRIs), increase the level of serotonin in the brain and improve mood. Talking therapies, such as cognitive behavioural therapy, counselling or psychotherapy, may be recommended. Light therapy involves sitting beside a light box (a special lamp that gives out bright light). This imitates natural sunlight and stimulates the production of serotonin, while reducing the production of melatonin (a hormone that induces sleep).

 ## NATURAL REMEDIES

The following remedies may help you to feel better and relieve the symptoms of SAD.

AROMATHERAPY For an energising and stimulating air freshener, add 18 drops of orange and 12 drops of grapefruit essential oils to a spray bottle containing 90ml distilled water.

REFLEXOLOGY Try massaging the pads of the big toes. These areas correspond to the parts of the brain responsible for regulating mood.

ACUPUNCTURE This treatment regulates energy flow and rebalances your body to relieve the symptoms of depression.

 ## HEALING FOODS

The following nutrients may help to reduce symptoms.

- The body needs tryptophan to make serotonin. It occurs in chicken, dairy products, eggs, fish, nuts and seeds. It can also be taken as a supplement in the form of 5-hydroxytryptophan (5-HTP).
- Vitamin D is very important. You get this from the action of sunlight on your skin, but it is also found in oily fish, eggs and fortified foods.
- Omega-3 fatty acids are found in oily fish, flax seeds and walnuts.

 ## HERBAL REMEDIES

You may find the following herbs and supplements useful for treating SAD.

- Take 300mg St John's Wort three times daily to treat mild to moderate depression.
- Take 1000mg Korean ginseng three times daily to reduce stress and improve your mood.
- Take 500mg dl-phenylalanine (DPLA) daily to stimulate the production of 'feel good' chemicals in your brain.
- Lemon balm is a natural antidepressant – drink it as a tea or use it in salads and soups.
- Many culinary herbs are uplifting and stimulating, so try to cook with them every day. Choose from basil, parsley, mint, thyme, rosemary, sage, ginger and cinnamon.

 ## SEE YOUR DOCTOR

If you think that you have seasonal affective disorder, you should see your doctor, who will be able to advise you about helpful treatments.

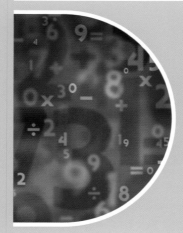

Dementia

Dementia is characterised by emotional, mental and physical deterioration caused by damage to the brain. Symptoms of dementia can develop very suddenly or more slowly over a long period of time, and the risk of dementia increases as you get older. There are different ways of treating the symptoms and improving quality of life.

 SYMPTOMS

▷ Difficulty concentrating and planning things
▷ Memory loss and confusion
▷ Short attention span and lack of motivation
▷ Depression
▷ Personality, mood and behavioural changes
▷ Delusions or hallucinations
▷ Incontinence
▷ Muscle weakness, stiffness or paralysis
▷ Slow and unsteady movements
▷ Trembling in arms and legs
▷ Sleeping difficulties
▷ Aggression and frustration
▷ Difficulty communicating

 PREVENTION

To prevent dementia in later life, it helps to keep physically and mentally active. There are other factors to consider regarding your general health and wellbeing. Pay attention to the following.

- Eat a healthy balanced diet with plenty of fruit and vegetables.
- Limit foods that are high in saturated fat.
- Reduce your salt intake to no more than six grams a day.
- Don't drink alcohol excessively. Men should have no more than four units of alcohol a day, and women no more than three.
- Maintain a healthy body weight – obesity can cause high blood pressure.
- Take regular exercise to maintain good circulation.
- Avoid smoking.

 Did you know?

There are different types of dementia, including Alzheimer's disease, vascular dementia, dementia with Lewy bodies and frontotemporal dementia. Each type of dementia affects the brain in different ways.

 CONVENTIONAL REMEDIES

If you are diagnosed with dementia, a health care plan will be drawn up, and treatment options to manage your symptoms will be discussed. Psychological treatments include cognitive stimulation, behavioural therapy, reality orientation therapy, multisensory stimulation and exercise therapy. Medications may be helpful, such as acetylcholinesterase inhibitors (AIs) or antipsychotics.

NATURAL REMEDIES

The following natural remedies may help to relieve the symptoms of dementia.

AROMATHERAPY Add a few drops of calming lavender essential oil to a vaporiser to relieve stress, agitation and depression.

HERBAL REMEDIES Take 60mg gingko biloba twice daily to support the central nervous system, increase blood circulation to the brain, and improve memory.

MUSIC THERAPY Despite the deterioration of mental function associated with dementia, people with the condition are often able to enjoy music. Music therapy can reduce agitation and improve mood, thus enhancing quality of life.

 HOMEOPATHIC REMEDIES

The following remedies may provide some support, depending on the symptoms.

Alumina 6C: Take two tablets four times daily for sluggishness and staggering.

Argentum nitricum 30C: Take two tablets three times daily for loss of control and trembling.

Cicuta 6C: Take two tablets four times daily for strange or violent behaviour.

 SEE YOUR DOCTOR

See your doctor if you suspect that you or your partner may have some of the symptoms of dementia. Symptoms associated with dementia can be caused by other conditions, such as anaemia, diabetes, kidney problems, thyroid disorders or vitamin B12 deficiency, so you need to get an accurate diagnosis.

Nutritional supplements

The following supplements may help slow the advancement of dementia.

- Phosphatidylserine may improve memory and concentration, increase awareness and relieve depression. Take 100mg three times daily.
- Vitamin E is an antioxidant important for the protection of cell membranes. Take 400 IU per day.
- Coenzyme Q10 is an antioxidant important for normal cell function. Take 100mg each day.
- Omega-3 fatty acids support the heart and blood vessels, protect cell membranes and enhance mental function. Take 1000mg of omega-3 fish oil each day.
- B vitamins are important for the healthy functioning of the brain and nervous system.
- Zinc is important for good mental function. Take 25mg per day.

Relaxation and meditation techniques

Relaxation and meditation are two important ways of relaxing the body and releasing stress and tension. They have been used in Eastern health systems for thousands of years, to help people maintain a healthy body and mind and cope more efficiently with stress. Both relaxation and meditation are easy to learn – here are some ways in which you can incorporate them into your daily life.

MUSCLE RELAXATION TECHNIQUE

Relaxing all the muscles in your body is a great way of releasing tension and stress. You can do it at any time of the day, but it's particularly good at night just before going to bed, as it can help you drift off into a deep sleep once your body is fully relaxed.

1 Lie down flat on your back, wearing loose clothing, and cover yourself with a light blanket. Close your eyes and become aware of your breathing. Take a deep breath and slowly breathe out. If you're breathing fast, try and slow down your breathing into a steady rhythm, pausing briefly as you exhale and before you take another breath.

2 Start by focusing on the muscles in your legs and feet. Tense and hold the muscles in your left foot for a few seconds, then release. Repeat by tensing and releasing the muscles in your left calf and left thigh, before repeating the sequence with your right leg and foot.

3 Next, clench each of your fists in turn and release them, wiggle your fingers, then let them relax. In turn, tense the muscles in your arms and each buttock, then release them.

4 Move onto your shoulders, lifting them up, then lower them back down. Gently move your neck from side to side to release tension, then focus on your face. Raise your eyebrows and move your mouth for a few seconds, then release to your relaxed state.

5 All the major muscles in your body should now be relaxed. Continue to lie still, breathing slowly, and enjoy the relaxed feeling. When you're ready, open your eyes and slowly get up.

SIMPLE OBJECT MEDITATION

Meditation is good for clearing the mind, relieving stress and aiding relaxation. It can also help you think more clearly. Meditating regularly, for a few minutes each day, can have positive effects on your health.

1 Choose a quiet place and find a comfortable chair to sit on. Put your arms by your side or in your lap. Find an object to focus on – it could be a lit candle, a picture, a photograph, a vase of flowers or a piece of art.

2 Breathe slowly and deeply, inhaling through your mouth, exhaling through your nose. Focus your attention on the object.

3 It's natural for your mind to wander, but when it does, bring it back to the object of your meditation and your breathing. Stay still, keep breathing, and relax. If you feel like closing your eyes, then do so.

4 Continue with your meditation until you feel ready to end. Open your eyes and slowly get up.

Men's health problems

We hear far more about women's health than men's in the media, and, traditionally, many men have been reluctant to take preventative measures, adopt self-help remedies, or consult their health professional when they do experience problems. However, many men today, especially young ones, not only value good health, physical fitness and general wellbeing but also equate it with their sexual health and virility, and they're not prepared to suffer in silence any more.

With the exception of shaving problems, most exclusively male health disorders relate to their sexual health and reproductive organs. Serious reproductive health issues include impotence (erectile dysfunction), infertility, and prostate problems (enlarged prostate and prostate cancer).

A healthy lifestyle plays a big part in preventing these problems, and regular exercise, not smoking or taking recreational drugs, drinking alcohol in moderation, good stress management, maintaining a healthy weight, and eating a diet that is rich in fruit, vegetables and omega-3 oils are all helpful. They will also increase your life expectancy and reduce the likelihood of heart disease, high blood pressure, diabetes and high cholesterol. And, as you get older, it becomes even more important to check out your weight, diet, cholesterol levels, alcohol consumption and overall fitness to maximise your chances of staying healthy for as long as possible.

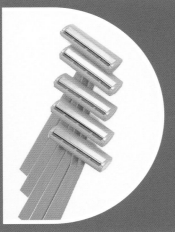

Shaving problems

Some men are prone to shaving problems while others can suddenly develop irritated skin after years of problem-free shaving. Fortunately, there are lots of things you can do to prevent bad reactions and to treat them successfully with commercial and natural remedies if they do occur.

 SYMPTOMS

▷ Sore raised lumps and bumps
▷ Dry, irritated skin
▷ A red 'razor' rash on the skin
▷ In-growing hairs

 PREVENTION

The most effective way to prevent shaving problems is to shave correctly.

- Rub your face and neck briskly with a flannel before shaving to remove dead skin cells and lift the hairs. Alternatively, use an exfoliating facial cleanser or scrub to open the pores of the skin.
- Always use a sharp razor blade to avoid catching your skin.
- Go with the grain, shaving in the direction in which your hair grows naturally – this creates less pull on the hairs and minimizes skin irritation.
- If you are prone to shaving problems, use a specially formulated razor for sensitive skin.
- Do not shave too close – you'll be less likely to cut your skin and will avoid in-growing hairs – when the hair curls and grows back into the skin.
- Never stretch or tighten the skin excessively when shaving – try to keep it relaxed.
- For preference, use a razor with disposable blade cartridges and change them regularly.
- Use a shaving gel or cream to minimise friction and irritation.
- If you find that using an electric razor is irritating your skin, switch to wet shaving, or vice versa. Alternate between the two to minimise irritation.
- Avoid highly scented shaving products and harsh aftershaves containing alcohol, which can actually dry, sting and irritate the skin. It is better to use a moisturiser after shaving.

 Did you know?

Shaving problems are most common among men of Afro-Caribbean descent with curly facial hair – about 80 per cent are affected at some time or another. The hairs curl under and grow into the follicle, causing red bumps, which are tender and can lead to scarring.

CONVENTIONAL REMEDIES

To treat shaving rashes and inflammation, you can use a hydrocortisone cream but take care and only apply it sparingly and not for long periods. If the rash does not clear up, see your doctor.

 NATURAL REMEDIES

There are many self-help treatments that you can try for razor burn, including drinking chamomile tea. Eating plenty of fresh fruit and vegetables containing vitamin C will help to clear it up quickly.

HERBAL REMEDIES Choose a shaving cream or gel with added aloe vera to soothe sensitive skin. If your skin is very sore after shaving, apply pure aloe vera gel to the affected area or pat your face with a little soothing witch hazel. Calendula (marigold) cream can also be very effective in treating shaving rashes.

AROMATHERAPY Aromatherapy shaving oils can be beneficial for men with sensitive skin – avocado and lemon oils are commonly used in these products.

 HOME-MADE REMEDIES

Some of the kitchen medicine ingredients in your refrigerator can be used to soothe irritated skin and bring welcome relief. Try the following:

- Cut a few thin slices off a cucumber and place on the irritated skin for a few minutes.
- Mash up some ripe avocado and apply to sore patches of skin for instant relief. Leave for a few minutes and then wash off.

 SEE YOUR DOCTOR

Most shaving rashes and problems clear up by themselves, but if they persist over a period of time you may have an allergy or an infection and should seek your doctor's advice.

 Quick fix

You can try rubbing in some baby rash cream after shaving – it's soothing, moisturising and is unlikely to irritate your skin.

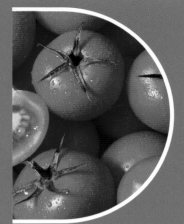

Prostate problems

The prostate is a walnut-sized sex gland, located under the bladder and encircling the urethra. Its function is to supply chemicals that are important in producing semen. However, it can become swollen, inflamed, enlarged or even infected, especially in men over 50. As they grow older, the prostate gland may enlarge due to an overgrowth of cells, thereby putting pressure on the urethra.

 SYMPTOMS

▷ Slow, reduced urination

▷ Need to urinate more frequently

▷ Delay in starting to urinate

▷ Dribbling and weak flow of urine

▷ Sensation that bladder is not fully emptied

▷ Incontinence

▷ Possible urine infections

 PREVENTION

There is a lot of conflicting advice on how to prevent prostate problems, especially prostate cancer. This disease develops slowly – and often invisibly without any symptoms – making it quite difficult to diagnose in many sufferers. For a healthy prostate, follow the advice listed below.

• Eat a healthy diet that includes lots of fresh fruit, green leafy vegetables and omega-3 oils (found in salmon, mackerel and other cold-water oily fish and flax seed oil), which reduce the risk of cancer.

• Watch your weight and don't over-eat, especially fatty foods.

• Cut down your alcohol intake, and choose wine and beer rather than spirits, which can irritate the prostate.

• Try to eat foods that contain zinc (the prostate contains more zinc than any other organ in the body). Meat, liver, seafood, wheatgerm, brewer's yeast, pumpkin seeds, eggs and mushrooms are all good sources.

 Did you know?

The risk of prostate cancer increases if you are over 50, have a family history of the disease (or of breast or ovarian cancer), are of African descent or obese. The symptoms are similar to those for an enlarged prostate but may also include pain or burning while urinating, passing urine more often and pain or stiffness in the pelvis, hips and lower back.

- Eat tomatoes or tomato products every day. The lycopene in tomatoes is a natural oxidant and some researchers think that it can help reduce swelling of the prostate gland.
- Drink plenty of fluids, especially water, but not later in the evening before going to bed.
- Reduce your consumption of caffeine – it's a diuretic. Switch to green or herbal tea and decaf coffee, and avoid caffeinated cola drinks.
- Stop smoking – as well as all its other detrimental effects on health, nicotine irritates the bladder.

CONVENTIONAL REMEDIES

If you have an enlarged prostate, your doctor may prescribe medication, such as alpha-blockers to increase the flow of urine, and/or 5-alpha-reductase inhibitors to reduce the size of your prostate. Surgery may be another option.

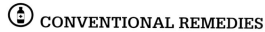 NATURAL REMEDIES

Relaxation, regular exercise and a healthy diet are all important factors in treating an enlarged prostate.
- Try to relax in a warm bath for at 20 minutes at least once a day to reduce swelling.
- Make love frequently and always ejaculate fully to remove prostatic fluid.

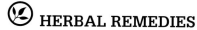 HERBAL REMEDIES

- If urination is difficult, try taking a cleansing diuretic, such as chamomile tea.
- Stinging nettle may help to reduce prostate symptoms – you can make it into a tea or take it in capsule or extract form.
- Supplements of dried nettle root, hydrangea, saw palmetto and pygeum may all be helpful in reducing swelling.

HOMEOPATHIC REMEDIES

Homeopathy may have a role to play but you should always consult a qualified homeopath and discuss your symptoms before taking homeopathic medicines. The most common remedies for prostate problems are Chimaphilia, Conium maculatum, Hepar sulphuris, Staphysagria and Thuja. Seek professional advice on which remedy is best for your symptoms.

SEE YOUR DOCTOR

If you suspect that you may have an enlarged prostate or are experiencing any problems with urination, especially if you are over 50 years old, you must consult your doctor and get it checked out immediately.

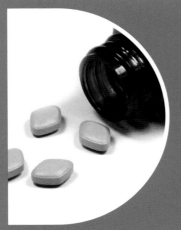

Impotence

Impotence (or erectile dysfunction) is the inability to achieve or sustain an erection that enables penetration and satisfactory sexual relations. This problem is relatively common, and 50 per cent of all men over the age of 40 experience it at some time or another. There are a number of reasons for impotence, ranging from physical problems affecting blood supply to the penis to psychological ones, such as anxiety, depression and stress.

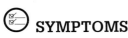 SYMPTOMS

▷ Failure to achieve or sustain an erection

 PREVENTION

The ability to achieve an erection can be influenced by many psychological and physical factors, but lifestyle and the quality of your relationship play an important role. If there are no serious underlying health issues or a physical reason for your problem, you may wish to consider the following possibilities.

- Eating a healthy diet that is low in saturated fats and contains all the essential nutrients for good health can be helpful. Make sure you get your 5-a-day portions of fruit and vegetables as well as omega-3 oils (found in oily fish and flax seeds), which improve blood flow.

- Do you exercise enough? Regular exercise will improve blood flow, make you feel more energetic and is a good way to relax and decrease stress. Working out in the gym, or going for a run, cycle or even a brisk walk can all help to put your worries and problems in perspective and make you feel better about yourself.

- Take a candid look at your alcohol intake: too much alcohol can affect sexual performance, so limit your consumption to a maximum of two drinks per day

- Some alternative practitioners think that too much caffeine can affect erectile function, so try cutting out regular cola, coffee and tea and opting for decaf instead.

 Did you know?

Although many men experience impotence, most are embarrassed and suffer in silence; only about 10 per cent of them seek medical or professional help. The good news is that 95 per cent of men can be treated successfully.

- There is evidence that smoking can affect a man's capacity to achieve a lasting erection. Nicotine constricts blood vessels, so stop smoking.
- Examine your life and your relationships to see if there are any areas that might be stressful and making you feel anxious, guilty or depressed. Try to resolve any conflicts with your partner, family members or work colleagues. Are there positive steps you can take to improve your lifestyle, reduce worries or stressful situations and make you feel generally more content and relaxed?
- To help prevent impotence, do not be afraid to discuss your worries openly with your partner. With their support, you can avoid misunderstandings and overcome your problem.
- Some medications can have an effect on the capacity to achieve a sustained erection. These include some prescribed drugs for high blood pressure, heart problems and depression.

CONVENTIONAL REMEDIES

The best-known drug for treating impotence is Viagra, but your doctor can prescribe other similar medicines, such as Cialis and Levitra. These all work by relaxing the blood vessels in the penis, so more blood flows into it, thereby creating an erection. Talking therapies, such as cognitive behavioural therapy, may be preferable to medication.

NATURAL REMEDIES

Some natural therapies may be helpful, including herbal medicine and acupressure.
ACUPRESSURE Governing vessel 20, a point on top of the head halfway between the ears, is recommended for treating impotence.

 ## HERBAL REMEDIES

- Ginkgo biloba helps to boost blood flow and you could try taking 40 to 80mg three times a day. However, don't take more than the recommended dose as there may be an increased risk of serious side effects.
- Ginseng is believed to enhance vitality and sexual function; take up to 150mg three times daily.
- Evening primrose oil is recommended for healthy blood vessels, so you could try taking a daily supplement.

SEE YOUR DOCTOR

If you have problems achieving an erection and this has been the case for at least a couple of months, see your doctor. The condition is nearly always treatable. Impotence may also be linked to other health conditions, including poor cardiovascular fitness, coronary heart disease, diabetes, Parkinson's disease and hormonal imbalance. Early and accurate diagnosis is important, so check it out.

Caution
Viagra is not suitable for everyone and it can have unpleasant side effects, so never buy it from friends or over the internet. Only take it if prescribed and monitored by your doctor.

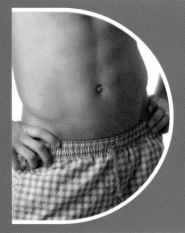

Fertility problems

You may have a fertility problem if you have been having sexual intercourse with your partner for more than twelve months without using any contraception and she has not conceived. Male infertility is usually caused by abnormal semen, damaged testicles or a blockage during ejaculation. There are several reasons for abnormal semen, including a very low sperm count, decreased sperm mobility and abnormally shaped sperm.

 SYMPTOMS

▷ Failure to conceive

▷ Possible pain or swelling inside the scrotum

 PREVENTION

You can increase your chances of conceiving by ensuring that both you and your partner are in good health and are following the advice below.

- Eat a healthy diet and watch your weight – being seriously overweight or obese with a BMI of over 29 can affect your fertility, making it more difficult to conceive.

- Keep your alcohol intake to a minimum – no more than the recommended three to four units a day maximum. Too much alcohol can damage the quality of your sperm.

- If you smoke, think about stopping. Smoking can affect your fertility.

- Have intercourse at least three times a week so it is more likely that you won't miss your partner's fertile days in the monthly cycle, which are usually halfway between her periods.

- Wear loose-fitting underpants made of cotton or natural fibre – tight underpants can increase the temperature within your scrotum, reducing fertility.

- Some conventional and herbal medicines can affect sperm production, so check with your doctor if you are taking medication and avoid a Chinese herb called Tripterygium wilfordii.

- Try to relax and not to worry about the time it's taking to conceive. Stress can reduce your sex drive and limit sperm production.

(i) Did you know?

About 85 per cent of couples having regular unprotected intercourse at least three times a week will conceive naturally within 12 months.

- Illegal drugs, such as marijuana or cocaine, can also affect male fertility, so don't take them.
- Some recent studies have suggested that excessive laptop computer use and carrying a mobile phone in a trouser pocket while speaking on an earpiece may damage sperm, but this is not proven. However, you may wish to check out safety standards in your workplace if you use a computer for long periods or work with potentially hazardous chemicals.

 CONVENTIONAL REMEDIES

The treatment for male infertility will depend on the cause of the problem. The available options include medications to improve fertility and assisted conception. Your doctor may arrange for to have a male fertility test, such as a sperm count. If you have a blockage in your testicles that prevents you ejaculating sperm normally (epididymal blockage), you may need surgery to correct it.

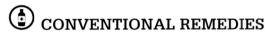 **NATURAL REMEDIES**

Improving your quality of life and cutting out all the unhealthy elements in your diet and daily routine is a natural way to improve your chances of you and your partner conceiving.

NUTRITIONAL MEDICINE Zinc is especially beneficial in aiding healthy functioning of the male reproductive system. You can include foods that are rich in zinc in your daily diet – pumpkin seeds, mushrooms, seafood, meat, liver – or take a daily supplement.

 HERBAL REMEDIES

- Saw palmetto, astragalus root and tribulus are often used to treat male infertility.
- Ginseng is thought to increase sperm motility and you can try taking a supplement of 100 to 200mg per day.

 HOMEOPATHIC REMEDIES

The following remedies are used to treat male fertility problems. Use the appropriate one for your symptoms.
Sepia 6C, for low sex drive
Medorrhinum, for impotence.

SEE YOUR DOCTOR

If you and your partner have been trying to conceive for a year without any success, make an appointment to see your doctor. You should go sooner if you have had an STI (sexually transmitted infection), such as chlamydia, or have received treatment for cancer and are concerned about your fertility.

Traditional Chinese medicine

As the name suggests, Traditional Chinese Medicine (TCM) is one of the world's oldest medical systems and it has been used for thousands of years. It is based on a holistic approach and uses a combination of therapies, including acupuncture, Chinese herbal medicine and tuina, a form of massage.

KEY IDEAS

At the heart of Traditional Chinese Medicine is the belief that the body should be treated holistically. Rather than starting with a symptom and looking for a particular disease or illness that is causing it, Traditional Chinese Medicine practitioners diagnose an individual pattern of symptoms.

Practitioners believe that a series of meridians run throughout the body which help qi, or life energy, to flow through. Other key concepts include yin and yang, which represent certain organs of the body and the five elements – fire, wood, water, metal and earth – that relate to symptoms and parts of the body.

When identifying the pattern of illness and the treatment or herbal remedy that could help, a practitioner makes their assessment by looking at yin, yang and the five elements.

ACUPUNCTURE

A full medical history is taken by an acupuncturist and, as well as conventional details, they will test your pulse and look at your tongue, as it's believed that the tongue can hold important information about your health.

The meridian system is central to the work of an acupuncturist, who uses fine needles to stimulate the acu-points that exist on the channels throughout the body. It does not usually hurt and the needles are left in place for a few minutes, or in some cases up to an hour; they work by stimulating or suppressing the flow of qi.

A special herb called moxa is often used, too, particularly in instances where the acupuncturist needs to create heat over a certain point. The herb is burnt over the acupuncture point for a short time.

CHINESE HERBAL MEDICINE

Chinese herbal medicine is often practised on its own or in conjunction with other aspects of Chinese medicine. For example, it is not unusual for an acupuncturist to also prescribe you herbs to take between sessions to continue healing and treatment at home.

After taking notes on your medical symptoms, and analysing your tongue and pulse, herbal remedies are prescribed. Herbs are classified according to whether they are sweet, sour, pungent, bitter, salty, hot or cold. Mixtures of herbs are tailored to individual needs and may be taken as teas, powders, pills, creams or lotions.

It is important to find a qualified Chinese herbal medicine practitioner and to never try taking herbs without proper advice, as some can cause ill effects if used inappropriately.

TUINA

Tuina is a therapeutic form of Chinese massage. Like acupuncture, it focuses on using the meridians and points where qi typically gets stuck to release discomfort and aid healing.

As with other forms of Traditional Chinese Medicine, a full case history is taken and a practitioner will identify a pattern of symptoms before working out how best you can be treated.

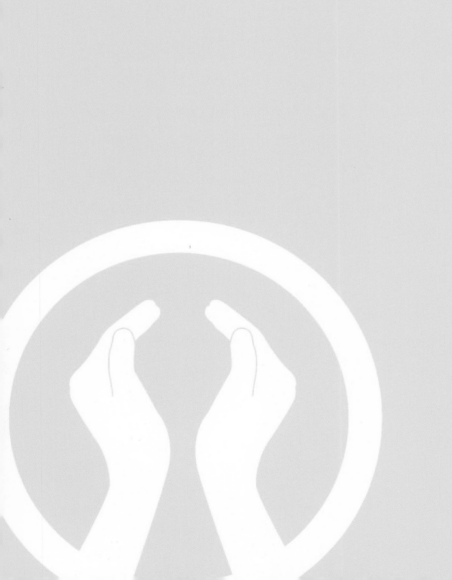

Women's health problems

A woman's body changes as she progresses from puberty and adolescence through her child-bearing years to menopause and old age, and specific health problems are associated with these different stages in her life. During her reproductive years, there are also monthly variations in hormone levels in the body, which can also affect her physical and psychological health.

This chapter focuses on some of the things that go wrong, and how to treat them with conventional, self-help and natural remedies. There is also practical advice on preventing common health problems and, as always, the emphasis is on the essential components of a healthy lifestyle: diet, weight control, exercise, relaxation and stress management, quitting smoking and not drinking more alcohol than the recommended guidelines.

By being well informed, you can take preventive action to protect your health, recognise and respond quickly to symptoms when they occur, and treat your problem with natural or conventional remedies. Self-examination and listening to your body can help alert you to the early-warning signs of poor health.

Your sexual health is important for your wellbeing, self-esteem and your relationship with your partner. The most common health problems associated with the reproductive system are difficulties with periods (premenstrual tension, pain and irregular or heavy bleeding), pregnancy and menopause. For many women, vaginal discharge, infection and thrush can be debilitating and recurring. As well as conventional medical wisdom, there are many tried and tested natural home remedies that offer effective treatment or relief from the symptoms of these women's health conditions.

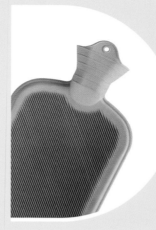

Premenstrual tension (PMT)

Premenstrual tension, also known as premenstrual syndrome, is a term covering a wide range of symptoms from which women can suffer during the week or two before a period. For some, these symptoms can become so severe that they seriously affect their quality of life.

 SYMPTOMS

▷ Depression, tearfulness and anxiety
▷ Irritability
▷ Insomnia
▷ Sugar cravings and increased appetite
▷ Fatigue
▷ Fluid retention and weight gain
▷ Confusion and forgetfulness
▷ Lack of concentration
▷ Clumsiness
▷ Swollen, bloated abdomen
▷ Breast tenderness
▷ Headaches

 PREVENTION

• Avoid alcohol in the week or two weeks before a period is due, as it can exacerbate symptoms.
• Cut down on caffeine-containing drinks and sip herbal teas instead.
• Drink plenty of water.
• Avoid sugary foods that can cause blood sugar peaks followed by dips. Eat regular, small healthy meals and snacks to keep blood sugar levels as level as possible.

 CONVENTIONAL REMEDIES

Your doctor might prescribe hormone treatments, such as the contraceptive Pill, or oestrogen or progesterone-only pills or intrauterine devices, to help balance your hormones. Antidepressants may be offered to treat depression. Alprazolam has been shown to be effective in treating all the psychological symptoms of PMT. Diuretics can be prescribed for water retention. Bromocriptine, danazol or tamoxifen can be prescribed for breast tenderness and diphenhydramine for sleep disturbances. GnRH (Gonadotrophin-releasing hormone) analogues might be offered for severe PMT; they stop your normal cycle and plunge you into a temporary menopause.

NATURAL REMEDIES

There are several natural remedies you can try to tackle PMT symptoms.

FLOWER REMEDIES Australian Bush Flower's She Oak and Women's Essence help to balance hormones.

AROMATHERAPY Clary sage essential oil helps lift the mood and balance your hormones, while fennel can be used to treat water retention. Jasmine may ease depression and anxiety, and juniper is excellent for bloating.

 HERBAL REMEDIES

- The best-known herbal treatment is evening primrose oil. It's especially good at improving mood, lessening breast pain and easing sugar cravings. You may need to take it for three months before the effects are seen.
- Agnus castus is a hormone-balancing herb that can help to even out mood swings and irritability, as well as easing breast tenderness.
- St John's wort is useful for women who get very depressed and anxious, but check with your doctor first if you take any other medication.

 HOMEOPATHIC REMEDIES

A homeopath would treat you constitutionally, but you could try one of the following remedies.

Nux vomica 30C, if you crave sweets or fatty foods and are irritable

Natrum mur 30C, if you are sad and irritable, have fluid retention, swollen breasts and migraines

Pulsatilla 30C, if you are feeling tearful, have painful breasts, and a tendency to irregular periods and nausea

Sepia 30C, if you crave sweets or salty foods, are tearful, depressed and/or generally irritable.

HEALING FOODS

- Magnesium deficiency can be a contributory factor in PMT. Take a daily 300mg supplement.
- Vitamin B6 is useful for counteracting the emotional effects of PMS. Take a supplement containing 2mg a day.
- Soya foods, such as soya milk, soya yoghurt, soya beans and tofu, contain phytoestrogens, which mimic the action of oestrogen in the body and can help to balance the body's oestrogen levels when eaten regularly.

SEE YOUR DOCTOR

Most women find their own solutions to dealing with their PMT, however annoying the symptoms, but if it becomes severe and affects your well-being to such an extent that it interferes with your everyday routine, you should seek help and see your doctor.

Quick fix

When you are about to explode with temper, drink 10 drops of avena sativa (oat straw) in a glass of water. It's a potent source of vitamin B6 and works almost instantly to calm you down and reduce irritability.

Heavy bleeding

Heavy periods (menorrhagia) can be dangerous if they make you anaemic, and they can seriously affect the quality of your life. If you find yourself turning down invitations during your period for fear of flooding, it's time to take action.

 SYMPTOMS

▷ Heavy and/or prolonged periods
▷ Can be accompanied by pain, nausea, diarrhoea and dizziness

 PREVENTION

- Low levels of essential fatty acids, iron, zinc, and vitamins A, C and K are all linked to menorrhagia, so it's worth taking supplements.
- Avoid hot baths during your period, as these may make the bleeding worse. Don't take aspirin-containing drugs for the same reason.

 CONVENTIONAL REMEDIES

Your doctor might prescribe a hormone treatment, such as a progesterone-releasing IUD, or the contraceptive pill. Tranexamic acid tablets taken for the first four days of a period can help to reduce blood loss in many cases.

 NATURAL REMEDIES

Heavy periods can be caused by your liver not eliminating old hormones efficiently, so any remedies that stimulate liver function can be helpful.
AROMATHERAPY Fennel, geranium and rose oils are used to regulate periods and blood flow.

 HERBAL REMEDIES

- Take milk thistle tablets or tincture, and drink dandelion tea or coffee to improve liver function.
- The hormone-balancing effects of agnus castus tincture can be helpful.
- Lady's mantle has an astringent effect on the womb, drying up excretions. You can take it as a tea or a tincture.

 HOMEOPATHIC REMEDIES

Chamomilla 30C, for heavy periods with cramping; blood may look dark or clotted.
Lycopodium 30C, for long, heavy periods accompanied by digestive upsets.
Veratrum album 30C, for heavy periods, cramping and feeling exhausted.

 SEE YOUR DOCTOR

You should seek medical advice if your complexion looks very pale, you are unusually tired, you find it hard to walk up hills you would normally manage without a problem, or if you experience heart palpitations. All these can be symptoms of anaemia.

Period pain

Period pain (dysmenorrhoea) can range from a mild, dull ache in the lower abdomen through to sharp pain that is so severe it causes you to pass out. The pain is usually caused by cramping of the muscles of the uterus.

 ## SYMPTOMS
▷ Pain in the lower abdomen
▷ Lower back pain
▷ Nausea and vomiting
▷ Diarrhoea
▷ Dizziness and fainting

 ## PREVENTION
- Eat a balanced diet, including three servings of oily fish a week. If you don't like fish, take a supplement of Omega-3 essential fatty acids, because dysmenorrhoea is much worse for those who have low levels of essential fatty acids.
- Keep life as stress-free as you can during your periods.
- Take gentle exercise and get plenty of sleep.

 ## CONVENTIONAL REMEDIES
There are plenty of over-the-counter painkillers, but avoid any containing aspirin, which could increase bleeding. Mefenamic acid is often prescribed to treat painful periods; it has a mild anti-inflammatory action as well as painkilling effects.

 ## NATURAL REMEDIES
A traditional remedy is to soak a muslin cloth in castor oil, then wrap it in clingfilm before placing it on your lower abdomen. Put a hot water bottle on top and relax for half an hour. This decongests the womb and relaxes the muscles.

 ## HERBAL REMEDIES
Take wild yam capsules to reduce painful spasms. Crampbark tincture is an effective anti-spasmodic and muscle relaxant.

 ## NUTRITIONAL MEDICINE
- Vitamin E (300iu per day) has been shown to relieve menstrual cramps in 70 per cent of women within two menstrual cycles
- Magnesium (300 mg per day) has a beneficial effect on painful periods and lower back pain.

 ## SEE YOUR DOCTOR
If your symptoms are severe, see your doctor. You may be referred for a scan to rule out other possible causes of the pain, such as endometriosis.

Caution
If you take painkillers to ease your symptoms, take care not to exceed the maximum daily dosage, as stated on the packet instructions.

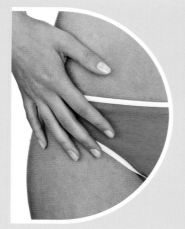

Thrush (candida)

Thrush is an infection caused by a yeast (fungus) known as candida albicans, which occurs naturally in the gut, skin and vagina. Under normal circumstances, it is kept under control by other 'friendly' bacteria in the body, but it can overgrow after antibiotics, when you're rundown, or if you take hormones such as the contraceptive pill.

 SYMPTOMS

▷ Itching of the vulva

▷ Soreness and irritation of the vulva

▷ Pain or discomfort during sex or urination

▷ Odourless vaginal discharge, usually thin and watery or thick and white

▷ Oral thrush affects the mouth, causing white patches that are red and sore underneath

 PREVENTION

- A healthy diet that is low in sugar can help to prevent thrush; sugar feeds the candida fungus.
- Wear cotton undergarments, which can help the area to 'breathe' and prevent over-heating.
- Avoid wearing tight-fitting clothing, such as tights, bathing suits, exercise clothes or trousers for long periods of time, as this can cause irritation.
- Alcohol can contribute to an increased risk of thrush, as can bubble baths, so try to avoid them if you are prone.

 CONVENTIONAL REMEDIES

Thrush is normally treated with antifungal medication, such as fluconazole or itraconazole. Medication can be taken orally or as pessaries, and topical creams can be used for the sore parts of your vulva.

 Did you know?

Stress can also exacerbate the problem of thrush, as can natural hormonal changes (around the time of your period, for example).

NATURAL REMEDIES

Thrush can be treated with a wide range of natural remedies. A healthy diet is very important, and you should also eat plenty of live yoghurt, which is full of healthy bacteria. Take a probiotic regularly, particularly if you suffer from recurrent thrush. Look for one that contains at least four million bacteria per dose; acidophilus is a good choice.

NUTRITIONAL MEDICINE Vitamin C (1000mg per day) helps your body to form collagen, which maintains the structural integrity of your vagina, making infestations and infections less likely. It also works to boost your immune system. B vitamins are often deficient in women with chronic yeast or bacterial infections. Take 50mg of each B vitamin daily.

 ## HERBAL REMEDIES

- Calendula tincture has antimicrobial properties, and is useful to combat vaginal infections and infestations, and promote healing. Echinacea will boost your immune system, making easier for your body to fight off invaders.
- Increase your intake of fresh, raw garlic or take garlic capsules. One of the ingredients in garlic, known as 'allicin', can prevent the overgrowth of yeast.
- Goldenseal tincture contains a substance called 'berberine', which stimulates the immune system and combats yeast and bacteria.
- Pau d'arco has immune-boosting properties, and is also antifungal; take as a tincture or decoction.

 ## AROMATHERAPY

- Tea tree oil is ideal for treating fungal infections. Buy tea tree pessaries to insert in your vagina, or add 5 to 10 drops to your bath water.
- Lavender oil can help to destroy fungi; use in your bath water, or place a few drops on a clean moist flannel and wash the area regularly.
- Thyme oil boosts immunity and can also help to fight yeasts.

 ## HOMEOPATHIC REMEDIES

For vaginal thrush, you can try one of the following:

Pulsatilla 30C, for cloudy or watery discharge which causes smarting and soreness

Graphites 30C, if the vagina is sore, with small ulcers on the labia

Calcarea 30C, if there is vaginal itching, yellow or milk discharge and increased itchiness around periods.

Oral thrush may respond to one of the following:

Borax 30C, at the first sign of an outbreak

Capsicum 30C, for sore, hot patches

Arsenicum 30C, for burning pains, mouth ulcers and feeling worn out.

 ## SEE YOUR DOCTOR

If your vaginal discharge has an unpleasant odour, you are likely to have a viral or bacterial infection rather than a fungal infestation. See your doctor or visit a sexual health clinic for an accurate diagnosis.

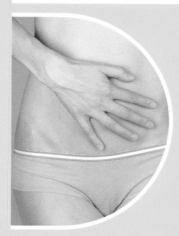

Fibroids

Fibroids are benign tumours that grow in and around the uterus. They are fed by oestrogen, so they tend to occur in women of childbearing age and decrease in size after the menopause. Many women do not even realise that they have them, but, for others, fibroids can cause a host of troublesome and potentially dangerous health problems.

 SYMPTOMS

▷ Heavy, prolonged periods, which can lead to anaemia
▷ Acute pain during periods
▷ Abdominal pain and bloating
▷ Discomfort during sex
▷ More frequent urination; waking several times a night to urinate
▷ Constipation
▷ Pain in the lower back and legs
▷ Can cause infertility or complications during pregnancy

 PREVENTION

One in four women has fibroids and most do not have any associated problems, but if the growths get very large, or are in an awkward position, they will become symptomatic. You can help to avoid them growing huge by doing the following things.

• Don't let yourself get overweight.
• Don't drink too much alcohol.
• Make sure you get enough exercise.
• Eat only organic dairy produce and meat to avoid ingesting the artificial hormones that are routinely fed to farm animals.

 CONVENTIONAL REMEDIES

Your doctor may prescribe hormone treatments, either as a progesterone coil or the contraceptive pill. Tranexamic acid is commonly prescribed to deal with heavy periods, while mefanemic acid can be effective in treating period pains. In severe cases, you may be recommended to have injections of Gonadotropin-releasing hormone agonist (GnRHa), which temporarily stops your menstrual cycle and can bring on some menopausal symptoms. Alternatively, there are a number of surgical procedures used, with hysterectomy at the extreme, and non-surgical procedures, such as MRI-focused ultrasound treatment or uterine artery embolisation.

NATURAL REMEDIES

A useful home-made remedy is to make a castor oil pack to help relieve congestion in the womb.

 ## HERBAL REMEDIES

- Herbs that strengthen the liver, such as milk thistle tablets or tincture, will help it to eliminate old hormones from the blood.
- Agnus castus is useful for hormone balance. Take 25 drops of tincture in a glass of water every morning, or as prescribed by your herbalist.
- Lady's mantle can be effective at reducing excessive bleeding and lowering oestrogen dominance, as is chaste tree. Take them as a tincture or in teas.

 ## AROMATHERAPY

- Ginger oil is a powerful circulation stimulant, and it improves liver function. Put a few drops in the bath, or use in massage.
- Marjoram can help to relieve cramping and discomfort.
- Rose oil helps to ease tension. It also has mild hormone-balancing properties and is believed to work as a uterine tonic.

 ## SEE YOUR DOCTOR

If you are worried that you may have fibroids, see your doctor. Most cases do not require medical intervention, but if the symptoms are severe and troublesome you may need medication or even surgery as a last resort.

 ## NUTRITIONAL MEDICINE

- Eat foods containing phytoestrogens, such as soya products, lentils and chickpeas, which can help to reduce excessive levels of oestrogen in your blood.
- Reduce your intake of saturated fat but get plenty of essential fatty acids from eating oily fish, nuts and seeds.
- Make sure you include plenty of fibre in your diet to ease constipation. Choose whole-grain products, brown rice and oats, as well as lots of fruit and vegetables.
- Dark chocolate with at least 80 per cent cocoa is a good source of iron, for those who are worried about anaemia, or take a daily teaspoonful of black strap molasses.
- Vitamins A, B, C, plus zinc, calcium, magnesium and iron are all essential for hormone balance. Choose a good-quality multivitamin that contains them all.

 ## HOMEOPATHIC REMEDIES

There are dozens of remedies that could be appropriate, according to your individual constitution and symptoms, of which the following may be useful:

Calc carb 30C, for fibroids causing very heavy bleeding, fatigue or chills

Sabina 30C, for fibroids causing lower-back pain and heavy bleeding with clots

Phosphorus 30C will help with heavy bleeding and clots.

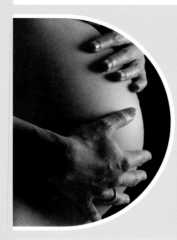

Pregnancy health problems

Many women sail through their pregnancy without any uncomfortable symptoms, while others seem to be plagued constantly. Symptoms are caused by many factors, such as changing hormones and the impact they have on your body, as well as the extra demands of your growing baby.

 ## SYMPTOMS

▷ Nausea (morning sickness)
▷ Fatigue
▷ Heartburn
▷ Oedema (swelling) of the feet, ankles and face
▷ Backache
▷ Headaches
▷ Breast tenderness
▷ Sleep difficulties
▷ Constipation and haemorrhoids
▷ Mood swings

 ## PREVENTION

A healthy diet, with plenty of fresh, whole foods, will help to ensure that your body has the fuel it needs to operate at optimum level, and provide your baby with everything it needs to grow and develop.

- Gentle, regular exercise has been shown to reduce symptoms by improving circulation and by increasing endorphins, the 'feel-good' hormones.
- Relaxation and restful sleep can also help, as many symptoms are exacerbated by fatigue.
- It's also important to drink plenty of water, as dehydration can make symptoms worse.

 ## CONVENTIONAL REMEDIES

Most doctors are reluctant to prescribe medication to pregnant women unless strictly necessary. However, in extreme circumstances you may need some medical intervention. Chronic, debilitating morning sickness (known as Hyperemesis Gravidarum) may be treated with serotonin antagonists or even steroids. Paracetamol is considered to be safe during pregnancy for any related aches and pains. Fibre supplements or glucose syrup may be recommended for constipation.

NATURAL REMEDIES

Many natural remedies are available to treat problem ailments and symptoms during pregnancy. If you are unsure as to their safety, consult your doctor.

FLOWER REMEDIES Olive is ideal for exhaustion. Use Walnut to relieve anxiety and mood swings. Impatiens helps when you are feeling irritable.

HERBAL REMEDIES

- Ginger is a traditional remedy for morning sickness and can be taken in tablet form, or added to foods or drinks. You can also chew crystallised or candied ginger.
- Slippery elm powder mixed with water or milk will protect the mucous membranes lining your digestive system, and ease symptoms.
- Nettle tea can reduce leg cramps, haemorrhoids and swelling.
- Dandelion root tea or coffee has a strong effect on your liver, which can help to ease digestive symptoms and hormone imbalances. The leaf is a mild diuretic, which can reduce water retention.

AROMATHERAPY

- Lavender oil can be added to a bath to encourage restful sleep, or dabbed neat on your temples to soothe headaches.
- Have a warm (not hot bath) about 30 minutes before bedtime, and add 8 to 10 drops of Roman chamomile oil to encourage sleep.
- Lemon oil can be inhaled to ease morning sickness.

NUTRITIONAL MEDICINE

- Vitamin B6 deficiency has been linked with morning sickness, so take a regular B-complex supplement with 50mg of each of the B vitamins.
- Fibre is very important in preventing constipation and ensuring that the vitamins and minerals from the food you eat are assimilated by your body. Psyllium or ispaghula husks (plantain seeds) are effective unblockers, and safe during pregnancy.
- If you suffer from oedema, include lots of natural diuretics in your diet, such as asparagus, pumpkin, onions, grapes, beets, parsley, green beans, pineapple and garlic.

HOMEOPATHIC REMEDIES

Treatment will be based on your individual symptoms, but the following remedies may be helpful.

Ipecacuanha 30C, for morning sickness characterised by continuous nausea and vomiting.

Symphoricarpus 30C, for morning sickness made worse by food and any sort of motion.

Nux vomica 30C, for constipation, with a frequent urge to pass a bowel movement, but only managing a little a time; also itching, bleeding haemorrhoids.

Sulphur 30C, for constipation with haemorrhoids that itch and burn and are worse for heat.

SEE YOUR DOCTOR

If you are worried about any health problems or unfamiliar symptoms that you may experience during your pregnancy, make an appointment to see your doctor or mention it to your midwife or the medical staff at your regular check-ups.

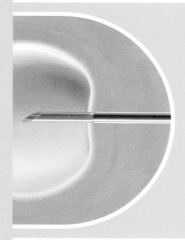

Infertility

Infertility is a general diagnosis given when you are unable to conceive after 18 months of unprotected sex. Many cases are treatable, particularly when the cause is established. Common causes include endometriosis, ovulation problems, poor egg or sperm quality, polycystic ovaries, tube blockages (male or female) or sperm allergy. However, most cases of infertility are unexplained.

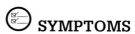 ## SYMPTOMS

▷ Inability to conceive

 ## PREVENTION

- Both you and your partner should eat a healthy diet, which is crucial to a successful pregnancy and a healthy baby, and can help to balance hormones that may be at the root of the problem.
- Avoid drinking alcohol and coffee, which can reduce your fertility by half.
- Smoking has also been linked with infertility in women, and can even bring on an early menopause. If you are a smoker and trying to conceive, stop smoking now.
- Eat organic food whenever possible to avoid consuming the environmental oestrogens that are found in some pesticides used on many vegetables and fruit.

 ## Did you know?

About one in six couples has difficulty conceiving. Research indicates that women's fertility begins to decline in their late 20s, and men's in their late 30s.

CONVENTIONAL REMEDIES

There are a number of options available, including assisted fertilisation and medication. Your treatment will be undertaken according to the cause of your infertility. Some options include:

- Intrauterine insemination (IUI), a procedure that puts your partner's sperm directly into your womb using a fine catheter
- IVF (in vitro fertilization), which involves placing a fertilised egg into your uterus, usually after drug therapy
- Stimulatory drugs (such as clomiphene), which can encourage several eggs to mature at a time
- Follicle-stimulating hormone (FSH), which makes the ovaries begin the process of ovulation
- Human menopausal gonadotropin (hMG), which is used for women who don't ovulate due to problems with their pituitary gland
- Bromocriptine is often used for women who have trouble ovulating because of high levels of the hormone prolactin.

 NATURAL REMEDIES

There are many natural remedies that you can try to help maximise your chances of conception.

 NUTRITIONAL MEDICINE

- Vitamin B6 can help women who have trouble conceiving, whereas vitamin B12 is useful for men. Take 50mg per day.
- Zinc is crucial for successful fertilization, and it also reduces the risk of miscarriage. Both you and your partner should take 40mg per day.
- Eat plenty of essential fatty acids (in nuts, seeds, oily fish). Consider taking a fish oil supplement.
- Vitamin E (400iu per day) is a powerful antioxidant and can increase fertility in men and women.
- Vitamin C (1000mg per day) encourages the production of healthy sperm.

 HERBAL REMEDIES

- Agnus castus helps to restore hormonal balance and increases fertility – take in tincture form.
- Lemon balm can help to reduce the impact of stress, which may be at the root of the problem. Take as an infusion.
- False unicorn root is traditionally used to regulate the ovaries – look for it in tincture form.

AROMATHERAPY

- Rose oil is frequently used to treat fertility problems. Use for massage or in the bath.
- Geranium has oestrogenic properties, and can help to balance your hormones.
- Melissa (lemon balm) helps to regulate your menstrual cycle, and is also very relaxing.

HOMEOPATHIC REMEDIES

Your treatment will be constitutional, working to address anything that may be causing fertility problems. Some commonly used remedies include:

Sepia 30C, for irregular or absent ovulation

Aurum 30C, for low sex drive and depression

Phosphorus 30C, when stress is causing problems

Sabina 30C, when you suffer from recurrent miscarriage

Silica 30C, which is an overall remedy to boost your chances of becoming pregnant.

SEE YOUR DOCTOR

Consult your doctor if you haven't had any success conceiving after trying for a year. You may be referred to a specialist fertility clinic for treatment.

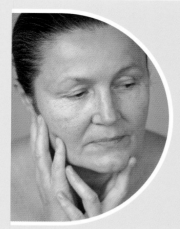

Menopause

The hormonal and biological changes that lead up to the cessation of menstrual periods can cause a number of physical and emotional symptoms that vary from woman to woman. Most get through it without recourse to medical treatments but there's no need to suffer in silence, as there are a number of natural remedies that can be tried.

 SYMPTOMS

▷ Hot flushes and night sweats
▷ Mood swings
▷ Depression and anxiety
▷ Weight gain
▷ Insomnia
▷ Headaches
▷ Tiredness and lack of concentration
▷ Vaginal dryness
▷ Loss of skin elasticity
▷ Increased frequency of urination
▷ Reduced sex drive

PREVENTION

- Hot flushes can be triggered by eating spicy foods, drinking alcohol or caffeine-containing drinks, or hot climates, so avoid these.
- Wear light natural-fibre clothing and try to keep rooms cool, especially the bedroom.
- Exercise regularly and eat sensibly to keep your weight under control.
- Avoid sugar-laden foods that cause blood sugar peaks and troughs that affect your emotions.
- Use lots of moisturiser on your skin, reapplying throughout the day.

 CONVENTIONAL REMEDIES

Hormone replacement therapy (HRT) can be taken as a tablet, cream, gel or skin patch. It provides oestrogen to replace the falling natural levels. Tibolone works in the same way but, unlike HRT, your periods will stop when you take it. Clonidine may be prescribed to treat hot flushes and night sweats. Your doctor might even suggest taking antidepressants or sleeping pills if you have severe problems with depression or insomnia.

 Did you know?

The adrenal gland can help to balance your hormones during the period leading up to and after menopause, so long as you are not too stressed. This is a good time to take up relaxation therapies such as yoga or tai chi, which can help to maintain muscle strength, improve breathing and alleviate stress.

NATURAL REMEDIES

Many women prefer to treat the annoying symptoms of menopause with a range of natural treatments rather than resort to conventional medicine. There are many over-the-counter remedies available in pharmacies and health food stores.

FLOWER REMEDIES Impatiens is ideal for mood swings and irritability, while Walnut is perfect for this time of life. Cherry Plum helps when you are feeling irrational, or ready to explode.

NUTRITIONAL MEDICINE Regularly eating foods containing phytoestrogens, such as soya products, can significantly reduce menopausal symptoms. Eating a well-balanced diet with plenty of essential fatty acids from oily fish, nuts and seeds, and a full range of vitamins and minerals is vitally important.

 HERBAL REMEDIES

- Black cohosh is the best-known treatment, and in several tests it has emerged as being at least as effective as HRT in treating menopausal symptoms (see cautionary note).
- Drink sage tea to combat hot flushes and night sweats. Keep a cup of cold tea by your bedside to sip during the night as required.
- St John's wort is extremely effective at combating depression and anxiety, and it can also boost your sex drive. Consult a qualified professional before taking it if you are on any other medications.
- Dong quai, liquorice, sage and yarrow can help to counteract hot flushes and night sweats. Blend tinctures together, if you wish.

 SEE YOUR DOCTOR

If gentle natural remedies do not appear to be working and your symptoms are severe, consult your doctor.

AROMATHERAPY

- Lavender, marjoram and Roman chamomile can be added to the bath to soothe anxiety and irritation, and to encourage restful sleep.
- Clary sage helps to balance hormones, which can ease symptoms.
- Anise, fennel and angelica oils all contain oestrogen-like substances that can provide relief from many menopausal symptoms. Use two or three drops in the bath.

HOMEOPATHIC REMEDIES

Treatment should be constitutional but the following remedies are commonly used.

Sepia 30C helps with hot flushes, a low libido, irritability and feelings of weakness.

Lachesis 30C helps with hot flushes that feel like a rush of blood to the head, headaches, and left-sided pain

Pulsatilla 30C is great for tearfulness, irritability and symptoms that seem to change constantly.

Caution

Don't take black cohosh if you have any liver problems. Talk to your doctor about this.

255

TOP 20
aromatherapy oils

Aromatherapy uses aromatic essential oils, extracted from plants, to promote good health and treat many common ailments. The essential oils can be used in massage, baths, warm compresses, steam inhalations, sprays and vaporizers. For massage, a few drops are added to a carrier oil, such as sweet almond, grapeseed, jojoba or sunflower oil.

1 BERGAMOT
Scent citrus, fresh
Used for calming, healing; depression, stress; acne, boils, psoriasis; colds, coughs

2 CEDARWOOD
Scent woody
Used for stimulating, toning; eczema; dandruff

3 CHAMOMILE (ROMAN)
Scent pungent
Used for calming, soothing; insomnia, stress; skin irritations and inflammations, acne; digestive problems; children's ailments; headaches; sprains and strains

4 CYPRESS
Scent Spicy, balsamic, sweet
Used for astringent; chest infections; dandruff; varicose veins; eczema; cramp; haemorrhoids

5 EUCALYPTUS
Scent camphor, woody
Used for antiseptic; colds, flu, catarrh, sinusitis, upper respiratory tract infections; muscular pain; headaches; chicken pox, shingles

6 FRANKINCENSE
Scent balsamic, sweet
Used for calming, soothing; promotes skin healing; asthma; coughs, bronchitis

7 GERANIUM
Scent floral, sweet
Used for relaxing, calming; hormonal imbalance, premenstrual syndrome, menopause; acne, eczema; depression, stress; headaches; cramp; haemorrhoids; varicose veins

8 GINGER
Scent spicy
Used for stimulating, warming; muscle aches and pains; digestive problems, nausea, motion sickness, constipation, indigestion, heartburn; arthritis, rheumatism

9 LAVENDER
Scent sweet, floral
Used for calming, sedative, antiseptic; insomnia, stress, depression; burns; acne, eczema; back ache, muscular pain, sprains and strains; nausea; catarrh, sinusitis, colds, coughs, chest infections; dandruff

10 **LEMON**
Scent refreshing, citrus
Used for astringent, antiseptic; warts, verrucae, athlete's foot; bad breath; flu

11 **LEMON GRASS**
Scent fresh, citrus
Used for sedative, antiseptic; fatigue, ME, stress; insect repellent, restless legs; digestive problems, constipation; acne

12 **MANDARIN**
Scent fresh, fruity, citrus
Used for relaxing, calming, refreshing, gentle, safe; suitable for babies

13 **MARJORAM**
Scent Herby, sweet, camphor
Used for calming, antiseptic; chest infections, coughs and colds; constipation, flatulence; headaches; insomnia; muscular pain, backache; arthritis, rheumatism

14 **NEROLI**
Scent sweet, floral
Used for calming, sedative; stress; insomnia; diarrhoea, irritable bowel syndrome; premenstrual syndrome

15 **ORANGE**
Scent fresh, citrus
Used for astringent, uplifting; constipation; stress

16 **PEPPERMINT**
Scent minty, fresh
Used for stimulating, decongestant; catarrh, sinusitis, coughs, colds, chest infections; headaches; nausea

17 **ROSEMARY**
Scent herby, fresh
Used for invigorating, refreshing, antibacterial, decongestant; backache, muscular pain, sprains and strains; catarrh, sinusitis, coughs, colds; headaches, dandruff

18 **SANDALWOOD**
Scent sweet, woody
Used for calming, soothing, anti-inflammatory, antiseptic; skin problems, eczema; sore throats, coughs, colds, chest infections, sore throat

19 **TEA TREE**
Scent fresh, spicy
Used for antifungal, antiviral, antibacterial, antiseptic; boosting immune system; warts, verrucae; acne, boils, dermatitis; bad breath, gum disease; insect bites; cuts; colds, coughs, sinusitis, sore throat, tonsillitis; fainting, fever

20 **YLANG YLANG**
Scent exotic, floral
Used for sedative, soothing, antidepressant; depression; premenstrual sydrome

Children's health problems

Babies and children experience rapid physical growth and emotional development. Their fast-growing bodies require healthy nutrients and exercise, and they also need to develop a wide range of everyday skills, mobility and social behaviours. As they grow and develop individually, they will not only pass many milestones but will also come into contact with common health problems and infectious childhood illnesses. This is perfectly natural and your child needs to be vaccinated against some diseases, such as mumps, measles, rubella and whooping cough, and exposed to a range of minor infections and viruses in order to build up immunity.

Even the common cold or a cough is distressing for babies and, and it is always sensible to err on the side of caution and to consult your doctor if you are worried or in any doubt. The younger your baby or toddler is, the more vigilant you must be in spotting the symptoms of poor health or illness and taking action or seeking medical advice as soon as possible – your child cannot tell you what is wrong or describe the location and nature of the pain. Especially in their first year, when their immune system is not well-developed, children are very susceptible to infections, and fevers, dehydration and breathing difficulties are potentially more serious, so don't adopt a 'wait and see how it is in the morning' policy – act fast and play safe.

Not all health problems are a cause for concern: all babies will suffer from teething problems, nappy rash and sleepless nights to a lesser or greater degree, and many of these problems can be treated with some traditional self-help measures or natural remedies and a large pinch of common sense.

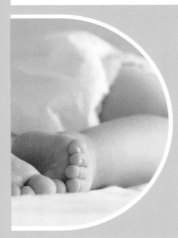

Nappy rash

Nappy rash is caused by contact with either urine or faeces, which makes the skin produce less protective oil and therefore provide a less effective barrier to further irritation. Friction may also exacerbate this distressing condition, which can be very painful and may make your baby irritable and prone to waking up during the night.

 SYMPTOMS

▷ Redness in the nappy area, sometimes spreading up to the abdomen or down your baby's legs

▷ Redness may be blotchy, spotty or appear as a uniform, raised red rash covering a large area

▷ White patches on the nappy rash may indicate thrush (candida), which is a fungal infection.

▷ In a candida rash, the skin may be inflamed with extra spots around the edges, and these are called 'satellite lesions'

 PREVENTION

Although most babes will get nappy rash at some time or anther, there are many things you can do to try to prevent it occurring.

- Change your baby as soon as the nappy becomes wet or soiled. Use a barrier cream, such as zinc oxide, which will protect his/her bottom from contact with faeces and urine.

- If your baby is prone to nappy rash, you might consider using disposables some of the time as they tend to be better than reusable nappies at keeping urine away from the skin.

- If you prefer using reusable nappies, put them through an extra rinse cycle to be sure that there are no traces of detergent.

- Avoid using soap or other detergents on the nappy area. Rinse carefully with clean water at each nappy change.

- Allow your baby to spend as long as possible with a bare bottom, to allow it to dry and heal.

CONVENTIONAL REMEDIES

Your doctor will recommend changing your baby more frequently and allowing periods of time without a nappy. In severe cases, an ointment containing a mild corticosteroid drug may be prescribed to suppress the inflammation. This might be prescribed in combination with an antifungal drug to kill any candida present.

 HERBAL REMEDIES

- Rub a little calendula (marigold) ointment on to the cleaned nappy area to soothe and to reduce inflammation.
- Powdered goldenseal can be applied to a clean nappy area before you put on the nappy.
- Give your baby lots of soothing drinks, such as very diluted, cooled chamomile tea, to reduce the acidity of the urine. There are many herbal formulas available for newborn babies, but make sure there isn't any sugar in the preparation. If you are breastfeeding, continue to do so, ensuring that your baby remains well hydrated and that his/her urine is not too concentrated.

 HOMEOPATHIC REMEDIES

Homeopathic remedies may be helpful, but see a homeopath if your baby suffers from regular rashes in the nappy area, or if you suspect thrush.

Rhus tox 6C: Use for an itchy, blistered rash.

Sulphur 6C: This may be appropriate if the skin is dry and scaled.

Merc sol 6C: This can help to reduce the acidity of the urine.

Cantharis 6C: Use when the urine is scalding and the skin is raw.

 SEE YOUR DOCTOR

Any nappy rash that does not heal within a week or so should be seen by a doctor. Rashes that are accompanied by white patches, sores or yellow spots should also always be investigated.

Flower remedies

Rescue Remedy cream may be gently massaged into the affected area to reduce inflammation and ease any pain or itching. A few drops of Rescue Remedy on the pulse points will help to calm down a baby who is distressed.

Aromatherapy

- A drop of lavender or rose oil in a peach kernel carrier oil can be gently rubbed into the nappy area. Use this to protect against nappy rash as well as heal it.
- A drop of oregano or thyme oil in a light carrier oil, such as olive oil, can be used to discourage thrush.

Traditional remedies

- Egg white can be painted on the baby's sore bottom and allowed to dry before putting on a nappy. This will encourage the skin to heal and prevent further irritation.
- Live yoghurt can be spread on the nappy area to soothe, and to prevent thrush from occurring in the skin folds.
- Some people swear that using powdered cornflour or arrowroot instead of talcum powder is soothing to a baby's skin.
- Blend a little baking soda with some warm water and use to wash your baby's bottom.

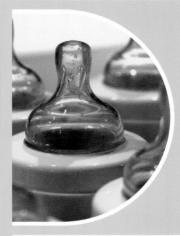

Infant colic

Colic is characterised by apparently unending frantic crying, usually at around the same time of the day or night. Your baby's legs will be drawn up to the abdomen, and he may appear to be in severe pain. Excessive crying causes him to swallow air, which can lead to abdominal bloating and exacerbate the problem. Most cases of colic resolve themselves at around three or four months of age.

 SYMPTOMS

▷ Seemingly endless crying, usually at the same time of day or night

▷ Legs drawn up to abdomen

▷ Belching and other symptoms of wind

▷ Abdominal bloating

▷ Arched back

 PREVENTION

- If you are bottle-feeding, consider changing the brand of formula – you can ask your doctor about hypoallergenic or lactose-free formulas. You can also purchase 'anti-colic' feeding bottles, which reduce the amount of air that your baby takes in while feeding. Winding your baby several times during feeding may also help, as well as giving a massage before a feed.

- If you are breastfeeding, avoid eating dairy produce for a few days to see if this helps. Your baby could have an allergy or intolerance that is making him or her react to something in your milk. Other foods to be avoided are very spicy dishes, citrus fruits, gas-producing foods (beans, cabbage, etc.) and sugar, all of which may make your baby uncomfortable

- Some mothers who breastfeed their babies find that abstaining from eating onions and garlic helps to prevent colic.

 Did you know?

The causes are unknown, but colic may be linked with contractions of the colon, an intolerance to formula (if bottle-fed) or the mother's diet (if breastfed), or simply excessive air which is gulped in during repeated bouts of crying. There is some evidence that a difficult birth can lead to colic.

CONVENTIONAL REMEDIES

There are a variety of over-the-counter, anti-spasmodic drugs that may be suggested for your baby. Simeticone, which is used to relieve trapped air, may help. Babies over three months can be given paracetamol to ease discomfort.

 ## NATURAL REMEDIES

You may need to experiment to find out which natural remedies work best for your baby.

HERBAL REMEDIES Because colic in babies is exacerbated by tension, relaxing herbs are often suggested – used in the bath, or infused, cooled slightly and drunk from a bottle. Chamomile, lemon balm and limeflower are most effective. A warm bath with an infusion of dill, fennel, marshmallow or lemon balm will usually soothe a colicky baby.

FLOWER REMEDIES Rock Rose flower essence is excellent for distress and fright, and Rescue Remedy can be used to calm and help to reduce any spasm. Place a drop or two on your baby's pulse points.

 ## HOMEOPATHIC REMEDIES

Make sure you use the appropriate homeopathic remedy for the symptoms presented.

Chamomilla 30C is useful for babies who seem better when they are held.

Pulsatilla 30C is suggested for babies who are better in the fresh air, and when they are rocked.

Cuprum met 30C is appropriate when your baby's tummy rumbles, and fingers and toes are curled in discomfort.

 ## SEE YOUR DOCTOR

Colic is distressing for you as well as your baby, and you may well find it very difficult or even impossible to comfort your screaming child. However, colic is rarely a serious problem and if your baby is healthy, putting on weight and sleeping well, you need not worry. If your baby begins to resist feeding or suffers from vomiting, diarrhoea or a fever, then you must contact your doctor and get professional medical advice.

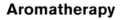

Aromatherapy

- A gentle massage of the abdominal area with one or a blend of essential oils of chamomile, dill, lavender or rose, will help to ease symptoms and calm a distressed baby. Try massaging before feeding. A drop of each in a warm carrier oil, such as grapeseed, should be adequate.

- Try a drop of lavender or chamomile oil in a warm bath just before evening feeds.

Teething

Babies get their first teeth between four and six months of age, but there can be problems with teeth coming through until they reach two or three. The majority experience some discomfort, which can range from being clingy and fractious to dribbling, loosened stools and problems sleeping.

 SYMPTOMS

▷ Irritability and fussiness as the gums become sore
▷ Drooling
▷ Coughing or gagging, as a result of extra saliva
▷ A rash on the chin
▷ Gnawing and biting everything put into the mouth
▷ Rubbing cheeks and pulling ears, as the pain travels to the ear area and around the jaw
▷ Mild diarrhoea
▷ A slightly raised temperature
▷ Poor sleep
▷ A runny nose

 PREVENTION

You can't do much to prevent the discomfort, but you can make your baby more comfortable by offering a cool teething gel to gnaw on, or a flannel soaked in freezing-cold water. Rub the gums with a clean finger.

 CONVENTIONAL REMEDIES

Use a gentle teething gel to rub into the gums, but many contain paracetamol, so don't use them at the same time as any oral doses for pain relief.

 NATURAL REMEDIES

AROMATHERAPY A few drops of chamomile and lavender essential oils can be added to the bathwater to calm a distressed baby.

FLOWER REMEDIES Rub a little Rescue Remedy directly into the gums, or apply to pulse points if your baby is crying inconsolably. A few drops at night-time will encourage sleep, as will a few drops of lavender oil on a hanky tied to the head of the cot.

 HOMEOPATHIC REMEDIES

· Chamomilla is standard for teething, and 6C can be taken as required up to six times a day to ease symptoms and relieve the distress.
· Homeopathic teething granules are also available in many good pharmacies, and they will help to ease the symptoms.
· If your baby has bright-red cheeks and a high fever, offer Belladonna, 6C.

 HERBAL REMEDIES

Syrup made from the marshmallow root will soothe inflamed gums, and a few teaspoons can be added to your baby's meals. You can also offer infusions of chamomile or fennel to calm, and to soothe.

 SEE YOUR DOCTOR

High fever and vomiting are not symptoms of teething. Always see your doctor without delay if your baby seems unwell.

Catarrh

This is over-production of thick phlegm by the mucous membranes of the air passages. Inflammation of the membranes, as a result of a cold or flu, is the usual cause, but other triggers include passive smoking, inhalation of dust, chronic sinusitis, upper respiratory tract infection or allergy.

 SYMPTOMS
▷ A blocked and stuffy nose.
▷ An excessive discharge of mucus from the nose, or down the back of the throat
▷ An irritating, persistent cough
▷ Headaches or facial pain

 PREVENTION
- Ensure that your house is free of dust and smoke.
- Chronic catarrh is a common symptom of food allergy, so assess your child's diet carefully (see pages 148–149).

 CONVENTIONAL REMEDIES
Antihistamine or steroid nasal sprays, cough suppressants, decongestants and paracetamol are the usual conventional remedies for treating pain. Antibiotics are used to treat any bacterial infection.

 NATURAL REMEDIES
If the problem is recurrent, it's worth getting an individual opinion from a qualified therapist.
HERBAL REMEDIES Herbs such as golden rod, elderflower and eyebright are anti-catarrhal and astringent. Take them as an infusion, several times each day.
AROMATHERAPY Eucalyptus, chamomile and mint oils are decongestant and expectorant. Rub into the child's chest and temples in a light carrier oil, such as grapeseed, or place several drops in a vaporiser and encourage your child to inhale.

 NUTRITIONAL MEDICINE
- Beta-carotene helps to strengthen mucous membranes of the respiratory system; choose red, orange and yellow fruits and vegetables.
- Cut down on mucus-forming foods, such as dairy produce.

 HOMEOPATHIC REMEDIES
Choose the most appropriate remedy for the symptoms presented.
Arsenicum 30C, for thick, yellow discharge that makes the nose and the surrounding area sore.
Pulsatilla 30C, for yellow or green catarrh that is not painful; accompanied by weepiness.
Natrum mur 30C, for catarrh like raw egg white, with a dry nose and loss of taste and smell.

 SEE YOUR DOCTOR
If the catarrh becomes very thick and yellow or green, see your doctor to rule out an infection.

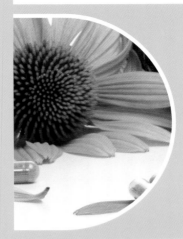

Colds

The common cold is an infection of the upper respiratory tract, which may be caused by any one of up to 200 strains of virus. These are spread either by inhaling droplets coughed or sneezed by others, or more probably by direct contact when your child touches something that has been touched by someone with the virus. The incubation period is from one to three days, after which symptoms start to occur, and most colds run their course in three to ten days.

 SYMPTOMS

▷ Running or stuffy nose
▷ Headache
▷ Sometimes a cough
▷ Sometimes throat discomfort
▷ Fevers of up to 39°C (102°F) in infants and children
▷ General malaise

 PREVENTION

Small children are more susceptible than adults to the viruses that cause colds and flu because their immune systems are immature. Don't be surprised if your children seem to contract every cold they come into contact with. Keeping their immune system strong by feeding a healthy diet and making sure that they get plenty of sleep can help. Teach them to wash their hands regularly with hot soapy water.

 CONVENTIONAL REMEDIES

In conventional medicine, colds are usually treated with rest and fluids, in addition to antihistamines, decongestants, and cough medicines as required. Paracetamol or ibuprofen may be suggested to lower your child's temperature and relieve any pain.

 Did you know?

Babies and children can have a temperature of up to 39°C (102°F). Such a high fever in an adult would indicate flu but it is less to worry about in children who become hotter faster.

NATURAL REMEDIES

Natural remedies work to heal a cold gently, while boosting your child's overall vitality.

FLOWER REMEDIES Rescue Remedy is the traditional way to soothe any distress – rub the cream into your child's chest area to calm them. Olive flower essence will help with fatigue.

 ## HERBAL REMEDIES

- Goldenseal and elecampane are useful for clearing mucus from the lungs and nasal passages in chronic colds.
- Elderflower, drunk as an infusion, will reduce catarrh and help to decongest.
- Chamomile infusion will soothe an irritable child and help him to sleep. Chamomile also has antiseptic action, which will help to rid the body of infection, and it works to reduce fever and feverish symptoms.
- Herbs to strengthen the immune system, such as echinacea, can be taken throughout a cold, and in the period afterwards to stimulate healing and prevent subsequent infection.

Aromatherapy

- Place your child's head over a steaming bowl of water with a few drops of added essential oil of cinnamon. Drape a towel over his head to make a tent, and let him sit there for four or five minutes to ease congestion. Take great care that the water is not boiling and that it cannot be knocked over
- Try adding a few drops of lavender or tea tree oil to a warm bath to encourage healing and help to open up the airways.

 ## HOMEOPATHIC REMEDIES

If your child gets recurrent colds, it would be a good idea to try a constitutional homeopathic treatment and perhaps consult a qualified practitioner. In the short-term, however, the following remedies should help, according to the symptoms presented.

Aconite 30C in the first stages of a cold, particularly if it seems to have come on suddenly, after your child has been outside, for example.

Belladonna 30C, for colds with a high temperature, and great thirst.

Natrum mur 30C, for watery colds, particularly if they are accompanied by cold sores.

Arsenicum 30C, for watery colds, especially if your child is prone to frequent colds.

Pulsatilla 30C is useful if your child is clingy and irritable, and when there is thick yellow discharge from the nose.

Bryonia 30C helps an irritable child who is thirsty and wants to be left alone.

 ## SEE YOUR DOCTOR

Most colds can be treated at home with plenty of rest, regular fluids and conventional over-the-counter medications formulated for children. However, if your child also has a sore throat or fever and it lasts for more than 48 hours, or if your baby has a fever for more than 24 hours or is struggling to feed, you must see your doctor without delay.

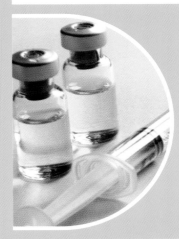

Infectious childhood illnesses

The majority of childhood illnesses are on the wane as a result of mass immunisation but children who have not been immunised, and even a proportion of those who have been vaccinated, can still contract these conditions, which include mumps, measles and whooping cough.

 ## PREVENTION

The MMR vaccine is offered to prevent the likelihood of acquiring mumps and measles; immunisation against whooping cough (pertussis) is routinely offered to infants, and is given in three doses from two months of age. If you have any concerns about immunisation, talk them over with your doctor.

 ## CONVENTIONAL REMEDIES

Drinking lots of fluids and getting plenty of rest are the main recommendation for all these infectious childhood illnesses, as well as paracetamol for pain relief and treating fever. Antibiotics are not prescribed unless there is a secondary infection. If whooping cough is diagnosed early enough, erythromycin can be given to reduce your child's infectivity to others and also to reduce the duration of the illness.

 ## NATURAL REMEDIES

Many of the natural treatments for childhood illnesses are similar. Suggested remedies are given for each of the infectious diseases on the following pages.

FLOWER REMEDIES Rescue Remedy is excellent for calming a child who is frightened by any of the three illnesses (mumps, measles and whooping cough). A few drops applied to the pulse points, or sipped in a glass of cool water, will help to soothe an upset child. Cherry Plum will help if there is serious spasmodic coughing, and Mimulus and Olive are good in the later stages of whooping cough.

 ## SEE YOUR DOCTOR

If you suspect that your child may have any of these infectious diseases, you must call out a doctor to confirm the diagnosis.

 ## Did you know?

Mumps and measles are viral illnesses, whereas whooping cough is bacterial, and all these diseases are highly infectious.

INFECTIOUS CHILDHOOD ILLNESSES

Mumps

This viral infection is highly contagious, and children are more commonly affected than adults. There is no cure for mumps and the aim of treatment is always to relieve the symptoms, which usually pass within two weeks.

 SYMPTOMS

▷ Swollen salivary glands, producing a characteristic chipmunk appearance
▷ Fever and general malaise
▷ Headache
▷ Pains in the neck area

 NATURAL REMEDIES

Try the following natural remedies to alleviate the symptoms of mumps.

HERBAL REMEDIES Red clover and marigold can help to reduce congestion and swelling. Add tinctures of these to any drink, or offer them to your child as a tea.

AROMATHERAPY Very gently massage the child's neck and jaw with one drop each of chamomile, eucalyptus and lavender oils in 6 tablespoons of olive oil.

 HOMEOPATHIC REMEDIES

If your child has not had mumps, the homeopathic remedies Phytolacca 30C or Parotidium 30C can be taken during an epidemic to reduce severity of symptoms. If he does succumb, try the following.

Rhus tox 30C when the left glands are more severely affected than the right.

Belladonna 30C when there is high fever, shooting pains, and a bright red face and throat.

Merc sol 30C is useful when there is heavy sweating and a coated tongue.

Pulsatilla 30C may help to prevent orchitis, and is useful if fever continues.

 SEE YOUR DOCTOR

If mumps is followed by a severe headache, stiffness or fever, see your doctor immediately.

Caution

Teenagers and adults have a higher risk of developing complications, such as swelling of the testicles (in boys and men), hearing loss, meningitis and encephalitis. Always consult your doctor.

INFECTIOUS CHILDHOOD ILLNESSES

Measles

Another highly infectious viral disease, measles can occasionally have serious complications and you should check this out with your doctor.

 SYMPTOMS

▷ A rash characterised by flat, brown-red spots, which usually begins behind the ears and on the face
▷ High fever
▷ Swollen lymph nodes
▷ Little or no appetite
▷ Occasionally vomiting and diarrhoea

 NATURAL REMEDIES

Try the following natural remedies to alleviate the symptoms of measles.

HERBAL REMEDIES A compress of crushed ginger may be placed on the rash to encourage the release of toxins from the body. Heat it a little and wrap it in several layers of gauze to protect the skin.

AROMATHERAPY Lavender oil can be dropped on the bedclothes or on a hanky by the bed to calm. It can also be applied neat to spots, to encourage healing. When there is a build-up of phlegm, a gentle chest massage with a few drops of tea tree oil in a light carrier oil base will help.

 HOMEOPATHIC REMEDIES

If your child has not been immunised, a homeopath would offer Morbillinum, a nosode that works to reduce the harmful effects of the condition and, in some cases, to infer immunity against it. In the short-term, offer on of the following.

Aconite 30C and **Belladonna 30C,** for high fever.

Pulsatilla 30C when there is diarrhoea, yellow discharge and a cough.

Bryonia 30C when there is a hard, painful cough and a high temperature accompanied by thirst.

Stramonium 30C when there is a high fever, a red face and convulsions.

 SEE YOUR DOCTOR

With measles, you should see your doctor if the fever recurs several days after the spots have begun to heal.

Caution

Keep your child in a darkened room when they have measles. Many children are sensitive to bright light during measles, and their eyes can be damaged.

INFECTIOUS CHILDHOOD ILLNESSES

Whooping cough

This is an infection of the lining of the respiratory tract. The name is derived from the cough, followed by an intake of breath that sounds like a 'whoop'.

 SYMPTOMS

▷ A runny or snuffly nose for about a week
▷ Paroxysms of coughing, which can cause a blue or red face and bulging eyes
▷ There may be a whooping sound as the child draws breath between coughs
▷ Coughing fits may cause vomiting

 NATURAL REMEDIES

Try the following remedies to alleviate the symptoms of whooping cough.

AROMATHERAPY Mix a few drops of lavender and chamomile oils in a light carrier oil and massage into the chest and back area to calm your child, and to relax tensed muscles. Tea tree, lavender, chamomile and eucalyptus can be used in a vaporiser to help open the lungs.

 HERBAL REMEDIES

• A few drops of thyme tincture can be taken to loosen and expel mucus.
• Elecampane is commonly used for children's coughs, and can be purchased in easy-to-use syrup form.
• After a bath, you can massage a little comfrey ointment into the chest and back to relax and expand the lungs.

 HOMEOPATHIC REMEDIES

Treatment should be constitutional, but the following homeopathic remedies could be useful. Use the appropriate one for the symptoms.

Aconite 30C can be taken during an attack, or at the beginning of the illness.

Ant tart 30C is particularly good when there is a rattling cough with gasping.

Drosera 30C is useful when the cough is made worse by lying down, and there are pains below the ribs.

Bryonia 30C is suggested when there is a dry, painful cough and vomiting.

Pertussin 30C may be given in one dose towards the end off the disease to prevent an 'echo' effect.

 SEE YOUR DOCTOR

Most cases of whooping cough in older children and adults can be treated at home, but you must call your doctor immediately if your child becomes blue around the lips. Babies are most at risk of developing complications and sometimes they are admitted to hospital for treatment.

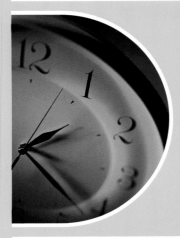

Sleep problems

Many children have difficulty sleeping, suffering from nightmares or night terrors, sleepwalking or sleeptalking, struggling to get to sleep at night or waking in the early hours and being unable to settle again. Sleep is essential for a child's emotional and physical health and wellbeing, so it is important that you investigate the underlying causes of sleep disturbances before attempting treatment.

 SYMPTOMS

▷ Night-waking
▷ Inability to fall asleep – or stay asleep
▷ Nightmares or night terrors
▷ Sleepwalking
▷ Sleeptalking
▷ Sleep apnoea

 PREVENTION

How you prevent sleep problems depends to some extent on your child's age. It takes babies a while to get into a regular pattern of sleeping and waking, and many parents expect them to sleep more than they actually need to, thereby creating a problem for themselves. Most toddlers and pre-school children sleep between 10 and 12 hours per night

- Do ensure that your child has plenty of regular exercise and fresh air, so that he is physically tired enough to fall asleep.
- A healthy diet that is low in processed food and sugar, focusing instead on good-quality proteins and whole grains, can help to prevent your child's blood sugar from soaring and dipping, which can exacerbate sleep problems.
- Establish a simple, reassuring bedtime routine and modify it as your child gets older. This should include: a bath, brushing teeth, a bedtime story, a goodnight cuddle and a kiss. A favourite cuddly toy and soothing music or a warm milky drink may also be helpful in encouraging sleep.

 Did you know?

Doctors and psychologists estimate that roughly 30 per cent of children will suffer from a sleep disorder at some point in their childhood. In many cases, the problems are only temporary, caused by illness, a change in routine, or even growth spurts.

CONVENTIONAL REMEDIES

Your child will be treated according to the cause of any sleep problems, but most doctors are reluctant to offer medication except in severe cases. Behavioural modification would be offered first.

 NATURAL REMEDIES

There are several types of remedy to try, depending on the specific problem. A common-sense approach is to get your child into a relaxing bedtime routine (see Prevention opposite), so that going to bed becomes a pleasurable experience.

AROMATHERAPY A few drops of chamomile, geranium, rose or lavender can be added to the bathwater to calm and soothe, or placed on a hanky by the bed. A gentle massage before bedtime, with a little lavender or chamomile blended into a light carrier oil, may ease any tension or distress.

 HERBAL REMEDIES

- Vervain infusion is a gentle sedative and can help children fall asleep – particularly, if they are fighting it.
- An infusion of limeflowers is useful for children who are nervous and sensitive.
- A crying baby may be soothed with an infusion of chamomile, offered an hour or so before bedtime, or on waking in the night.
- A strong infusion of chamomile, hops, lavender or limeflowers can be added to a warm bath to soothe and calm a baby or child.

 HOMEOPATHIC REMEDIES

Remedies should be taken an hour before going to bed, for up to 14 days. Repeat the dose if your child wakes in the night and cannot get back to sleep.

Calcarea 30C and **Ant tart 30C**, for night terrors.

Colocynth 30C or **Bryonia 30C**, for constant crying.

Arsenicum 30C, when your child wakes between midnight and 2am, restless, worried and apprehensive.

Rhus tox 30C when your child cannot sleep, is irritable, restless and wants to walk around.

Aconite 30C, for restlessness and nightmares.

Pulsatilla 30C, for a weepy, clingy child.

Chamomilla 30C if sleep is disturbed by teething, or if your child cannot settle without being hugged, rocked or patted to sleep.

Nux vomica 30C, for irritability, and after a busy day or too much food or fun.

 SEE YOUR DOCTOR

If the sleep difficulties last longer than a couple of months, your child is very sleepy during the day, or seems distressed by chronic nightmares or night terrors, you should see your doctor.

Flower remedies
- White Chestnut will be helpful for children with overactive minds.
- Offer Rock Rose for night terrors.
- Aspen is useful for fear of the dark, and Mimulus is good for other 'known' fears.

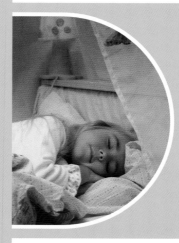

Bedwetting

Bedwetting (enuresis) is not considered a problem until your child is at least five years old. Many children, boys in particular, are slow in getting the message that they should get up to use the lavatory at night, but that is no reflection on the state of their health – emotional or otherwise. Some children are naturally deep sleepers and may take several years to stay dry at night; many children manage it by the age of two or three.

 SYMPTOMS

▷ Night-time urination

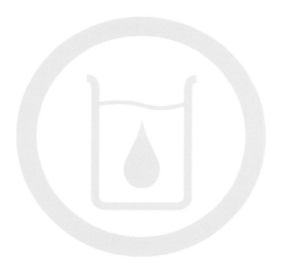

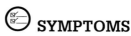 **Did you know?**

Bedwetting almost always stops as children get older because their bladder capacity increases as they grow and they learn to wake up if their bladder is full.

 PREVENTION

- Limit drinks in the hour or so before bedtime.
- Some parents find it helps to 'lift' their children to the toilet partway through the night.
- Reassure your child, as embarrassment can exacerbate the problem.
- Don't be tempted to carry on using nappies – it can be belittling for older children, and younger children will continue to wet them.
- A resumption of bedwetting in children who have already established a pattern of dry nights is often caused by stress or trauma of some sort, such as moving house, changing schools, family problems or even a new sibling. In most cases, the problem is resolved by age eight

CONVENTIONAL REMEDIES

Your doctor may prescribe antidepressants (not for depression, but because they have an impact on urination) and antidiuretic hormone medication (known as desmopressin), which concentrates the urine at night. A bedtime alarm (known as an enuresis alarm) can waken your child when he begins to urinate, giving him time to get to the lavatory. This has the impact of conditioning him to waken at the first signs of urination.

NATURAL REMEDIES

Treatment should be undertaken according to the likely cause of the enuresis.

HERBAL REMEDIES Offer St John's wort in a cup of water and sweetened with honey, sipped throughout the day, to encourage control of the bladder. If the bedwetting stems from an emotional upset or disturbance, infusions of vervain and lemon balm will relax and soothe.

HOMEOPATHIC REMEDIES

The following remedies may have some success.

Equisetum 30C when the wetting occurs during dreams.

Belladonna 30C when it occurs early in the night.

Kreosotum 30C when wetting occurs during dreams in early night, and deep sleep.

Causticum 30C, for wetting in first sleep, worse in clear weather or when your child has a cough,

Plantago 30C when all else fails.

 ## FLOWER REMEDIES

- Wild Rose if your child seems to drift through life.
- Walnut will help if the bedwetting is brought on by change, such as a new house, school or baby.
- Vervain may help if your child is stressed.
- Star of Bethlehem if bedwetting is related to a trauma or shock.
- Mimulus, when the problem is linked to fear.

 ## SEE YOUR DOCTOR

If your child is still bedwetting at the age of five, consult your doctor. In some cases, physical illness can be at the root, including food allergies, diabetes, a urinary tract infection, constipation and sleep apnoea. If your previously dry child wets the bed consistently for six months or more, there may be an underlying physical or emotional cause and it's worth seeking professional advice.

Self-help remedies

Try not to become angry with your child as this will only exacerbate the problem and affect their self-esteem. Instead, use a star chart and plenty of praise for dry nights, and don't comment if you find a wet bed. If your child is slightly older, you could suggest a sleepover at a friend's. Many children will not wet the bed under these circumstances, and it can help to break a long-term habit.

Caution

Never punish your child for wetting the bed, however troublesome it may be for you. This could lower their self-esteem and harm them psychologically. Try to be patient.

TOP 20
Healing herbs

Safe and gentle herbal remedies can offer a holistic approach to healing and help maintain our wellbeing. Here are the top 20 healing herbs with information on their properties and which common ailments they can be used to treat.

1 ALOE VERA

Properties antiseptic, blood purifier, laxative, purgative.

Used for acne and skin problems, burns, minor cuts, insect bites, digestive problems.

2 BASIL

Properties energy stimulant, respiratory decongestant, reduces mucus, aids digestion.

Used for fatigue, hay fever, headaches, insomnia, PMS, sinusitis.

3 CHAMOMILE

Properties carminative, anti-inflammatory, aids digestion, reduces mucus, calming.

Used for insomnia, stress, nervous tension, digestive problems, sore throat, colds, catarrh, asthma, eczema, teething problems in babies.

4 COMFREY

Properties tonic, demulcent, arrests bleeding, heals tissue, respiratory system, anaemia.

Used for soothing coughs, bronchial inflammation, healing cuts and burns.

5 DANDELION

Properties diuretic, purifies blood, liver tonic, aids digestion, nutritive.

Used for anaemia, constipation, fluid retention, diabetes, hepatitis, heart disease, excess weight.

6 ECHINACEA

Properties antibiotic, antiviral, antifungal, immune tonic, blood purifier, fever reducing.

Used for colds, flu, sore throats, acne, athlete's foot, kidney infections, candida and vaginal yeast infections.

7 GARLIC

Properties antiseptic, antibacterial, antifungal, blood purifier, circulatory stimulant, digestive stimulant.

Used for good digestion, lowering blood cholesterol, hypertension, heart disease, respiratory infections, strengthening immune system.

8 GINGER

Properties circulatory stimulant, antiseptic, analgesic, antispasmodic, expectorant.

Used for colds, flu, fever, nausea and vomiting,

9 GOLDEN SEAL

Properties antibiotic, astringent, blood purifier, laxative.

Used for treating inflammation and infection, colds, flu, catarrh, ulcers, nausea, colitis, IBS, gastroenteritis, urinary tract infections, boils.

10 LAVENDER

Properties sedative, cooling, antibacterial, aromatic.

Used for anxiety, stress, headaches, migraines, insomnia, stress, indigestion, coughs, colds, burns, stings, minor cuts, sunburn.

⑪ LEMON BALM

Properties calming, antibacterial, anti-depressant, antiseptic, blood purifier and regulator, insect repellant.

Used for depression, easing menstrual cramping, digestive upsets, infections, fever, insect bites, wounds.

⑫ MARSHMALLOW

Properties astringent, anti-inflammatory, demulcent, blood purifier, nutritive.

Used for irritable bowel, colitis, kidney stones, urinary inflammations, coughs, catarrh, boils, abscesses, drawing splinters and pus

⑬ MEADOWSWEET

Properties calming, antacid, antiseptic, anti-inflammatory, analgesic, diuretic, astringent, source of natural aspirin.

Used for gastritis and digestive upsets, arthritis, rheumatism, headaches, urinary infections.

⑭ PLANTAIN

Properties antibacterial, diuretic, blood purifier, astringent, demulcent.

Used for insects stings, cuts, abrasions, burns, eczema, IBS, cystitis, heavy menstrual bleeding, thrush, vaginal discharge, gum disease, fever.

⑮ ROSEMARY

Properties restorative, antiseptic, circulatory stimulant, blood regulator, aromatic.

Used for PMT, depression, headaches, migraine, indigestion, constipation, arthritis, rheumatism, colds, flu, fever,

⑯ SAGE

Properties astringent, antiseptic, diuretic, stimulant, clears mucus.

Used for respiratory problems, ulcers, sore throat, hot flushes in menopause.

⑰ ST JOHN'S WORT

Properties anti-depressant, sedative, restorative, anti-inflammatory, tonic and pain relieving, soothing, antiseptic.

Used for wounds, inflammations, ulcers, sciatica, neuralgia, rheumatism, anxiety, depression, post-operative pain, period pain, burns, cuts and scrapes.

⑱ TEA TREE

Properties antiseptic, antifungal, treating infections.

Used for acne, cold sores, insect stings and bites, warts, abscesses, gum and tooth infections, ringworm, athlete's foot, thrush.

⑲ THYME

Properties antiseptic, stimulant, respiratory cleanser, expectorant.

Used for colds, flu, coughs, bronchitis, sore throat, diarrhoea, wounds.

⑳ YARROW

Properties anti-inflammatory, astringent, digestive tonic, blood regulator.

Used for fever, wounds, urinary problems, colds, flu, infections, excessive menstrual bleeding, cramping.

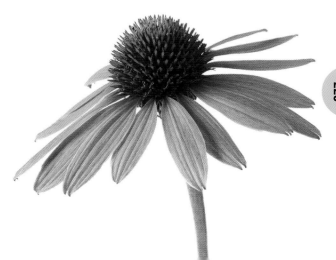

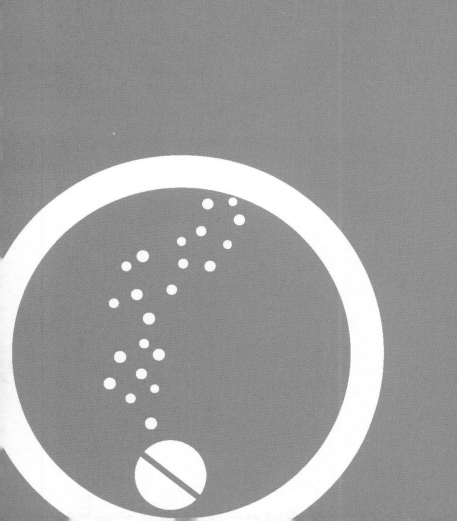

First aid and emergencies

You can treat most minor accidental injuries yourself at home with conventional treatments and first-aid measures or natural remedies. Featured in the following pages is practical advice on treating a wide range of problems, ranging from insect bites and stings to nosebleeds, splinters and fainting. If you know how to treat them fast and effectively, you are less likely to suffer from complications and you can prevent the condition worsening and speed up the healing process.

However, if you have to deal with a serious accident or life-threatening injury, you must contact the emergency services immediately and, if necessary, carry out emergency life-saving first aid, such as resuscitation, which does not come within the scope of this book. It is a good idea to familiarise yourself with these techniques and go on a first-aid course to enable you to deal with emergencies if they arise.

Common sense and good judgement are essential, even when dealing with common injuries, and it is extremely important to stay calm, to reassure your patient and protect them from further danger. You should also have a first-aid box at home and keep it stocked up with conventional medications, bandages, dressings, plasters and antiseptic creams as well as natural remedies, such as arnica cream, Bach Rescue Remedy liquid or cream, witch hazel, aloe vera gel and marigold cream. Eucalyptus, lavender and tea tree essential oils are also useful. Tweezers, scissors and safety pins are essential items.

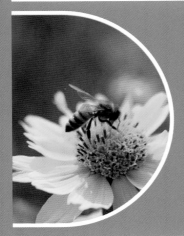

Bites and stings

If your skin is punctured by an animal bite, you must act quickly as bite and puncture wounds can become infected if they are not treated promptly. Insect bites and stings are seldom serious but they may trigger allergic reactions in some people. Conventional first aid and natural remedies can treat the problem and alleviate the symptoms.

 ## SYMPTOMS

▷ Puncture marks in the skin
▷ Bleeding from wound
▷ Pain and swelling from snake bites
▷ Itching, pain, redness and swelling from insect bites and stings
▷ In rare cases, an allergic reaction with difficulty breathing, pale and clammy skin, sweating, nausea, fainting, mental confusion

 ## PREVENTION

You can't prevent bites and stings happening but you can minimise their likelihood.

- If you live in an area where there are snakes, wear trousers and do not go barefoot in the summer. In the UK, watch out for adders in long grass and on heaths.
- If mosquitoes are commonplace, use an insect repellent. You can buy non-toxic natural products as well as chemical repellents. Cover up any exposed skin.
- If you are travelling to a tropical country where malaria is a problem, seek medical advice before you go. You can take a course of anti-malaria medication. Be sure to sleep under a mosquito net and check that all doors and windows have insect-proof screens.
- Don't use strongly perfumed cosmetics and deodorants – these can attract insects.
- Check there are no wasp nests in your garden.
- Keep your tetanus injections up to date.

 ## Did you know?

If you are stung by a jellyfish, remove any visible stings and treat with calamine lotion or antihistamine cream. Apply cut tomato slices or sit in a warm bath. A Portuguese Man-of-War sting may cause more severe reactions and shortness of breath; seek medical help.

FIRST AID

The conventional remedies for dealing with bites and stings are as follows.

ANIMAL BITES Wash the wound carefully with soap and warm water. Pat dry with a clean tissue, then cover with a sterile dressing or plaster. For wounds with severe bleeding, using a clean pad or dressing, apply direct pressure to the wound to control the bleeding. Cover it with a sterile dressing and bandage and seek medical attention immediately. You may need an anti-tetanus vaccination or, in some countries, anti-rabies injections.

SNAKE BITES In the British Isles, the only poisonous snake is the adder, which is easily identifiable from the distinctive dark zigzag pattern along its back and dark V- or X-shaped marking on the head. Adder bites are rare and most cases are very mild. If you are bitten by a snake, don't panic – stay calm. Keep the bitten area as still as possible, wash the wound gently with soap and water if available, and seek immediate medical attention.

INSECT BITES Most gnat and mosquito bites can be treated locally with soothing calamine lotion or antihistamine cream. Or apply a cold compress and take painkillers, such as paracetamol. For severe swelling, your doctor may prescribe oral steroids. If you have a severe allergic reaction, seek immediate medical assistance.

INSECT STINGS If the sting is visible, try to remove it with a clean finger or tweezers. Wash with soap and warm water and apply a cold compress to reduce the swelling. If the sting is painful, take paracetamol or another painkiller. If the pain and swelling persist for 48 hours or you experience a severe allergic reaction, seek expert medical help.

 # NATURAL REMEDIES

There are many traditional remedies for insect bites.

- Cut a clove of garlic and rub onto the skin surrounding mosquito bites, or blend a crushed clove with honey and apply to bites and stings.
- Rub a slice of raw onion onto flea bites, bee and wasp stings.
- Make a paste with bicarbonate of soda and vinegar and dab onto bee stings.
- Make a paste with salt and vinegar and dab onto wasp stings.

AROMATHERAPY Apply a drop of neat lavender oil to the insect bite or sting.

 # HERBAL REMEDIES

- Apply the soothing sap of the aloe vera plant or a little gel to the insect bite.
- Rub the affected area with some plantain leaves or lemon balm.
- For bee and wasp stings, bathe with an infusion of sage or marigold.

 # HOMEOPATHIC REMEDIES

The remedy used will depend on the symptoms.

Apis mel 30C, for burning and rapid swelling from bee and wasp stings and insect bites, take one tablet every hour for three doses.

Ledum 30C, for immediate swelling from animal and insect bites and stings, take one tablet hourly for three doses.

 # SEE YOUR DOCTOR

If you are bitten by an animal or snake, or develop a severe reaction to an insect bite, see a doctor as soon as possible.

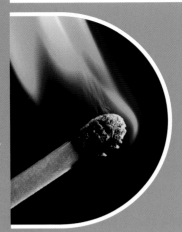

Burns and scalds

Burns are damage to the skin's tissues, caused by dry heat (fire), corrosive chemicals, electricity, radiated heat (from the sun) or friction. Scalds are caused by moist heat (hot liquids or steam). Both burns and scalds are treated in the same way with first aid measures, although natural remedies may be used to relieve pain and speed up healing.

 ## SYMPTOMS

▷ Sore, red skin

▷ May be blisters (pockets of clear fluid)

▷ Pain and swelling

▷ In severe cases, skin may be broken, severely blistered or charred (black) with intense pain

 ## PREVENTION

To minimise the risk of burns and scalds, be aware of potentially dangerous situations and substances and follow common-sense safety guidelines.

- Always take care when filling hot water bottles, pouring boiling water out of kennels and handling hot liquids.
- Use coiled safety cables on kettles and never leave any wires and cables hanging down within reach of young children.
- Never put your hand over steam.
- Take special care when using or carrying hot chip pans.
- Be careful when handling chemicals or electrical wires. Always unplug appliances and turn off the electric current before tackling DIY jobs.
- Protect open fires and gas fires with a sturdy fireguard.
- Wear a strong sunscreen in hot, sunny weather to protect your skin from burning.

Caution

- Do not try to remove any clothing that may be stuck to the burnt skin.
- Do not burst any blisters that form.
- Do not apply cream, ointment or butter to the burn.
- Do not attempt to cool it with ice.

FIRST AID

The conventional advice for dealing with minor burns and scalds is to treat them immediately without delay.

1 Stop the burning process by dousing the flames with water or smothering them in a blanket.

2 Remove any jewellery or clothing near the burnt skin but not if it is sticking to it. If it has been soaked in boiling water, hot fat or chemical agents and is not sticking to the burnt area, you should remove it.

3 Cool the burn with cold or tepid water for at least 10 minutes or until the pain stops. You can do this by immersing the burnt area in cold water or holding it under a running tap.

4 Cover the burn with cling film or a clean transparent plastic bag or clean, non-fluffy material to protect it from infection.

5 Keep warm if the burn is extensive to prevent your body temperature dropping and hypothermia.

NOTE For burns to the mouth and throat, sip some cold water.

 # NATURAL REMEDIES

Severe burns should always be treated by a medical professional but there are some natural remedies that may be helpful for healing minor burns after the first aid measures outlined above.

HERBAL REMEDIES When healing is underway, you can soothe minor burns with aloe vera sap or gel. Alternatively, smooth in a little calendula ointment. Diluted witch hazel promotes healing and helps prevent infection.

AROMATHERAPY Apply a drop of neat lavender oil to minor burns where there is no blistering or broken skin after immersing the area in cold water and patting it dry.

 # HOMEOPATHIC REMEDIES

The remedy used will depend on the symptoms.

Aconitum 30C, for initial trauma and shock.

Cantharis 30C, for raw burns with severe pain and possibly blisters.

Urtica urens 30C, for red skin with minor stinging.

 # SEE YOUR DOCTOR

You can treat most minor burns yourself at home but severe burns will require immediate medical attention. These include the following:

- Burns affecting an extensive area with seriously blistered skin
- Burns to the mouth and throat, which cause swelling and inflammation
- Deep burns with broken, charred skin
- Chemical and electrical burns.

NOTE Pregnant women, babies and young children should also see a doctor.

Self-help remedies

- Always keep the burnt area clean and dry.
- If the burn is extensive, drink additional fluids
  to prevent feeling dehydrated.
- Eating foods that are good sources of vitamin
  C (citrus fruits, strawberries, tomatoes, peppers, blackcurrants and leafy green vegetables) and zinc (pumpkin seeds, mushrooms, seafood, meat, eggs) will promote repair of damaged skin tissue. Or you can take supplements.

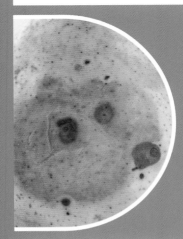

Bruises

A bruise is a discoloured area of skin caused by damaged tiny broken blood vessels leaking blood underneath into the dermis. It is usually caused by a blow or pressure and gradually fades as it heals. Severe bruising and swelling of the eye socket and eye lids is known as a black eye.

 ## SYMPTOMS
▷ Blue, purple or black patch of skin
▷ Fades to yellow or green before disappearing
▷ Pain, tenderness and swelling
▷ Movement may be restricted

 ## PREVENTION
You can't prevent bruising but if you have a tendency to bruise easily and frequently you should take extra care to avoid knocks, falls and other injuries.

FIRST AID
Treat a bruise as soon as possible after injury to minimise the swelling and bruising.
1 Apply an ice pack to the bruised area. A bag of frozen peas is ideal for this – wrap it in a cloth or towel first. Keep it in place with a bandage or cloth. Cooling the area with ice packs will help limit the bleeding under the skin.
2 Alternatively, apply a cold compress – soak a towel or flannel in cold water, wring it out and apply to the bruise, changing it every 10 minutes for 30 minutes.
3 Elevating the bruised limb, especially if it is a leg or foot, may promote healing.
4 If necessary, take a painkiller, such as ibuprofen.

 ## Did you know?
You may have a tendency to bruise more easily if you are very slim and don't have much 'padding' and fat covering your arms and legs.

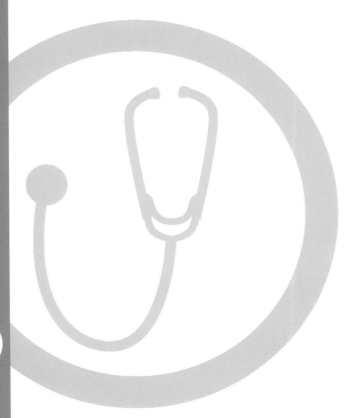

NATURAL REMEDIES

Bruises usually respond well to old-fashioned, natural remedies. Some people believe that the best remedy for a black eye is to hold a raw steak against it.

HERBAL REMEDIES Apply a cold compress soaked in an infusion of comfrey or rue; or gently smooth some comfrey, chickweed or arnica lotion or cream into the bruised area. Or you can rub some aloe vera gel or sap into the bruise.

AROMATHERAPY Add 2 drops each chamomile and lavender essential oils to some ice-cold water and use as a compress.

SELF-HELP REMEDIES For a black eye or any other form of bruising, drink several glasses of pineapple juice daily. It contains enzymes that help to speed up healing. Apply a vitamin E cream to the bruised skin.

 ## HOMEOPATHIC REMEDIES

The remedy used will depend on the symptoms.

Arnica 30C, for all bruising.

Ledum 30C, for dark bruises that feel cold and black eyes with swollen skin.

Bellis perennis 30C, for deep bruising and sore muscles.

Aconite 30C, for shock after the blow of a black eye.

 ## SEE YOUR DOCTOR

Most bruising is minor and does not need medical attention, but you should consult your doctor for any of the following:

- You have two black eyes – may indicate a fractured skull
- Bruises appear for no apparent reason without injury
- You have a tendency to bruise easily and often
- Bruising is accompanied by severe pain and difficulty moving.

NOTE There may be an underlying medical condition that is causing unexplained bruising, possibly linked to blood clotting or liver problems, so check it out without delay. In addition, not all bruises are visible. Deep, internal bruising after an injury or accident may cause pain and swelling – if in doubt, always check with your doctor.

 ## Quick fix

If you hit your skin, injure yourself or at the first sign of a bruise appearing, quickly rub in some arnica cream.

Caution

- Never rub or vigorously massage the bruise – this will only make it worse.
- Never apply arnica cream to broken skin.

Cuts and grazes

You can treat most minor cuts and grazes yourself. They may bleed and feel painful at the time but they will soon heal. However, deeper cuts with greater blood loss may damage blood vessels, nerves and tendons below the skin.

 ## SYMPTOMS

▷ Bleeding and pain
▷ Surface layer of skin is scraped off (graze)

 ## PREVENTION

Obviously you cannot prevent cuts and grazes happening from time to time but you can take extra care when you are using sharp kitchen knives, saws, axes and gardening implements. A lot of accidents involving cuts occur in the home and garden.

 ## FIRST AID

1 Stop any bleeding by applying pressure to the cut with a clean, dry towel or cloth.
2 Wash the cut area under running tap water or bathe with warm water to clean the wound and remove dirt.
3 Gently pat dry with a clean towel.
4 Cover with a sterile dressing or plaster.

 ## NATURAL REMEDIES

Cuts and grazes have been treated with natural therapies and remedies for centuries.

HERBAL REMEDIES Chamomile, echinacea, calendula (marigold) or St John's wort cream may aid the healing process for cuts and grazes.

AROMATHERAPY When cleaning a cut or graze, add antiseptic lavender or tea tree oil to the warm water. To speed up healing, apply diluted essential oil of lavender or cloves.

 ## HOMEOPATHIC REMEDIES

The remedy used will depend on the symptoms.

Hypericum 30C, for all deep and painful wounds, especially with dirt.

Ledum 30C, for clean puncture wounds and cuts.

Calendula 30C, for profuse bleeding and likely infection.

 ## SEE YOUR DOCTOR

Seek medical help in the following instances:

- You have a deep wound and cannot stop the bleeding after applying direct pressure for 10 minutes. It may need stitching
- The cut is contaminated with substances you can't remove, such as glass
- It becomes infected and painful with swelling, redness and pus
- It will not close and opens up when you move.

NOTE Keep your tetanus injections up to date.

Self-help remedies

- To bathe cuts and grazes, add ordinary table salt to the warm water – this is a good disinfectant.
- Blend a spoonful of honey with a crushed garlic clove and smear over cuts and grazes before covering with a clean dressing.

Nosebleeds

Nosebleeds (epistaxis) are rarely serious and may be caused by minor injuries, infections, illness or cold weather. When the tiny blood vessels inside the nose rupture – perhaps due to cracked, dry mucous membranes – your nose bleeds.

 SYMPTOMS

▷ Bleeding from the nose
▷ Usually from one nostril but may be both
▷ Flow of blood may be heavy or light

 PREVENTION

You cannot prevent nosebleeds happening but you can make them less likely by not picking your nose or blowing it too hard.

 FIRST AID

1 Sit down, leaning forwards.
2 Breathing through your mouth, pinch the fleshy end of your nose (just above your nostrils) between your thumb and forefinger. Hold for 10–20 minutes, until the bleeding stops.
3 Wipe away any blood from around the nose and mouth with a cotton wool pad moistened with water.
NOTE Don't lie down – the blood will drain down the back of your throat.

 Did you know?

Nosebleeds are more common when you are pregnant as the increased blood supply in your body makes the tiny blood vessels in the nose more likely to rupture. You may also get them if you are taking aspirin or anticoagulants (such as warfarin) or have a blood disorder.

 NATURAL REMEDIES

The traditional natural approaches to dealing with nosebleeds are listed below. Applying an ice pack or cold sponge may help stop the bleeding.
HERBAL REMEDIES When the bleeding stops, plug the nostril with a little cotton wool or lint soaked in witch hazel.

 HOMEOPATHIC REMEDIES

The remedy used will depend on the symptoms.
Ferrum phos 30C, for bright red blood that oozes from the nose.
Phosphorus 30C, for nosebleeds in children and when blowing the nose.
Sabina 30C, for a general tendency to nosebleeds.
Arnica 30C, for nosebleeds resulting from a blow to the nose.

 SEE YOUR DOCTOR

If the bleeding continues for more than 30 minutes and will not stop, you should seek medical attention. Likewise, if it is accompanied by shortness of breath or palpitations, or you vomit from swallowing blood. See your doctor if you have frequent nosebleeds – more than once a week – for no apparent reason; they may be a symptom of an underlying medical condition, such as high blood pressure.

Fainting

Fainting is a brief loss of consciousness, caused by a sudden drop in blood pressure or abnormally low blood sugar levels. Emotional shock, stress, anxiety, exhaustion, standing for too long, dehydration and heat can interrupt temporarily the supply of blood to your brain, causing you to faint.

 ## SYMPTOMS

▷ Brief loss of consciousness
▷ May be preceded by feeling giddy, unsteady and light-headed
▷ Feeling weak, cold, sweaty or clammy
▷ Feeling nauseous
▷ Confusion
▷ Blurred vision
▷ A slow pulse
▷ May result in a fall

 ## PREVENTION

You can minimise the risk of fainting by makin sure you eat regular meals, drinking sufficient liquid (especially in hot climates), avoiding stuffy and overheated rooms, and not standing for long periods.

 ## FIRST AID

1 If you feel faint, sit or lie down immediately to prevent a fall and subsequent injuries.
2 Ideally, lie on your back with your legs raised above the level of your heart. Support them with some cushions or whatever is handy.
3 Alternatively, if there is no room to lie down, sit with your head between your knees.
4 Loosen any tight clothing and, if indoors, ask someone to open the windows to let in fresh air.
5 When you regain consciousness, stay lying down for a few minutes before trying to get up. You may feel weak and confused for up to 30 minutes.

 ## NATURAL REMEDIES

The old-fashioned remedy for fainting was smelling salts, and you can still buy these in most pharmacies. After regaining consciousness, sip some weak green or Indian tea sweetened with honey.
HERBAL REMEDIES To aid recovery, drink some chamomile tea.
AROMATHERAPY Sniffing rosemary or tea tree oil may help to bring a person round.
FLOWER REMEDIES Take three to four drops Rescue Remedy in water.

 ## HOMEOPATHIC REMEDIES

Crush a tablet and put a few grains on the tongue.
Ignatia 6C, for sudden emotional shock.
Lilium tigrinum 30C, for becoming overheated
Sepia 30C, for a general tendency to faint.

 ## SEE YOUR DOCTOR

Isolated episodes are not a cause for concern but if you have a tendency to faint, see your doctor. There may be an underlying medical reason for the problem, such as diabetes or heart disease.
NOTE If the person does not regain consciousness, call an ambulance immediately.

Sprains and strains

A sprain occurs when the ligaments around a joint, such as the wrist, thumb, ankle or knee, are over-stretched, twisted or even torn. A strain is when the tissues or fibres that make up a muscle become over-stretched or torn, usually due to a sudden movement. This is often referred to as 'pulling a muscle'.

 ## SYMPTOMS

SPRAINS
▷ Pain and tenderness around the joint
▷ Swelling, inflammation and bruising
▷ Inability to use a joint normally or put weight on it

STRAINS
▷ Sudden sharp pain and swelling in a muscle
▷ Bruising

 ## PREVENTION

Many sprains and strains are sports injuries: minimise the risk by stretching. Regular exercise in the gym, cycling, swimming, walking or whatever you enjoy, will keep you fit and supple. If you are prone to sprained ankles, strap them up when you exercise and wear supportive trainers. Don't wear really high heels!

 ## FIRST AID

The acronym for the recommended treatment for sprains and strains is PRICE.

1 Protect the injured joint or muscle from getting worse with a support if necessary.

2 Rest the injured area for at least 48 hours.

3 Ice packs should be applied to the injury to reduce the swelling for 15 to 20 minutes at a time. Repeat every three hours or so during the first couple of days.

4 Compression will limit movement and decrease swelling. Use a tubular, elastic or crepe bandage.

5 Elevation of the injured area, especially a knee or ankle joint, will also reduce the swelling.

 ## NATURAL REMEDIES

A warm bath will reduce the swelling and ease the pain – add a cup of Epsom salt or a spoonful of mustard powder.

HERBAL REMEDIES Make a poultice of comfrey or cabbage leaves and wrap around the injury in a towel or cloth. Leave for 20 to 30 minutes. Rub in a little arnica, comfrey or marigold cream.

AROMATHERAPY Add chamomile, cypress, eucalyptus or rosemary oil to a carrier oil and massage gently into the affected area, or add a few drops to a warm bath.

 ## HOMEOPATHIC REMEDIES

Choose a remedy according to the symptoms.

Arnica 30C, for bruising, pain and shock on the first day.

Ledum 6C, for sprains, especially ankles

 ## SEE YOUR DOCTOR

Because some sprains can be difficult to differentiate from a fracture, you must seek medical help if:
• The injured joint looks crooked or has unusual lumps and bumps
• The pain is severe and persistent
• You cannot put any weight on the injury or move it
• You experience numbness in the area.

NOTE Do not resume exercise until the injured joint is healed. Returning to sport too soon may cause further damage. If in doubt, check with your doctor or a sports fitness expert.

Heat exhaustion

This is when body temperature rises to 37–40°C (98.6–104°F). It should not be confused with heatstroke when your temperature rises above 40°C (104°F). Both conditions are more likely to happen in very hot, humid weather.

 SYMPTOMS

HEAT EXHAUSTION
▷ Feeling hot, flushed and sweating profusely
▷ Headache
▷ Feeling faint and dizzy
▷ Nausea and vomiting

HEATSTROKE
▷ Muscle cramps
▷ Rapid shallow breathing
▷ Mental confusion
▷ Seizures or fits
▷ Loss of consciousness

 PREVENTION

• Stay in the shade out of the sun, especially in the middle of the day, and wear a sun hat.
• Wear loose-fitting, light cotton or linen clothes.
• Don't drink alcohol or caffeinated drinks but have lots of cold drinks to stay hydrated.
• Keep your house cool.
• Don't leave babies, children, elderly people or pets in parked cars in hot weather.

 FIRST AID

Heat exhaustion leads to heatstroke if left untreated, so act fast.
1 Lie down in a cool place – preferably inside with a fan or air conditioning. Loosen any tight clothing.
2 Drink plenty of water or a sports rehydration drink.
3 Sponge your face and body with cold water or take a cold shower or bath to cool down.
NOTE If heatstroke is suspected, call an ambulance.

 NATURAL REMEDIES

In cases of heat exhaustion, common sense is the best remedy but the following may aid recovery.
HERBAL REMEDIES You can relieve a fever and headache by adding ½ teaspoon cayenne to 100ml boiling water. Dilute with cold water and sip slowly. Eating a raw or cooked onion may also help bring relief and protection.
FLOWER REMEDIES Add a few drops of Rescue Remedy to a glass of water and drink three to four times a day or apply directly to the tongue.

 HOMEOPATHIC REMEDIES

Choose a remedy according to the symptoms.
Belladonna 30C, for burning, hot, dry skin and dilated pupils.
Bryonia alba 30C, for a severe headache.

 SEE YOUR DOCTOR

Most cases of heat exhaustion do not require medical attention but heatstroke is a medical emergency and will require hospitalisation. Elderly people, babies, children and people with chronic health problems are most at risk of developing both conditions.

Sunburn

This is caused by the ultraviolet (UV) rays in sunlight. If you are fair skinned or have naturally blonde or red hair, you will have low levels of melanin – the pigment that protects your skin against burning and helps you to tan.

 ## SYMPTOMS

▷ Red, sore or painful skin
▷ Skin feels warm even in the shade
▷ May blister
▷ May peel or flake

 ## PREVENTION

- Apply sunscreen with an SPF of at least 15 at regular intervals, even if you are dark or olive skinned – you can still suffer sun damage.
- Use water-resistant sunscreen before and after swimming.
- Use a sunblock on your lips, nose and areas that burn easily or where the skin is very thin.
- Cover up with light, loose clothing and a sun hat.
- Wear sunglasses with UV filters to protect your eyes and the delicate skin around them.
- Stay indoors or in the shade between 11am and 3pm when the sun is at its strongest.

 ## FIRST AID

1 Cool sunburnt skin in a cool shower or bath, or sponge with some cold water and gently pat dry.
2 Apply an aftersun moisturizing cream.
3 If your skin is very itchy and sore, smooth on some calamine lotion.
4 Drink plenty of water or non-alcoholic fluids to rehydrate your body.
5 If it's very painful take paracetamol or ibuprofen.
6 If you go back in the sun, cover up and wear a hat.

 ## NATURAL REMEDIES

To relieve mild sunburn, blend two parts cider vinegar and one part olive oil and apply to the affected areas.
HERBAL REMEDIES To soothe sore skin apply aloe vera gel or some fresh sap. Calendula (marigold) cream is also soothing.
AROMATHERAPY Add a few drops of lavender, chamomile or peppermint oil to a tepid bath

 ## HOMEOPATHIC REMEDIES

Choose a remedy according to the symptoms.
Belladonna 6C, for red, sore, inflamed skin with throbbing headache.
Cantharsis 6C, for sunburn with blisters.

 ## SEE YOUR DOCTOR

Unless the sunburn is very severe or the blisters get infected, there is no need to seek medical advice.

Caution
You don't need to be in the sun to get sunburnt. Beware of hazy days with high cloud and a breeze at the seaside or even light reflecting off snow.

Shock

This life-threatening condition, usually associated with accidents, may be caused by large blood loss, severe burns or serious injuries. It is characterised by a dramatic drop in blood pressure and requires hospitalisation. Less severe emotional shock may follow bad news or a fright, triggering anxiety or fainting.

 SYMPTOMS

▷ Skin is pale, cold and clammy
▷ Rapid, weak pulse
▷ Shallow, fast breathing
▷ Thirst
▷ Yawning and sighing
▷ Drowsiness and confusion
▷ Loss of consciousness

 FIRST AID

For severe clinical shock, do the following:
1 Call an ambulance.
2 Lay the person down on their back with their legs slightly raised. Support them with cushions, pillows or whatever is available.
3 Loosen any tight clothing.
4 Talk reassuringly but do not offer anything to drink or eat.
5 Check the person's pulse and breathing often. If he or she becomes unconscious, they may need resuscitation.

 NATURAL REMEDIES

The traditional natural approach to dealing with lesser emotional shock is plenty of rest and relaxation.
HERBAL REMEDIES Sip a tea made with elderflower, rosemary, chamomile or lemon balm.
AROMATHERAPY Add lavender, geranium or chamomile oil to a carrier oil and use as a relaxing body massage or just work on the legs and arms.
FLOWER REMEDIES Take a few drops of Bach Rescue Remedy in water at regular intervals.
NUTRITIONAL MEDICINE Vitamin B and zinc may be beneficial. Take a daily supplement or eat foods that are rich in these nutrients.

 HOMEOPATHIC REMEDIES

The remedy used will depend on the symptoms.
Aconitum 30C, for a sudden fright, sweat and rapid pulse.
Arsenicum album 30C, for great anxiety, restlessness and weak pulse.

 SEE YOUR DOCTOR

For severe clinical shock, you must get medical assistance immediately. For lesser emotional shock, it may help to talk to your doctor or a therapist.

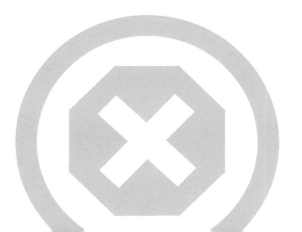

Splinters

Splinters are usually thorns or very small fragments of wood, glass or metal that become embedded in the skin, often when you are performing household chores or working in the garden. If the splinters are not removed, they can become infected and very painful.

 ## SYMPTOMS

▷ The end of the splinter may be visible
▷ Swollen and inflamed skin
▷ Discomfort and pain

 ## FIRST AID

1 Wash the area around the splinter with warm water and soap. If the splinter is embedded deeply, soak it in warm water for 10 to 15 minutes.
2 Squeeze the splinter out by applying pressure on the skin to both sides.
3 If it does not budge, pull it out with tweezers, grasping the end firmly and extracting it at the same angle it went in.
4 If the splinter is stubborn or embedded deeply, tease it out with a sterilised needle.
5 If the wound bleeds, cover it with a plaster.

 ## NATURAL REMEDIES

The traditional method of removing a splinter was to cover it with a hot bread poultice

HERBAL REMEDIES For deep splinters, rub some marshmallow, chickweed or slippery elm ointment into the skin, then cover with a dressing or plaster for an hour to two to draw out the splinter. You can then remove it in the usual way with tweezers or a sterile needle, and dab with tea tree oil or vervain tincture.

AROMATHERAPY After removing a splinter, add a drop of antiseptic lavender oil to the skin.

HOMEOPATHIC REMEDIES Try using Silicea 6C to expel glass shards and splinters, but take sparingly – no more than one tablet twice a day for a maximum of 14 days.

 ## SEE YOUR DOCTOR

Splinters rarely merit medical attention, but if they are really deep under the skin or a finger nail and become infected you may need to see a doctor. You may also wish to consider being inoculated against tetanus.

 ## Did you know?

To sterilise a needle or tweezers, you can pass it through a gas or candle flame, taking care not to burn your fingers.

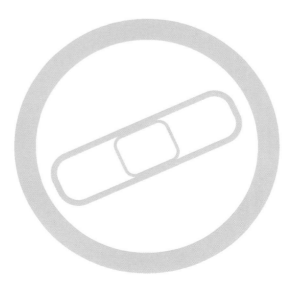

Motion sickness

This term is used to cover a range of symptoms that may be triggered by travelling by sea, air, road or rail. If you do have to go on a long journey or a sea crossing, there are conventional and natural remedies you can take.

 ## SYMPTOMS

▷ Feeling unwell
▷ Dizziness
▷ Cold sweat
▷ Nausea and sickness

 ## PREVENTION

To prevent motion sickness, you can buy over-the-counter tablets or patches in most pharmacies. You must follow the instructions and take them before you set out on your journey. You can also try the following.

- In a boat or car, get some fresh air. Go up on deck or open a window.
- Sit in the middle of a boat where it is more stable and moves less.
- Closing your eyes may help; otherwise try fixing them on a distant object and focus on that.
- Don't eat or drink before travelling.

 ## CONVENTIONAL REMEDIES

The usual remedy for dealing with nausea and sickness is hyoscine, which is widely available from pharmacists. It works by blocking nerve systems sent from the inner ear – which gives you your sense of balance – when they are in conflict with what your eyes can actually see.

 ## NATURAL REMEDIES

One of the simplest remedies is just to suck some liquorice sweets or eat a stick of candied liquorice.

HERBAL REMEDIES Make a chamomile, black horehound, lemon balm or licorice tea. Alternatively, put a couple of drops of tincture on your tongue.

AROMATHERAPY To settle an upset stomach, put a few drops of peppermint oil on a handkerchief and sniff frequently.

NUTRITIONAL MEDICINE Ginger supplements may help to prevent or alleviate the symptoms of motion sickness. Alternatively, steep some grated ginger in boiling water, then strain and sweeten with honey before sipping. Give children small pieces of crystallised ginger to nibble.

ACUPRESSURE You can try wearing an acupressure wristband; these are available from most health stores and pharmacies.

 ## HOMEOPATHIC REMEDIES

The remedy used will depend on the symptoms.

Cocculus 30C, for nausea and giddiness, worsened by watching moving objects.

Tabacum 30C, for nausea and headache, which improves in cold fresh air or with eyes closed.

 ## SEE YOUR DOCTOR

If over-the-counter medication does not work or you are over 70, have a history of heart disease, liver or kidney problems, have an overactive thyroid or are pregnant, see your doctor.

Hangover

This term is used to cover all the symptoms associated with drinking too much alcohol. Excessive alcohol dehydrates the body, dilates the blood vessels in your head and reduces blood sugar levels, causing a hangover.

 SYMPTOMS

▷ Feeling tired
▷ Throbbing headache and dizziness
▷ Dehydration and thirst
▷ Sensitivity to noise and light
▷ Sweating and interrupted sleep
▷ Nausea and sickness
▷ Diarrhoea
▷ Red, bloodshot eyes
▷ Shaking and tremors

 PREVENTION

• Drink plenty of water as well as alcohol, alternating them if possible.
• Always try to eat a meal before drinking alcohol.
• Avoid dark-coloured drinks, such as red wine, port and brandy – stick to white wine or clear spirits.

 CONVENTIONAL REMEDIES

Drink plenty of water and isotonic drinks to counter dehydration. Take paracetamol to ease headaches.

 Did you know?

Darker-coloured alcoholic drinks, such as red wine or port, may produce more severe hangovers, possibly due to the larger numbers of toxic 'congeners' that they contain.

 NATURAL REMEDIES

There are many traditional remedies for hangovers, including the 'hair of the dog' but drinking more alcohol will only make your symptoms worse.

HERBAL REMEDIES Make a soothing cup of dandelion or kudzu tea.

AROMATHERAPY Relax in a warm bath to which you have added a couple of drops of juniper and fennel essential oils.

NUTRITIONAL MEDICINE Have a large glass of fruit juice to rehydrate you. Orange, grapefruit and tomato juice all contain fructose, a natural sugar which helps your body to metabolise the alcohol faster. Sip some vegetable bouillon or clear chicken soup, or make a milkshake with a fresh banana, milk and honey.

HOMEOPATHIC REMEDIES The remedy used to treat headaches associated with too much alcohol is Nux vomica 6C.

 SEE YOUR DOCTOR

Most hangovers will get better within 24 hours. However, if you drink heavily and often wake up with a hangover, you have a serious problem and you should seek expert medical help.

NOTE Even the following day you may still be over the legal limit for driving, and it is also sensible not to operate any heavy machinery.

Glossary

Acupressure

In Traditional Chinese Medicine, pressure massage on the pressure points along the acupuncture meridians (the channels through which the body's motivating energy flows). Used to relieve tension-related ailments.

Acupuncture

Needles are inserted in the acupuncture points along the meridians running through the body to balance the flow of Qi (pronounced 'chee'), which is the vital motivating energy.

Alexander Technique

A technique, developed by F.M. Alexander, for improving posture, balance and respiratory function, and using muscles more efficiently

Analgesics

Pain-relieving drugs, including simple analgesics for mild pain (aspirin, paracetamol); anti-inflammatories for arthritis and muscular pain; and narcotic analgesics for severe pain (morphine).

Antibiotics

Drugs that destroy or inhibit the growth of bacteria in the body. They are not effective against viruses.

Antihistamines

Drugs that counteract allergic symptoms produced when histamine is released in the body.

Anti-inflammatories

Drugs that reduce inflammation, as in arthritis, gout and muscular problems. Include analgesics (see above); corticosteroids; and non-steroidal antu-inflammatory drugs (NSAIDs).

Antiseptic

A substance that controls infection and helps prevent tissue degeneration.

Antispasmodics

Drugs or natural substances for relieving cramp and bowel spasms.

Aromatherapy

The use of aromatic essential oils, which are extracted from plants, to treat many common health problems and illnesses. Used in massage, diffusers and inhalation.

Bach flower essences (remedies)

The 38 Bach flower essences (infusions of different plants) were developed by Dr Edward Bach and are used to correct emotional imbalances that can threaten our health, and to promote self-healing.

Chinese herbal medicine

A holistic branch of Traditional Chinese Medicine in which herbs are used to treat disease and health problems, by eliminating symptoms, rebalancing the body, and strengthening the individual. It emphasises the interaction between the body, mind and spirit.

Chiropractic

A form of manipulation whereby joints in the spine are manipulated to relieve not only back problems but also ones elsewhere in the body, as the spine carries the nerves to the rest of the body.

Cognitive behavioural therapy (CBT)

A term covering a number of talking therapies that are used to treat anxiety, depression and other psychological problems. It was developed from cognitive therapy and behavioural therapy.

Demulcent

A soothing agent that protects mucous membranes and relieves irritation.

Detoxicant

A substance that eliminates or counteracts poisons.

Distillation
Process of extracting essences of plants by heating to vapour, condensing by cooling, and collecting the liquid.

Essential oils
Concentrated essences extracted from plants.

Expectorant
A substance that removes excess mucous from the respiratory passages.

Herbal medicine
An ancient holistic system of medicine, which uses the healing properties of medicinal plants to treat a wide range of health disorders and common diseases.

Homeopathy
An ancient, natural system of medicine whereby minute amounts of diluted substances are used to treat various medical conditions on the principle that 'like cures like'. A qualified homeopath will address the patient's personality as well as their symptoms before prescribing an appropriate remedy.

Hydrotherapy
The therapeutic use of water in treating a range of health problems. Utilizes hot, cold and mineral baths; steam baths, vapour baths and Turkish baths; inhalation therapy; and hot and cold compresses.

Massage
An ancient hands-on therapy that is used to: induce mental and physical relaxation; eliminate toxins from the body; improve muscle tone and circulation; and help the digestive system to function effectively.

Meditation
Used to promote relaxation and spiritual growth and enlightenment. It is believed to be beneficial to health, relieving stress and treating high blood pressure.

Naturopathy
A holistic, preventive therapy emphasising the body's natural vitality and potential for self-healing. Encourages a healthy lifestyle, encompassing a natural, organic diet, relaxation, exercise and hydrotherapy.

Osteopathy
A therapy that involves massage and manipulation of the joints, especially in the spine, to promote self-healing and correct skeletal misalignment.

Pathogen
An agent that causes disease, such as bacteria, viruses, fungi and parasites.

Pilates
A system of body conditioning that improves posture, balance, alignment, flexibility and breathing.

Reflexology
An ancient therapy using foot massage, in which the soles of the feet mirror the rest of the body and pressure is applied to specific points that correspond to other body parts and organs.

Traditional Chinese Medicine (TCM)
A complete, integrated, holistic system of medicine, including acupuncture, acupressure, herbal medicine and food cores. Aims to promote health by restoring harmony to the body and balancing Yin and Yang.

Yin and Yang
The equal and opposite qualities of Qi (see above), the body's vital energy.

Yoga
An ancient Hindu system of exercises, postures, meditation, breathing and relaxation, designed to promote physical, mental and spiritual wellbeing by creating union between the body, mind and spirit.

Useful information

Acupuncture Association of Chartered Physiotherapists
Tel: 01733 390012
www.aacp.uk.com

Allergy UK
Information on allergies and allergic symptoms.
Helpline: 01322 619898
www.allergyuk.org

Aromatherapy Council
Regulatory body for aromatherapists in the UK.
www.aromatherapycouncil.co.uk

Arthritis Care
Charitable organisation working with and supporting people with arthritis.
Tel: 020 7380 6500
www.arthritiscare.org.uk

Arthritis Research UK
Information about arthritis and the latest research.
Tel: 01246 558033
www.arthritisresearchuk.org

Association of Reflexologists
For information on reflexology and finding a registered reflexologist.
Tel: 01823 351010
www.aor.org.uk

Association of Traditional Chinese Medicine (UK)
Regulatory body for TCM in the UK.
Tel: 020 8951 3030
www.atcm.co.uk

Asthma UK
Charity for improving health of asthma sufferers.
Tel: 0800 121 6255
Adviceline: 0800 121 6244
www.asthma.org.uk

The Bach Centre
Home of Bach flower remedies, and information on finding a Bach Foundation registered practitioner.
Tel: 01491 834678
www.bachcentre.com

British Acupuncture Council
Regulatory body for traditional acupuncture in the UK.
Tel: 020 8735 0400
www.acupuncture.org.uk

British Chiropractic Association
The largest association for chiropractors in the UK.
Tel: 0118 950 5950
www.chiropractic-uk.co.uk

British Complementary Medicine Association
Information on complementary medicine and finding registered practitioners.
Tel: 0845 129 8434
www.the-cma.org.uk

British Dental Health Foundation
Dental helpline: 0845 063 1188
www.dentalhealth.org.uk

British Heart Foundation
For information on heart disease and how to prevent it.
Tel: 020 7554 0000
www.bhf.org.uk

British Herbal Medicine Association
For information on herbal medicine.
Tel: 0845 680 1134
www.bhma.info

British Homeopathic Association
Association for medical doctors also trained in homeopathy.
Tel: 01582 408675
www.britishhomeopathic.org

British Medical Acupuncture Society
Organization of medical practitioners who use acupuncture in hospitals or general practice.
Tel: 020 7713 9437/01606 786782
www.medical-acupuncture.co.uk

British Medical Association
Professional medical association for UK doctors.
Tel: 020 7387 4499
www.bma.org.uk

British Nutrition Foundation
Information on nutrition and healthy eating.
Tel: 020 7404 6504
www.nutrition.org.uk

British Osteopathic Association (BOA)
Find a qualified osteopath in your area.
Tel: 01582 488455
www.osteopathy.org

British Reflexology Association
For information on reflexology.
Tel: 01886 821207
www.britreflex.co.uk

British Wheel of Yoga
Largest UK yoga organisation. Information on classes.
Tel: 01529 306851
www.bwy.org.uk

Cancer Research UK
For information about cancer and treatments.
Tel: 020 7242 0200
www.cancerresearchuk.org

Chartered Society of Physiotherapy
Professional and educational body for chartered physiotherapists in the UK.
Tel: 020 7306 6666
www.csp.org.uk

College of Naturopathic Medicine
Information on naturopathy and finding a practitioner.
Tel: 01342 410505
www.naturopathy-uk.com

Diabetes UK
Information on diabetes and how to prevent it.
Tel: 020 7424 1000
www.diabetes.org.uk

Food Standards Agency
Information on nutrition, healthy eating food safety and food-related diseases.
Tel: 020 7276 8829
www.food.gov.uk
www.eatwell.gov.uk

Foundation for Traditional Chinese Medicine
www.ftcm.org.uk

General Chiropractic Council

The regulating body for chiropractors in the UK.
Tel: 020 7713 5155
www.gcc-uk.org

General Council for Massage Therapies

The governing body for massage therapies in the UK
Tel: 0870 850 4452
www.gcmt.org.uk

General Osteopathic Council

Regulates osteopathy in the UK
Tel: 020 7357 6655
www.osteopathy.org.uk

Gut Trust

National UK charity for irritable bowel syndrome.
Tel: 0114 272 3253
Helpline: 0872 300 4537
www.theguttrust.org

Homeopathic Medical Association

Represents qualified homeopaths in the UK.
Tel: 01474 560336
www.the-hma.org

Institute for Complementary and Natural Medicine

Information on complementary medicine, best practice and how to find a registered practitioner.
Tel: 020 7922 7980
www.i-c-m.org.uk

Institute of Trichologists

For information on hair and scalp conditions.
Tel: 0845 604 4657
www.trichologists.org.uk

ME Association

Support and information for people with ME.
Tel: 0844 576 5326
www.meassociation.org.uk

Mind

Leading mental health charity.
Tel: 020 8519 2122
www.mind.org.uk

Mumsnet

UK website devoted to parenting tips and advice.
www.mumsnet.com

National Association for Colitis and Crohn's Disease

Information and support for people with inflammatory bowel disease.
Tel: 0845 130 2233
www.nacc.org.uk

National Childbirth Trust

UK charity offering antenatal and postnatal courses and advice on pregnancy, childbirth and childcare.
Tel: 0844 243 6000
Pregnancy and birth line: 0300 330 0772
www.nctpregnancyandbabycare.com

National Eczema Society

Eczema patient support organization.
Helpline: 0800 089 1122
www.eczema.org

National Institute of Medical Herbalists (NIMH)

Professional body of qualified medical herbalists.
Tel: 01392 426022
www.nimh.org.uk

National Osteoporosis Society
Charity for prevention and treatment of osteoporosis.
Helpline: 0845 450 0230
www.nos.org.uk

Nelsons Homeopathic Pharmacy
Supplier of homeopathic remedies.
Tel: 020 7629 3118
www.nelsonshomeopathy.com

NHS Direct
Health advice service and online self-help guide.
0845 4647
www.nhsdirect.nhs.uk

Pilates Foundation UK
A governing body for Pilates in the UK.
Tel: 020 7033 0078
www.pilatesfoundation.com

Prostate UK
Charity raising awareness of prostate diseases.
Tel: 020 8788 7720
www.prostateuk.org

Register of Chinese Herbal Medicine
Register of qualified practitioners in UK.
Tel: 01603 623994
www.rchm.co.uk

Royal College of Obstetricians and Gynaecologists
Leading organisation in obstetrics and gynaecology.
Tel: 020 7772 6200
www.rcog.org.uk

RSI Awareness
An online information resource for people with RSI.
www.rsi.org.uk

St John Ambulance
Advice on first aid and information about courses.
Tel: 08700 10 49 50
www.sja.org.uk

Seasonal Affective Disorder Association
For information on SAD, and support and advice.
www.sada.org.uk

Society of Chiropodists and Podiatrists
Information on finding a qualified practitioner.
Tel: 020 7234 8620
www.feetforlife.org

Society of Homeopaths
European organisation registering homeopaths.
Tel: 0845 450 6611
www.homeopathy-soh.org

Soil Association
Campaigning for organic food and certification.
Tel: 0117 314 5000
www.soilassociation.org

STAT
The Society of Teachers of the Alexander Technique.
Tel: 0207 482 5135
www.stat.org.uk

Vegetarian Society
UK charity promoting benefits of a vegetarian diet.
Tel: 0161 925 2000
www.vegsoc.org

Women's Health
Information on a range of women's health problems.
www.womens-health.co.uk

Index

A

abscesses 64, 65, 66
acid reflux 176
acne 17, 18–19
acupressure 89, 127, 139, 235, 294
acupuncture 21, 25, 27, 77, 80, 83, 85, 89, 95, 109, 119, 177, 207, 209, 211, 213, 219, 221, 223, 238
  electro- 217
adrenal gland 107, 254
Alexander Technique 77, 80, 81, 93, 95, 99, 125
allergies, 50, 63, 124, 125, 126, 127, 134, 138, 146–147, 231
  food 148–149, 170
anaemia 111, 112–113, 116, 186, 211, 219, 225, 244
anaphylactic shock 147, 149
angina 103, 104–105
antibiotics 19,, 268
antihistamines 35, 63, 126, 127, 148, 152, 266
antioxidants 22
anxiety 18, 111, 205, 210, 214, 215, 220, 222, 234, 242, 252, 292
arthritis 88–89, 90, 98
aspirin 105, 109, 112, 121, 150, 177, 182
asthenopia 58–59
asthma 20, 26, 50, 72, 123, 124–125, 126, 211
athlete's foot 36–37, 38, 42
ayurveda 40

B

back problems 72, 73, 76–79, 245, 250
bad breath 70, 186
bedwetting (children) 274–275
beta blockers 24, 107, 110, 119
biofeedback 195
bites 280–281
bladder 193, 198, 274
bleeding 286

blisters 30, 158, 162, 282, 291
blood clots 97, 105, 109, 117
blood pressure 106–107
  high 98, 103, 104, 106, 107, 109, 111, 229, 287
  low 107
body odour 42–43
body wraps 29
boils 33
bronchitis 123, 132–133
bruises 284–285, 289
burns 282–283
Buteyko Method 125

C

calluses 40
cardiovascular disease 103
cartilage 75, 76
catarrh 265
cellulite 28–29
chapped lips 31
chest pain 79, 81
chickenpox 156–157, 158
chilblains 103, 118–119
Chinese herbal medicine 239
chiropractic 72, 77, 80, 81, 83, 207
chlamydia 237
cholesterol 105, 106, 108
  high 98, 104, 108–109, 229
chronic fatigue syndrome (ME) 205, 211, 218–219
coeliac disease 112
cognitive behavioural therapy 205, 207, 213, 215, 219, 221, 223
cold(s) 125, 128–129, 134, 138, 259, 265
  in children 266–267
  sores 32, 162, 163
collagen 23
congestion 138–139
conjunctivitis 63, 160, 188
constipation 70, 167, 168–169, 180, 181, 214, 248, 250
corns 40
corticosteroids 18, 21, 85, 154
cough 123, 129, 130–131, 152,

259, 265, 266
counselling 205, 215, 221, 223
cranial osteopathy 57
Crohn's disease 112, 170, 178, 179
cryotherapy 41
cuts 286
cystitis 198–199

D

dandruff 47
deep vein thrombosis (DVT) 117
dehydration 107, 170, 171, 173, 174, 175, 250, 295
dementia 224–225
dental care 54, 64–65, 217
depression 210, 214, 215, 218, 220–221, 222, 224, 234, 242, 252
dermatitis 20, 2, 70
diabetes 15, 37, 41, 43, 70, 98, 104, 107, 109, 116, 199, 211, 225, 229, 235, 288
diarrhoea 146, 148, 167, 170–171, 174, 178, 179, 180, 185, 188, 214, 244, 245, 263, 264, 270, 295
digestion 75, 167
diuretics 197, 199
dry mouth 71
dry skin 14–15
dyspepsia 176–177

E

ear(s) 54, 56–57
  earache 56, 136
  infections 56
  wax 56, 57
eczema 20–21, 26, 148
emphysema 123
endermologie 29
endometriosis 245 252
exercise 15, 22, 24, 28, 29, 75, 77, 80, 84, 85, 88, 90, 96, 99, 104, 105, 106, 108, 110, 116, 117, 123, 130, 168, 180, 184, 200, 206, 208, 210, 212, 214, 220,

221, 222, 224, 234, 241, 245, 248, 250, 254
eye(s) 54, 126, 206, 208, 270
  conjunctivitis 63
  irritation 60–61, 127
  strain 58–59
  styes 62

F

fainting 107, 245, 288, 292
fatigue 88, 150, 153, 177, 178, 197, 202, 205, 210–211, 242, 250
Feldenkrais method 40
fertility problems: in men 236–237
  in women 248, 252–253
fever 56, 57, 65, 66, 79, 120, 121, 158, 160, 162, 178, 209, 263, 264, 266, 269, 270
fibroids 248–249
flower remedies 147, 150, 153, 154, 157, 161, 173, 177, 181, 187, 215, 243, 251, 255, 261, 263, 264, 267, 268, 273, 275, 288, 290, 292
food poisoning 167, 174–175
foot odour 42–43
foot pain 94–95
free radicals 22, 23
fungal infections 36, 42, 47, 246–247
  of nails 38–39

G

gastroenteritis 167, 170, 174–175
German measles 160–161, 259
glandular fever 154–155, 218
gout 88, 98–99
gum disease 54, 64–65, 67

H

haemorrhoids 188–189, 250
hair 13, 43–51
  dry 44–46
  greasy 48–49
halitosis 70
hangover 295
hay fever 20, 26, 126–127, 134, 147
head lice 50–51

headache 72, 73, 82, 83, 148, 152, 156, 160, 168, 174, 205, 206–207, 218, 242, 250, 252, 265, 266, 269, 290, 295
heart 103, 123
  disease 54, 98, 106, 108, 110, 129, 196, 229, 235, 288, 294
heartburn 176–177, 182, 250
heat exhaustion 290
heat rash 34–35
heatstroke 290
herbal: compresses 143
  decoctions 142
  infusions 142
  inhalations 143
  poultices 143
  tinctures 143
herpes simplex virus 32, 162–163
hiccups 140–141
hives 34–35, 148
Hopi ear candling 57
hormone replacement therapy (HRT) 254
hypertension 106
hypnotherapy 141
hypotension 107

I

ibuprofen 24, 83, 112, 121, 177, 182, 266
immune system 32, 33, 113, 129, 137, 145, 158, 163, 266
impotence 234–235
incontinence 194–195, 224
indigestion 176–177
infant colic 262–263
infertility: in men 236–237
  in women 248, 252–253
inflammatory bowel disease167, 170, 178–179
influenza 134, 138, 152–153, 265, 266
in-growing toe nails 38, 39
insomnia 205, 212–213, 242, 252
intestinal worms 186–187
iron deficiency 112, 113, 116
irregular heartbeat 110
irritable bowel syndrome (IBS) 180–181, 185

J

joints 75, 84, 88–89, 90, 98, 289

K

kidney(s) 193, 197
  disease 43, 98, 106, 109, 116, 196, 219, 225, 294
  stones 199, 200–201

L

laxatives 168, 169, 180, 186
ligaments 75, 76, 289
light therapy 223
liposuction 29
lips: chapped 31
  cold sores 32
liver disease 43, 109, 294
lungs 123, 124
lymphatic drainage 28, 29

M

massage 205
measles 259, 268, 270
meditation 24, 111, 179, 205
meningitis 269
menopause 112, 194, 241, 242, 254–255
menstruation 32
migraine 72, 73, 82, 205, 208–209
MMR vaccine 160, 268
motion sickness 294
mouth ulcers 68–69, 162
mumps 259, 268, 269
muscle(s) 75, 76, 90, 289
  cramps 96–97, 290

N

nails 37, 38–39
nappy rash 259, 260–261
nasal polyps 139
nausea 152, 158, 172–173, 174, 182, 208, 218, 244, 245, 250, 288, 290, 294, 295
neck problems 72, 73, 82–83
neural tube defects 113
neuralgia 216–217
nosebleed 287

O

obesity 98, 104, 108, 114, 117, 232, 236
oily skin 16–17
oral contraceptives 16, 18, 242, 244, 246, 248
osteoarthritis 88, 89
osteopathy 73, 80, 83, 125, 133
osteoporosis 84–85

P

palpitations 103, 110, 210, 214, 218, 244
parasites 50–51, 186–187
Parkinson's disease 235
pelvic floor exercises 194
peptic ulcers 182–183
periods 241, 242
  heavy 244, 248
  painful 245, 248
Pilates 80, 81, 93, 95, 101, 181
pneumonia 133, 153, 157
postnatal depression 113
posture 76, 78, 81, 82, 206
pregnancy 16, 112, 113, 161, 172, 188, 199, 210, 241, 248, 250–251, 294
premenstrual tension (PMT) 241, 242–243
prickly heat 34
progesterone 16
prostate 194, 232–233
psoriasis 24–25, 46, 47, 98
psychotherapy 223

Q

qi 238

R

reflexology 77, 177, 207, 213, 215, 223
relaxation 24, 179, 205, 210, 214, 218, 241, 254
repetitive strain injury (RSI) 72, 73, 92–93
respiratory system 123
restless legs 103, 116
Reye's syndrome 150, 160
rheumatism 90–91

rheumatoid arthritis 88, 89
rubella 160–161, 259

S

scalds 282¬–283
sciatica 72, 73, 80
seasonal affective disorder (SAD) 222–223
shaving problems 230–231
shin splints 86–87
shingles 156, 158–159
shock 107. 292
shoulder pain 82–83
sinusitis 138–139, 217, 265
skeleton 75
skin 13–35
  blisters 30
  boils 33
  brushing 29
  dry 14–15
  oily 16–17
  recipes 52–53
sleep problems (babies and children) 259, 272–273
smoking 241, 252
sore throat 123, 128, 130, 134–135, 137, 152, 160, 218, 267
spina bifida 113
spine 75, 76
splinters 293
split ends 45
sprains 289
steroids 35, 99, 124, 137
stings 280–281
strains 289
stress 18, 20, 24, 34 48, 96, 104, 106, 110, 111, 140, 179, 180, 182, 206, 207, 208, 210, 214–215, 218, 220, 222, 234, 236, 241, 245, 246
  fractures 87
  incontinence 194–195
stroke 54, 106, 108, 109
styes 62
sunburn 19, 21, 291

T

tai chi 111, 254

teeth 54
teething 259, 264
tendons 75, 90
testosterone 16
tetanus 280, 286, 293
throat: sore 123, 128, 130, 134–135, 137, 152, 160, 218, 267
thrush (candida) 241, 246–247, 260
thyroid gland 46, 97, 109, 111, 211, 219, 225, 294
tinnitus 73
toe nails 37, 38–39
tonsillitis 136–137
toothache 66–67
Traditional Chinese Medicine (TCM) 238–239
transcendental relaxation 107
trapped nerve 81
Tuina 239

U

ulcerative colitis 178
urinary system 193
urticaria 34, 148

V

vaginal discharge 241, 246, 247
varicose veins 103, 114–115
verrucas 41
vertigo 73
vomiting 121, 146, 148, 167, 172–173, 174, 182, 208, 209, 245, 263, 264, 270, 290

W

warts 41
water retention 196–197, 242
whooping cough 259, 268, 271
wind 168, 180, 184–185
wrinkles 14, 22–23

Y

yeast infections 31
yin and yang 238
yoga 45, 79, 80, 81, 89, 91, 93, 95, 105, 109, 111, 115, 125, 141, 179, 205, 254